KININS
Pharmacodynamics and Biological Roles

ADVANCES IN EXPERIMENTAL MEDICINE AND BIOLOGY

Recent Volumes in this Series

KININS
Pharmacodynamics and Biological Roles

Edited by

F. Sicuteri
University of Florence
Florence, Italy

Nathan Back
State University of New York
Buffalo, New York

and

G. L. Haberland
Pharmaceutical Research Center
Wuppertal-Elberfeld, West Germany

PLENUM PRESS • NEW YORK AND LONDON

Library of Congress Cataloging in Publication Data

Symposium on Vasopeptides, Fiesole, 1975.
  Kinins.

  (Advances in experimental medicine and biology; v. 70)
  Includes bibliographical references and index.
  1. Kinins—Congresses I. Sicuteri, Federico, 1920-   II. Back, Nathan. III.
Haberland, G. L. IV. Title.
QP552.K5S95 1975   574.3'1   76-7006
  ISBN 978-1-4684-3269-5   ISBN 978-1-4684-3267-1 (eBook)
  DOI 10.1007/978-1-4684-3267-1

Proceedings of the International Symposium on Vasopeptides "Kinin '75" held in
Fiesole–Villa Medici (Auditorium Hoechst), Florence, Italy, July 15–17, 1975

© 1976 Plenum Press, New York
Softcover reprint of the hardcover 1st edition 1976
A Division of Plenum Publishing Corporation
227 West 17th Street, New York, N.Y. 10011

United Kingdom edition published by Plenum Press, London
A Division of Plenum Publishing Company, Ltd.
Davis House (4th Floor), 8 Scrubs Lane, Harlesden, London, NW10 6SE, England

Preface

The tradition of meeting together periodically at Fiesole, in Florence, by now dear to those interested in the problems of Kinins, was respected once again. This year the Symposium "Kinin 1975" was held on the 15th - 17th of July.

Participation at the Symposium drew attention to the fact that 1975 was a particularly difficult year due to the delicate international economic situation as well as the time restrictions for organizing the Symposium as a satellite conference to the Sixth International Congress of Pharmacology held in Helsinki, Finland. Despite these difficulties, the "Kinin '75" Symposium was an unquestioned success, due, in great part, to the more than 40 contributors who presented their most current studies at the customary high scientific standard, presentations that provoked and stimulated considerable discussion and debate. While our family tree now includes new and active members, the presence of many members of our "Kinin" society unable to attend was missed. In particular, we mourne the death of Professor E. Werle, one of the most outstanding pioneers in the field of the kallikrein-kinin system. His friendship, participation and counsel was, and will continue to be, sorely missed by his many colleagues and students who are indebted to him for his voluminous and scientifically-expert contributions continued until the very end of his most full and productive life.

As in the past, the atmosphere of friendship and relaxation of the Symposium enhanced the very useful communication and exchange of ideas and information amongst the participants.

This volume contains the collection of studies presented at Fiesole which provide the most recent and progressive advances in the biochemistry, pharmacology, and clinical aspects of the kinins. The gradual expansion of our understanding and knowledge of these mediators has highlighted their relative importance in diverse biological systems, a purpose and goal well served by the tradition of yearly "kinin" meetings in different countries and periodically every 2-3 years at Fiesole. The "Academia Kininensis Faesulana" (this volume, page 2) which Professor Rocha e Silva has insisted

be established (with the support of other colleagues) is, indeed,
a practical and productive reality.

   The Organization Scientific Committee membership, reflecting
the international coloration of the Symposium, included Professors
N. Back, L.M. Greenbaum and J.J. Pisano (United States), Professors
G.L. Haberland and F. Sicuteri (Europe), Professor M. Rocha e Silva
(South America), and Professor T. Suzuki (Japan). Their assistance
and advice contributed greatly to the success of the Symposium.
Special thanks are extended to the highly competent and conscientious
work of the Symposium Secretariate, Professor G. Franchi, and
Professor M. Fanciullacci and to their very able assistants Mrs.
Mara Saccenti and Miss Joan L. Nonenbacher. The organization of
the locality, social and culinary arrangements and preparations are
attributed directly to the indefatigable efforts of our most gracious
Mrs. Maria Antoniette Sicuteri. Our thanks are offered to the
Bayer Company who published, in their customary elegant style of
typography, the attractive programme and abstracts of the Symposium.
The generosity of the Hoechst Italia is also acknowledged for
extending the use of their auditorium at the Villa Medici, which,
together with the enthusiastic collaboration of Dr. Biavati and
his assistants, facilitated the holding of the Symposium and assured
its success. The Organizing Committee offers its many thanks to
the Honorable Mayor of Fiesole, Mr. B. Latini, whose many courtesies
and customary interest in the cultural and scientific impact of the
Symposium made the tasks of the Committee much easier.

   The Symposium was under the patronage of the National Council
of Research of Rome, which, for many years, has followed with
interest and has provided financial support for the research in the
field of the Vasoactive Polypeptides and the Clinical Pharmacology
Society of Italy.

   The Editors wish to express their appreciation to Ms. Patricia
Poczkalski of the State University of New York at Buffalo for her
very skilled and dedicated transcription of the manuscripts to the
uniform type seen in this present volume, and to Ms. Phyllis Straw,
Editor of Plenum Press and her associates for providing, in the
most cooperative manner, this attractive and speadily published
volume. The editors also are indebted to Aaron I. Back for the
meticulous proofreading of the manuscripts.

   It is the hope of the Editors that this volume will help
maintain the tradition consolidated in the periodic encounters
with members of the "kinin" family who are linked together by
their mutual scientific interests and reciprocal feelings of
esteem and affectionate friendship.

Florence, Italy, March 1976   Federigo Sicuteri
                                             Nathan Back
                                             Gert Haberland

Contents

CONTENTS

PAST, PRESENT AND FUTURE OF KININS

Introductory Remarks(*)

Mauricio Rocha e Silva

Department of Pharmacology

Faculty of Medicine, USP, Ribeirao Preto, S.P., Brazil

It is a great pleasure to attend the demand of my friend Frederigo Sicuteri, to give a few Introductory Remarks to this Symposium that received the suggestive name of "Kinins-75". With such a title for the Symposium, and the title I gave to this address: Past, Present and Future of Kinins, I feel like Fellini, and would like to call it "Kinin Amarcord", to remind you of the early times of bradykinin, in the late 40's, to be precise, May 1948, when with Beraldo and Rosenfeld, we fell upon an intriguing substance appearing in the blood of dogs which received an injection of the venom of Bothrops jararaca. A few weeks later we observed the appearance of a similar principle in the defibrinated blood of the dog, in experiments of liver perfusion.

By that time we were interested in knowing whether the venom of Bothrops jararaca would release histamine, as a possible mediator or the profound circulatory shock observed in the dog and in humans by injection of the venom. What came out from the liver perfused with defibrinated blood was obviously not histamine, since it acted powerfully on the isolated guinea pig ileum treated with benadryl, and besides that, was rapidly destroyed by standing at room temperature in contact with serum and venom. We could also discard the liver, because by adding the venom directly to the defibrinated blood, we could observe an even more potent effect upon the isolated guinea pig ileum, desensitized (rendered tachy-Phylactic) to the venom itself.

(*) Address given to the Opening Session of the International Symposium, July, 15th, 1975, in Fiesole, Italy.

We had to give a name to this new principle that worked slowly upon the isolated guinea pig ileum, and was likewise slowly washed out from the preparation, about 7 times slower than histamine or acetylcholine. To translate into the Greek this "slow response" we combined the names <u>Kinin</u> (substance producing movement) and <u>bradys</u> (slow) and had <u>bradykinin</u>.

I insist upon the origins of bradykinin, which came to be known to the scientific world, by interference of a venom with the blood, and therefore an interference of a biblical power (a snake) with the mammalian blood. Then, followed the isolation of its pure form, which was done at the Biological Institute of Sao Paulo, in 1956, with Sylvia Andrade, after extensive preliminary work, with Beraldo, Diniz and Eline Prado; then, the elucidation of the sequence of amino-acids by Elliott, et al., at the National Research Institute, in London; and finally its synthesis by Boissonnas and his group, at Sandoz, in Basel. So ended, what I have called the pioneering time for bradykinin, that lasted exactly 10 years, as reported in the book recently published: "A Bradykinin Anthology", to commemorate the 25th anniversary of Bradykinin.

I don't know whether the name of Bradykinin was correct from a philological point of view; some spell it wrongly, using instead of a <u>k</u>, the phoneme <u>ch</u>, as in Italian <u>Chinine</u>, reminding you of the alkaloid quinine, or in Spanish, with a <u>qu</u>, with the same drawback, and sometimes in Portuguese, also with a <u>qu</u>, instead of the correct <u>c</u> or <u>k</u> as done in our first publication in Portuguese, or as in English or French. We know that this <u>k</u> of bradykinin, is the same as it appears in kinema, kinetics, kinesis and so-forth, and that became <u>c</u> in some of the Neo-Latin languages.

But, anyway, the name was appealing to the ear, considering the great success that it had in the literature, with thousands of papers and no less than 11 Symposia dedicated to this kind of polypeptides: the first one in Montreal, 1953; in London, 1959; in New York, 1963; in Florence, 1965; in Ribeirao Preto, 1966 and since then almost every two years in Fiesole, 1969, 1971; in San Francisco, 1972; in Ribeirao Preto, 1973, in Reston, Virginia, 1974; and this one again in Fiesole, 1975.

I remind you that Fiesole has been proclaimed the Capital of the kinins, and even an Academy on Kinins was founded in 1969-71, with the name of <u>Academia Kininensis Fiesolana</u>. I suppose that this Meeting on Kinins-75 could be forever quoted as the Third International Meeting of this Academy.

I have to stress the enormous creativity in the field, that
two meetings on kinins can be held within less than a ten month
interval, since the last one was in Reston, Virginia, in October
1974, sponsored by the Fogarty Center, and organized by Kinino-
logists of the NIH. However, there is a sad difference between the
last meeting and the one that starts today, and that is the absence
of Ernst Werle, who had been one of the Chairmen of the last
meeting. Those who were present then, remember that the whole
field was divided between Bradykinin and Kallikrein, by something
that I have named the "New Treaty of Tordesilhas", to remind the
division of the New World by the Pope in the beginning of the XVI
Century.

I don't know if the influence of the Pope induced my friend
Sicuteri to unify the field and call it Kinin-75, which simplifies
a great deal, and I suggest that from now on the meetings should
have such a denotation: Kinin-76, Kinin-77, 78 up to 99 and then
we have to change to Kinin-2000, to commemorate the entrance of
the New Century, if of course there will be survivors of so many
challenges, that are now under way. But, we can be sure, if a
race of humans or mammalians will survive any atomic or nuclear
holocaust, the Kinins will certainly survive _per secula seculorum_,
Amen.

BRADYKININ ANTAGONISM

A. Gecse, E. Zsilinszky, L. Szekeres

Department of Pathophysiology and Dermatologic Clinic

University Medical School of Szeged

Szeged, Hungary

Previously we have shown (1) that the C-phenyl-glycine-n-heptyl ester, henceforth abbreviated CPHE, is a potent inhibitor of mediators of allergic reactions both in vitro and in vivo.

It is well known that the basic amino acids (Arg, Lys) and amino acids containing aromatic ring (Phe) are very important in the receptor-bradykinin interaction (3). The exchange of the Arg^1 residue by neutral amino acids results in a very strong decrease in activity. The phenylalanine residue in position 5 and 8 can be replaced by other aromatic amino acids without loss in brady-kinin activity (4). It seems most reasonable that the pi electron clouds of aromatic amino acids both of receptor and peptide are responsible for the phenomenon.

On the basis of these observations we decided to synthetize hyptyl esters of aromatic and basic amino acids to determine their antibradykinin effect on different tests.

Isolated uterus of a rat was used for in vitro studies. Bradykinin (BRS 640, Sandoz), serotin creatinin sulfate (Sandoz), acetylcholin (La Roche) have been applied as agonists. Experiments were carried out on guinea-pig ileum and rat stomach strip, respectively.

Arginine-heptyl ester (AHE), phenylalanine-heptyl ester (PHE), d-CPHE and CPHE with mostly l-phenylglycine were used as antagonists.

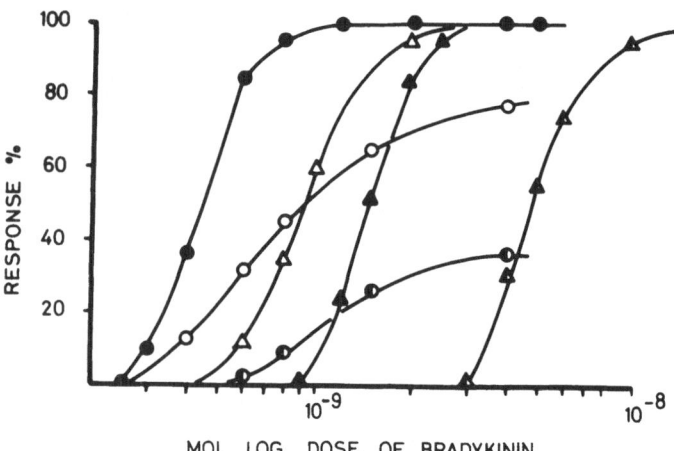

Fig.1. The dose-response curves of rat uterus to bradykinin. On the ordinate the percentage response induced
by bradykinin is indicated and log M dose of bradykinin on the abscissa. Control, without antagonist ● ,
2x 10^{-5} M CPHE ▲ , 4x 10^{-5} M CPHE ▲ , 1.6x 10^{-4} M
CPHE ▲ , 4x 10^{-5} M d-CPHE ○ , 8x 10^{-5} M d-CPHE ◑

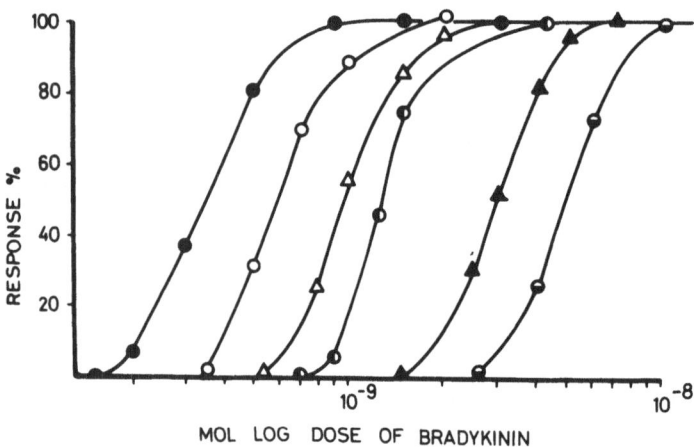

Fig.2. The dose-response curves of rat uterus to bradykinin. On the ordinate the percentage response induced
by bradykinin is indicated and log M dose of bradykinin
on the abscissa. Control, without antagonist ● , PHE
4 x 10^{-5} M ○ , PHE 8 x 10^{-5} M ◑ , PHE 3.6 x 10^{-4} M
◒ , AHE 5 x 10^{-6} M △ , AHE 1 x 10^{-5} M ▲ ,

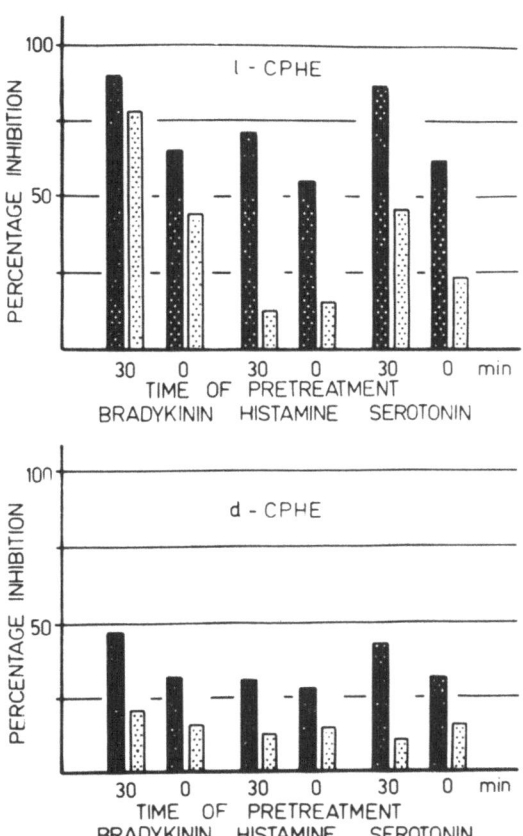

Fig.3. Effect of AHE and PHE on the dye exudate in rat skin induced by vasoactive substances. Ordinate : percentage inhibition of increased vascular permeability. Abscissa : time of pretreatment. Zero minute means that the i.p. injection of AHE or PHE and the intradermal application of permeability increasing materials took place nearly at once. AHE, PHE 2.5 mg/kg ⊞ AHE, PHE 7.5 mg/kg ▓

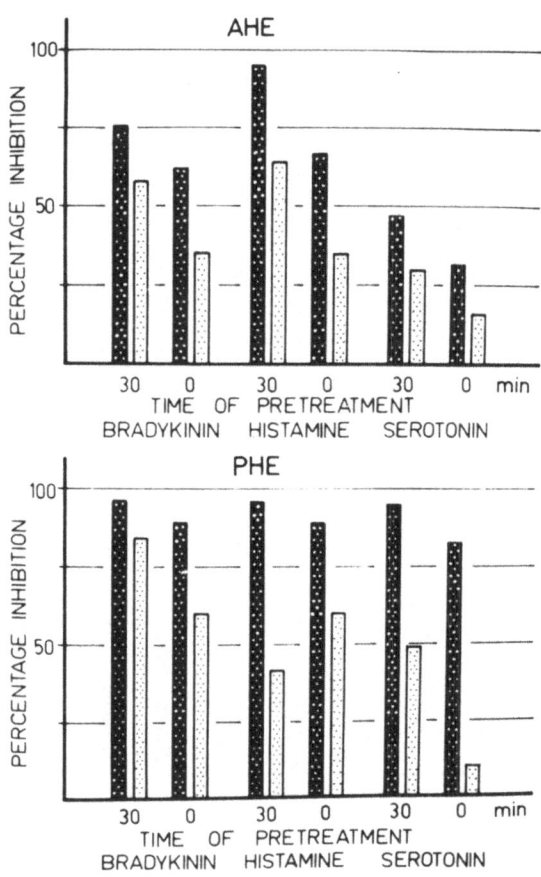

Fig.4. Effect of d-CPHE and l-CPHE on the dye exudate in rat skin induced by vasoactive substances. Ordinate: percentage inhibition of increased vascular permeability. Abscissa : time of pretreatment. d-CPHE, l-CPHE 2.5 mg/kg ▦ , d-CPHE, l-CPHE 7.5 mg/kg ▦

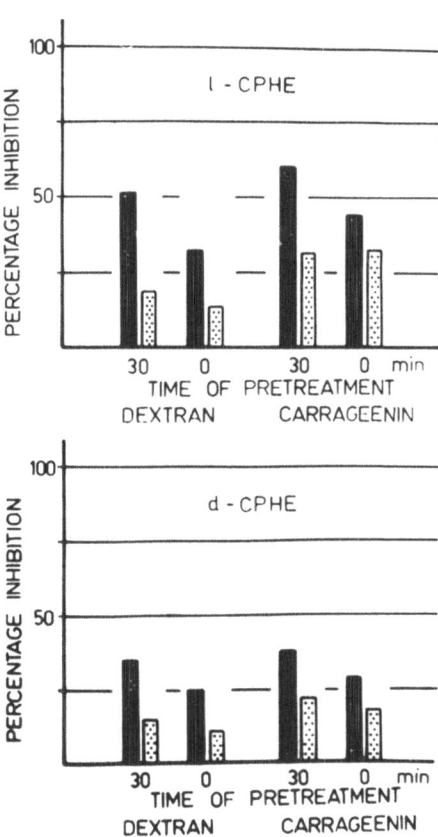

Fig.5. Effect of AHE and PHE on the dye exudate in rat skin induced by carrageenin or dextran. Ordinate : percentage inhibition of increased vascular permeability. Abscissa : time of pretreatment. AHE, PHE 2.5 mg/kg ▣ , AHE, PHE 7.5 mg/ kg ▦

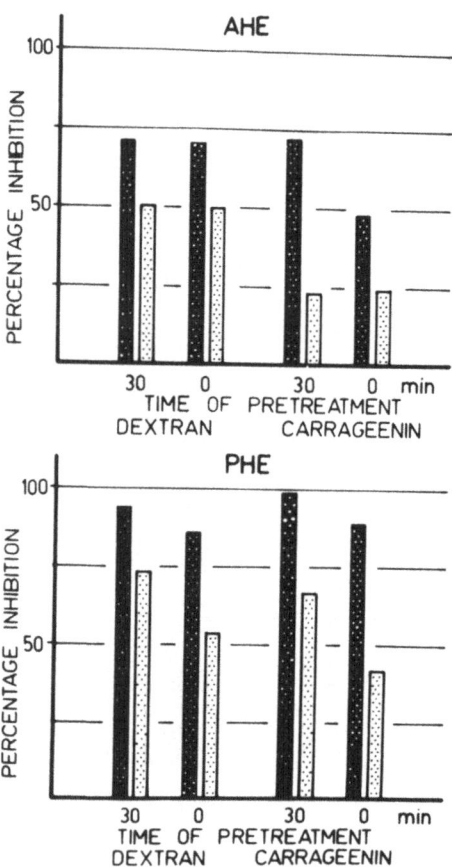

Fig.6. Effect of d-CPHE and l-CPHE on the dye exudate
in rat skin induced by carrageenin or dextran. Ordinate : percentage inhibition of increased vascular permeability. Abscissa : time of pretreatment. d-CPHE,
l-CPHE 2.5 mg/kg ⊞ , d-CPHE, l-CPHE 7.5 mg/kg ▓

Figure 1 shows the dose-response curves of the isolated rat uterus to bradykinin. 2×10^{-5} M 1-CPHE shifted the dose-response curve to the right. Increasing the dose of 1-CPHE the curve was shifted further to the right but maximal contraction was induced by bradykinin even if the concentration of antagonist was more than 10^{-4} M.

Higher amount of d-CPHE was needed to antagonize the effect of bradykinin on smooth muscle preparation. Using d-CPHE in a concentration of 4×10^{-5} M the dose-response curve declined, the bradykinin did not induce maximal contraction. Increasing the dose of d-CPHE (8×10^{-5} M) the dose-response curve was shifted to the right and less than 40% response was seen. Previously we found that the heptanol part is responsible for the spasmolytic effect found on rat uterus (1).

Further on we determined the antibradykinin potency both of Phenylalanine-heptyl ester and Arginine-heptyl ester. The PHE was not so effective as the AHE in vitro on rat uterus. 8×10^{-5} M PHE shifted the dose-response curve to the right as much as 5×10^{-6} M AHE. In both cases maximal contraction was induced by bradykinin. The dose-response curves were shifted to the right parallel with the control. On the basis of these results the action of PHE, AHE, 1-CPHE seemed to be a competitive antagonism. The AHE inhibited better the bradykinin effect in vitro than the CPHE.

Increased vascular permeability was induced in 350 female rats of R-Amsterdam strain weighing 180 to 200 g. Bradykinin (2.5 µg), serotonin (0.25 µg), histamine (10 µg) in 0.05 ml saline was injected intradermally into the depilated skin of rats, with Evans blue dye (10 mg/kg) in their circulation.

The rats were killed, their dorsal skin was removed, the Evans blue exuded into the injection places of vasoactive substances was extracted with Germanin (Bayer 205), according to Jancso's method (2) with the following modification. Only the inner surface of skin was extracted.

Two doses of antagonists (2.5 mg/kg and 7.5 mg/kg) were injected intraperitoneally 30 min. before or at the same time as the vascular permeability inducing substances were applied.

The bradykinin vascular permeability increasing effect was inhibited more than 80% after PHE pretreatment. When 2.5 mg/kg PHE was injected at the same time as bradykinin 60% inhibition was observed. The PHE was less effective against serotonin. In case of AHE the order of potency is histamine, bradykinin, serotonin. AHE effectiveness does not reach that of PHE. AHE has very little effect on serotonin induced vascular permeability.

The d-CPHE inhibition is less than 50% in each case. It is ineffective applying in a dose of 2.5 mg/kg against bradykinin, serotonin and histamine. The l-CPHE antagonizes the bradykinin action more than the AHE and less than the PHE. l-CPHE (2.5 mg/kg) is ineffective against histamine but shows inhibition in a dose of 7.5 mg/kg.

Further on, we determined the effect of heptyl esters when releasers of vasoactive substances (dextran 100 μg, carrageenin 50 μg) were injected in 0.05 ml saline intradermally. PHE was the most potent inhibitor from the investigated four materials, PHE (7.5 mg/kg) inhibited more than 80% both the dextran and carrageenin induced increased vascular permeability even if the PHE was injected at the same time as the releasers of vasoactive substances. When PHE (2.5 mg/kg) was administered together with carrageenin less than 50% inhibition was observed. Neither the dextran nor the carrageenin induced vascular permeability was inhibited more than 75% with AHE (7.5 mg/kg). AHE (2.5 mg/kg) inhibited the carrageenin induced reaction 25%.

d-CPHE was the less effective from the four esters when the permeability was induced by dextran or carrageenin. 7.5 mg/kg d-CPHE resulted the highest inhibition with 38% in case of carrageenin. l-CPHE (7.5 mg/kg) resulted 61%, or 45% inhibition when carrageenin was the agonist and 52%, or 33% when dextran was injected.

In vivo experiments were carried out on 52 male guinea-pigs weighing 280 to 350 g to reproduce asthmatic attack. Bronchus contraction was induced by histamine (0.24% base), serotonin (0.25% base), acetylcholine (0.6% base) aerosol. After the elicitation of coughing AHE, PHE, d-CPHE or l-CPHE was administered in aerosol, while the agonist aerosol was continued. When the concentration of heptyl esters varied from 0.2 - 0.4% the guinea-pigs recovered within 30-50 sec., the bronchus contraction was abolished. The d-CPHE was ineffective, the PHE was the most potent inhibitor, followed by l-CPHE and AHE.

Skin Reactive Factor (SRF) was isolated from induced lymphocytes through several purification steps. SRF induced increased vascular permeability was inhibited about 40% in guinea-pigs by PHE and AHE. CPHE was less effective than the AHE and PHE.

Summarizing our results we can say that in vitro the Arginine-heptyl ester is better bradykinin inhibitor than the Phenylalanine-heptyl ester or C-phenyl-glycine-n-heptyl ester.

In vivo the PHE showed better inhibition than the other three investigated esters. It seems probable that the esters might have some clinical significance in the treatment of inflammatory or allergic diseases.

Acknowledgement

We are very grateful to SOLCO BASLE, Ltd.

REFERENCES

1. Gecse, A., Zsilinszky, E., Lonovics, J., West, G.B.: C-phenylglycine-n-heptyl ester as an inhibitor of mediators of allergic reactions. Int. Arch. Allergy 41: 174-179, 1971.

2. Jancso-Gabor, A., Szolcsanyi, J., Jansco N.: A simple method for measuring the amount of azovan blue exuded into the skin in response to an inflammatory stimulus. J. Pharm. Pharmacol. 19: 486-487, 1967.

3. Schroder, E.: Uber Peptidsynthesen. XVII. Synthese von Gly^6-Bradykinin und Ala^5-Bradykinin. Justus Liebigs Ann. Chem. 673: 186-189, 1964.

4. Schroder, E.: Struktur-Aktivit-ts-Beziehungen bei brady-kinin-analogen Polypeptiden. In: Peptides. Proceedings of the 6th European Symposium, pp. 253, ed., L. Zervas. London, Pergamon Press, 1965.

A VASODEPRESSOR PEPTIDE IN COHN FRACTION III-0 OF HUMAN PLASMA PROTEINS

J. D. Horowitz and M. L. Mashford

Department of Medicine, University of Melbourne

St. Vincent's Hospital

Previous reports (1,2) have described the ability of human plasma to cause constriction in an isolated perfused vein from the rabbit ear. The activity emerges as a single peak from a Sephadex G200 column when high molality buffer is used, in a fraction suggesting a molecular weight of approximately 100,000. The original plasma and the eluate containing venoconstrictor activity are also vasodilator in the intact vascular beds of the guinea pig heart and the dog hind limb and on several other preparations behave very like bradykinin. Similar activity is also found in several Cohn fractions of human plasma proteins, the richest source being fraction III-0 the major components of which are partly denatured β-lipoproteins. The activity from this source is however readily dialysable and this paper describes the partial isolation of an active peptide from it.

MATERIALS AND METHODS

Cohn fraction III-0 was obtained from Commonwealth Serum Laboratories, Parkville, Australia. This had been prepared by standard cold ethanol prescription but had not been dialysed before lyophilization.

The columns used were: Sephadex CM_{25} 43 x 3 cm and 50 x 1 cm (Gradient column) and Sephadex G_{25} 90 x 1.75 cm. Buffers were as described with the results. Counter-current distribution was carried out in a Gallenkamp counter-current apparatus (Model Ev810/820) with 1% acetic acid as the lower phase and sec-butanol as the upper.

15

High voltage electrophoresis was performed on a Savant apparatus with a voltage gradient of 50 V/cm and 0.041 M pyridine/3.3% acetic acid pH 3.5 as buffer.

Amino acid analysis after 20 hours acid hydrolysis employed a Beckman 120B auto-analyser.

The assay preparation was the isolated perfused vein of the rabbit ear. This has been described in detail elsewhere (3).

RESULTS

In preliminary studies lyophilized Cohn fraction III-0 was dissolved in 5% acetic acid and applied to a Sephadex G_{25} column. The majority of material absorbing at 280 nm eluted in the void volume. Activity emerged in two peaks, the smaller in the void volume and the other, representing some 80%, was retarded to a degree suggesting a molecular weight of approximately 1500. (Fig. 1).

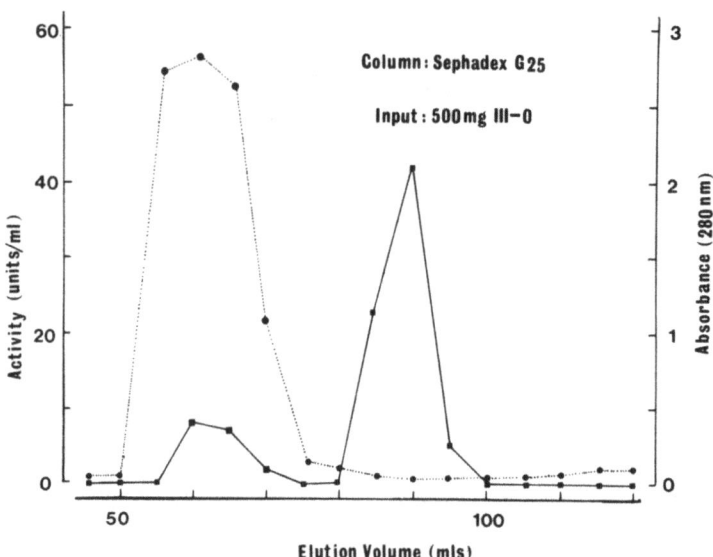

Fig. 1 Passage of III-0 in 5% acetic acid through Sephadex G_{25} column 90 x 1.75 cm

■━━■ = Venoconstrictor activity

●·····● = Absorbance (280 nM)

In preparative attempts, a total of 1 kg freeze-dried
fraction III-0, dissolved in 0.15 M NH_4 HCO_3, pH 8.0, was
applied in batches of 10-15 g to a Sephadex CM_{25} column and eluted
with the same buffer. The bulk of material absorbent at 280 nm
emerged with the void volume, while most venoconstrictor material
was eluted in later fractions (Fig. 2). Recovery of input
materials averaged 70-80% in this step with approximately 60 fold
purification.

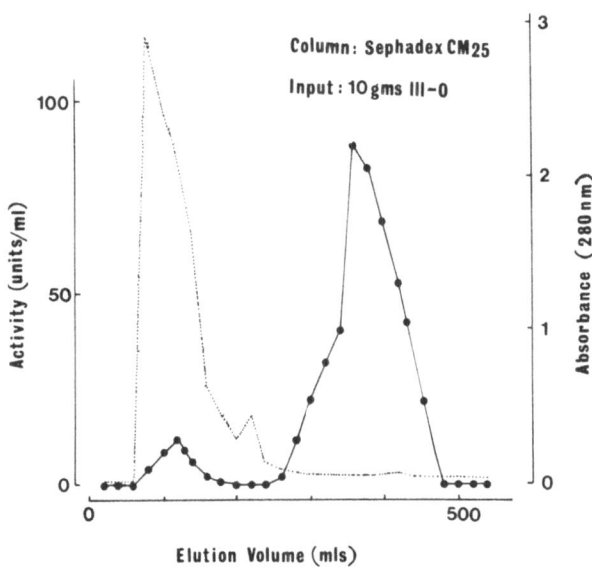

Fig. 2   Passage of III-0 in 0.15 M NH_4 HCO_3 through Sephadex CM_{25}
          column 43 x 3 cm
          ●———● = Venoconstrictor activity
          ·········· = Absorbance (280 nM)

This material was then further purified by passage through
a Sephadex G_{25} column using 5% acetic acid buffer. Venoconstrictor
material emerged in a single peak midway between the void volume
and the point of maximum elution of salts. This contained
40-50% of activity applied. The higher molecular weight
component of the activity of crude III-0 (Fig. 1) had been
eliminated by passage through Sephadex CM_{25}. Elution with 1%

acetic acid led to delay in appearance of active material from
the column, as might be expected from a basic peptide, with
consequently greater contamination with salts.

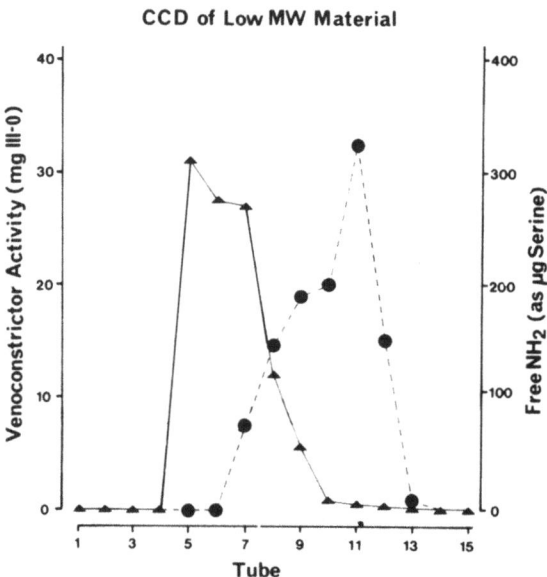

<u>Fig. 3</u> Distribution of venoconstrictor activity ● and ninhydrin
        positive material ▲ after 80 counter-current transfers
        in 1% acetic acid : 2-butanol.

        Lyophilized eluate from Sephadex G_{25} was redissolved in 1%
acetic acid and subjected to 80 transfers of counter-current extraction in a 2-butanol : 1% acetic acid system. Activity emerged
with a Kd of approximately 0.15 and the bulk of ninhydrin-positive
material remained near the origin (Fig. 3). Initial recovery of
activity indicated a purification of approximately 50,000 times
relative to original III-0; however, the resultant material was
unstable and activity fell over a 2-week period to 12% of that
found initially. The final material was thus only approximately
6,000 times purified.

This product was subjected to electrophoresis in pyridine :
acetic acid buffer, pH 3.5 with a voltage gradient of 50 V/cm.
Three ninhydrin positive spots were obtained (Fig. 4), that
with the lowest mobility containing the venoconstrictor activity.
The substance which migrated furthest had the mobility of arginine.

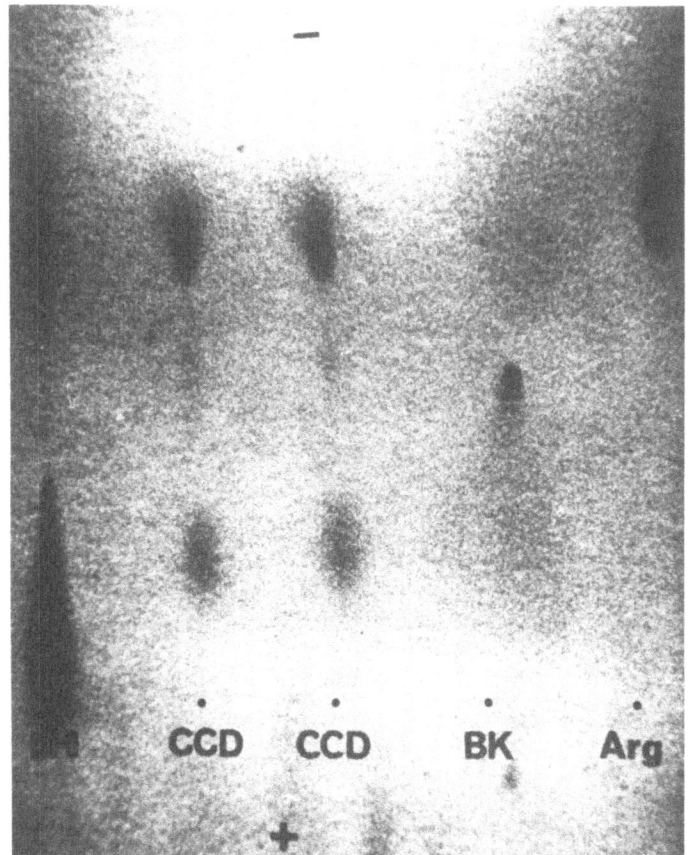

Fig. 4   High voltage electrophoresis (50 V/cm for 1 hr.) of
          III-0, CCD active fraction, bradykinin (BK) and arginine.
          Venoconstrictor activity was eluted from the region of
          the most proximal spot.

The segment of paper containing the activity was extracted
with 1 M acetic acid, lyophilized and then hydrolysed with 6 M
HCl for amino acid analysis. This detected five amino acids, viz.
glutamic acid, proline, alanine, glycine and arginine. However,
the total peptide available to be applied to the amino acid analyser
was insufficient to make an unequivocal assessment of primary
structure. The material having the highest electrophoretic mobility
was identified as arginine.

In view of the instability of the eluate from counter-
current separation and the small amounts of material available,
an alternative procedure for further purification of the G_{25}
eluate was attempted. This involved passage through a CM_{25} column
with a molarity gradient of 0.1 - 0.3 M ammonium bicarbonate at
pH 8.0. Activity was eluted in a narrow band and was subsequently
desalted on Sephadex G_{25}. The resultant freeze-dried material
exhibited a purification of approximately 25,000 relative to the
initial III-O.

Electrophoresis of this material revealed two ninhydrin-
positive spots. One was again arginine and the other contained
venoconstrictor activity. Amino acid analysis of this detected
eleven amino acids in mole ratios as detailed: Asp (1.1),
Thr (0.8), Ser (1.0), Glu (2.1), Pro (0.6), Gly (1.3), Ala (1.1),
Val (0.8), Leu (1.3), Lys (0.4) and Arg (0.4). This is clearly
not a pure material.

DISCUSSION

The venoconstrictor activity of Cohn fraction III-O has
identical pharmacological properties to the venoconstrictor
protein of plasma (2). Both are dilator in intact vascular beds.
The activity in fraction III-O comprises at least two components
which differ in molecular weight but which are both dialysable
and destroyed by chymotrypsin and carboxypeptidase B[4]. The
component with lower molecular weight has approximately 80% of
the total activity. It has been possible to produce a stable
preparation purified some 25,000 times by passage through
Sephadex CM_{25} and G_{25} columns. High voltage electrophoresis
revealed persistent contamination with arginine but the active
spot when eluted and hydrolysed was obviously still not completely
pure. Nevertheless several separate batches revealed similar
analyses.

The low mole ratios of arginine and perhaps lysine may be
explained by the apparent susceptibility of the peptide to acid
conditions. In all those steps where acetic acid has been employed
losses of activity have been considerable. The persistent reappearance of arginine after steps which should have removed it

suggests that loss of a terminal arginine is occurring with resultant loss of biological activity. The rapid destruction of activity by carboxypeptidase B is consistent with this suggestion.

While the precise constitution of this peptide has not been determined, the amino acids present differentiate it clearly from plasmakinins. Despite this, its pharmacological resemblance to them is most striking and suggests some common receptor mechanism.

REFERENCES

1. Horowitz, J.D. and Mashford, M.L. Vasoactivity of human plasma and plasma protein fractions, Experientia, 24, 1126, 1968.

2. idem: The occurrence in plasma of a protein with kinin-like activity, in Bradykinin and Related Kinins: Cardiovascular, Biochemical and Neural Actions, ed. N. Back, 1970, p. 117.

3. idem: A perfused vein preparation sensitive to plasma kinins, Naunyn-Schmiedebergs Arch. Pharm. exp. Path., 262, 332, 1969.

4. idem: Some properties of venoconstrictor peptide materials in Cohn Fraction III-0 of human plasma, Proc. Aust. Physiol. Pharmacol. Soc., 4, 146, 1973.

ACKNOWLEDGEMENTS

We are indebted to Dr. F.J. Morgan and Mr. G. Begg who performed the amino acid analyses, and to Mrs. S. Quaife for secretarial assistance.

The work was supported by grants from the National Health and Medical Research Council.

GENERATION OF KININ BY PLASMA KALLIKREIN AND PLASMIN AND THE EFFECT OF α_1-ANTITRYPSIN AND ANTITHROMBIN III ON THE KININOGENASES*

Flavio M. Habal**, Clement E. Burrowes, and Henry Z. Movat***

Division of Experimental Pathology, Department of Pathology, and Institute of Immunology, University of Toronto, Medical Sciences Building, Toronto, Ontario M5S 1A8, Canada

The two kininogenases of plasma are kallikrein and plasmin (1). Of these proteases kallikrein is more specific, acting almost exclusively on kininogen, whereas plasmin has a much wider spectrum of action, capable of degrading a number of non-specific proteins, e.g. casein. Both enzymes hydrolyse arginine esters, but while kallikrein has little effect on lysine esters, these synthetic substrates are readily hydrolysed by plasmin. Both enzymes are present in plasma as zymogens or proenzymes, kallikrein as pre-kallikrein (2) and plasmin as plasminogen (3).

A number of questions are not fully answered as yet concerning the two kininogenases. It is well known that kallikrein can act directly on kininogen. The mode of action of plasmin is somewhat uncertain. Some investigators presented circumstantial evidence that plasmin can generate kinin directly from plasma, by cleaving kinin from kininogen (4-8). Others were not able to release kinin by adding plasmin to partially purified kininogen (9-12). However, it has been known for some time that plasmin can activate prekallikrein to kallikrein when added to plasma. This was thought to represent a direct conversion of prekallikrein to kallikrein (10-12), but in subsequent studies it was shown that plasmin cleaves

* Supported by the Atkinson Charitable Foundation, The Ontario Heart Foundation and the Medical Research Council of Canada (MT-1251).

** Postdoctoral Fellow supported by the Ontario Heart Foundation.

*** Holder of an Associateship of the Medical Research Council of Canada.

23

factor XII to prekallikrein activator, which in turn converts prekallikrein to its active form (13, 14). Some of the discrepancies
in the literature may be due to the presence of plasma protease
inhibitors. It has been known for some time that α_2-macroglobulin
and $\overline{C1}$-inactivator inhibit both kallikrein and plasmin (15, 16),
but other inhibitors could have been likely contaminants of plasmin
preparations used in the past. Alpha$_2$-macroglobulin and $\overline{C1}$-inacti-
vator are readily separated from the kininogenases on the basis
of their size and charge. There are reports that α_1-antitrypsin
(17, 18) inhibits kallikrein and antithrombin III inhibits plasmin
(19). As will be discussed later these two inhibitors are difficult
to separate from each other and they are similar to plasminogen
with respect to size and charge. While kallikrein cleaves kinin
rapidly from high molecular weight kininogen, it does so at a
much slower rate when added to the low molecular weight substrate
(20). The effect of purified plasmin in this respect has not been
investigated, although older data indicate that plasmin generates
kinin at a much slower rate than kallikrein (1). Finally, the
nature of the peptide generated by plasmin has not been fully
investigated. Whereas plasma kallikrein is known to liberate
bradykinin (21), plasmin is believed to generate both the nonapeptide and the undecapeptide, mostly the latter (8).

Materials and Methods

Kallikrein was isolated as described before (20), by anion
exchange chromatography on QAE Sephadex and gel filtration through
Sephadex G-200. The plasma containing 10 µg/ml soy bean trypsin
inhibitor (SBTI) was dialysed against 0.1 M Tris HCl, containing
0.003 M EDTA. When applied to the QAE Sephadex column prekallikrein eluted in the excluded peak and SBTI with 0.12 M NaCl,
together with low molecular weight kininogen. After pooling of
the prekallikrein containing fractions, SBTI was again added to
prevent activation of prekallikrein. During gel filtration the
inhibitor was separated from the proenzyme, being retarded. A
small amount of prekallikrein was further purified by passage
through an immunoadsorbent anti-IgG column (20). The prekallikrein was activated with prekallikrein activator (22).

Plasminogen was obtained from the same plasma. From QAE
Sephadex it eluted immediately after the excluded peak with 0.075 M
NaCl. This material was passed through a lysine-Sepharose 4B
column (23), as described before (24). Sephadex G-200 was used
as a final purification step, yielding a highly purified preparation. By alkaline disc gel electrophoresis or isoelectric focusing
multiple bands and peaks respectively could be demonstrated.
However, the plasminogen was homogeneous by immunoelectrophoresis
and by disc gel electrophoresis in SDS (Fig. 1). The plasminogen
concentration was determined by radial immunodiffusion (M-Partigen,
Behringwerke, Hoechst Pharmaceuticals) or after activation to

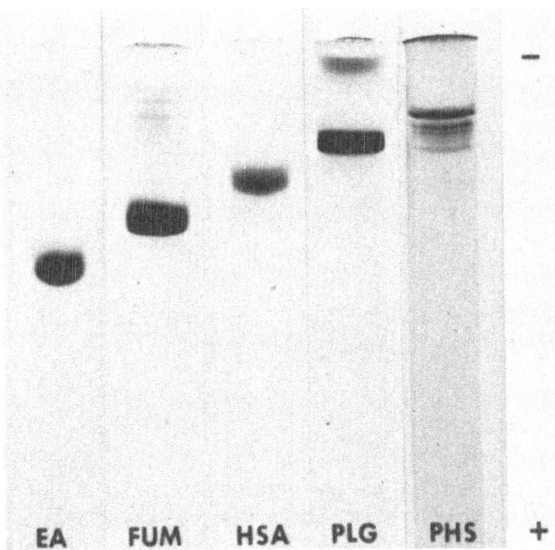

<u>Figure 1.</u>   Disc gel electrophoresis of plasminogen (PLG) in the
              presence of sodium dodecyl sulfate. Marker proteins:
              egg albumin (EA), fumarase (FUM), human serum albumin
              (HSA) and phosphorylase (PHS). Approximate molecular
              weight of plasminogen was 77,000.

plasmin, by the fibrin plate method (Hyland Laboratories).
Plasminogen (0.45 ml) was activated with streptokinase (0.05 ml;
400 units/ml; Lederle Laboratories) at 37° for 20 minutes.

    When, during QAE-Sephadex chromatography, the NaCl concentra-
tion was raised to 0.12 M low molecular weight (LMW) kininogen
eluted (20). This fraction contained the bulk of albumin, factor
XII, α_1-antitrypsin, α_2-macroglobulin, antithrombin III, C3 and
C5 and other unidentified proteins. Since the SBTI added to the
plasma eluted in this fraction and since this fraction contained
trypsin inhibitors, excess trypsin (100 µg) had to be added to
0.1 ml of fraction to detect the kininogen (20). The high molecular weight (HMW) kininogen eluted from QAE-Sephadex when the
NaCl concentration was raised to 0.35 M. Both kininogens were
further purified by a series of procedures as described elsewhere
(25). Highly purified preparations were obtained (Fig. 2).

    The inhibitors α_1-antitrypsin and antithrombin III were
isolated from both the plasma used for the isolation of prekallikrein, plasminogen and kininogens and from plasma samples
prepared exclusively for the isolation of the inhibitors. Alpha$_1$-
antitrypsin and antithrombin III eluted from QAE-Sephadex with

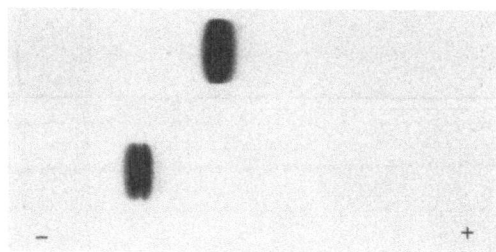

Figure 2. Alkaline disc gel electrophoresis of LMW-kininogen (top) and of HMW-kininogen (bottom).

0.12 M NaCl and during further purification of LMW-kininogen the inhibitors were recovered as by-products of this purification procedure in the supernatants of ammonium sulfate precipitation (20, 25). To obtain better yields of antithrombin III the procedure of Rosenberg and Damus (26) was followed. The prothrombin complex was removed from the plasma by adsorption with barium carbonate (50 mg/ml plasma). After centrifugation to remove the barium carbonate, concentrated aluminum hydroxide (Amphogel, unflavoured, Wyeth, Philadelphia) was added to the plasma in a ratio of 1:10. The Al(OH)$_3$ was washed free of entrapped plasma with 0.15 M NaCl and the antithrombin eluted from the gel by repeated washes with 0.35 M ammonium phosphate, pH 8.1. These washings were concentrated and chromatographed on QAE-Sephadex, Sephadex G-200 and Concanavalin A-Sepharose. In all these steps both inhibitors were eluted together. In order to separate them they were subjected to isoelectric focusing (Fig. 3). or passed through a column of heparin-Sepharose 4B (27). The inhibitors were quantitated by radial immunodiffusion (M-Partigen).

Assays for kinin-generating and arginine esterase activity (BAEe-hydrolysis) were carried out as described in detail before (20, 28). The two kininogenases were adjusted to hydrolyse approximately 200 mμmoles of BAEe per minute per ml. One tenth ml of kallikrein or plasmin was incubated for increasing time intervals with inhibitor or phosphate buffered saline (PBS), pH 7.4. For the kinin-assay 0.1 ml HMW-kininogen was added, the total volume adjusted to 1.0 ml with PBS and incubated at 37^0 for 10 minutes, followed by immersion of the tubes in boiling water for 10 minutes. After appropriate dilution with de Jalon solution the samples were tested on the estrous rat uterus. For the arginine esterase assay the enzyme-inhibitor or enzyme-buffer mixtures were mixed with 0.5 ml BAEe (0.003 M BAEe), adjusted to 3.0 ml with 0.1 M Tris HCl, containing 0.1 M NaCl (pH 8.0) and the increments in optical density were read at 253 mμ at 2 minute

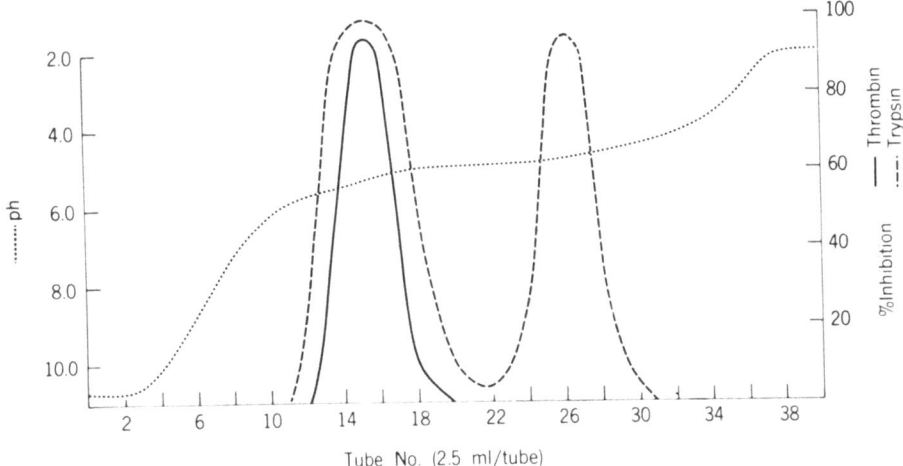

Tube No. (2.5 ml/tube)

<u>Figure 3.</u>   Separation of antithrombin III from α_1-antitrypsin
by isoelectric focusing (pH gradient: 4-6).

intervals for 12 minutes with buffer and BAEe as the blank. The
O.D. values were converted into mμmoles of BAEe hydrolysed per
minute per ml, from a calibration curve of known amount of
benzoyl arginine.

Results and Discussion

The LMW- and HMW-kininogens were adjusted (approx. 100 μg
protein/ml) to yield about the same amount of kinin when incubated
with excess trypsin (approx. 1.0 μg bradykinin equivalent). As
described before (20), under these conditions plasma kallikrein
(60 μg; BAEe hydrol. activity 275 mμmoles/min/ml) cleaved kinin
from HMW-kininogen at a much faster rate than from LMW-kininogen.
On the other hand plasmin (36 μg; BAEe-hydrol: activity 290
mμmoles/min/ml) cleaved the two substrates at about the same rate
(Fig. 4). Contrary to findings reported earlier (1), kinin-
generation by plasmin was only slightly slower than the peptide
formation from HMW-kininogen by kallikrein. As shown in Figure 1
the plasminogen was highly purified. By immunodiffusion and by
counterimmunoelectrophoresis the plasminogen and the kininogens
were free of all proteinase inhibitors. Traces of such inhibitors
could account for earlier reports of slow kinin-formation by
plasmin. The latter and LMW-kininogen could have been contaminated
by α_2-macroglobulin, α_1-antitrypsin and antithrombin III, whereas
a constant contaminant of HMW-kininogen was shown to be C$\overline{I}$-inacti-
vator (20, 25).

F.M. HABAL, C.E. BURROWES, AND H.Z. MOVAT

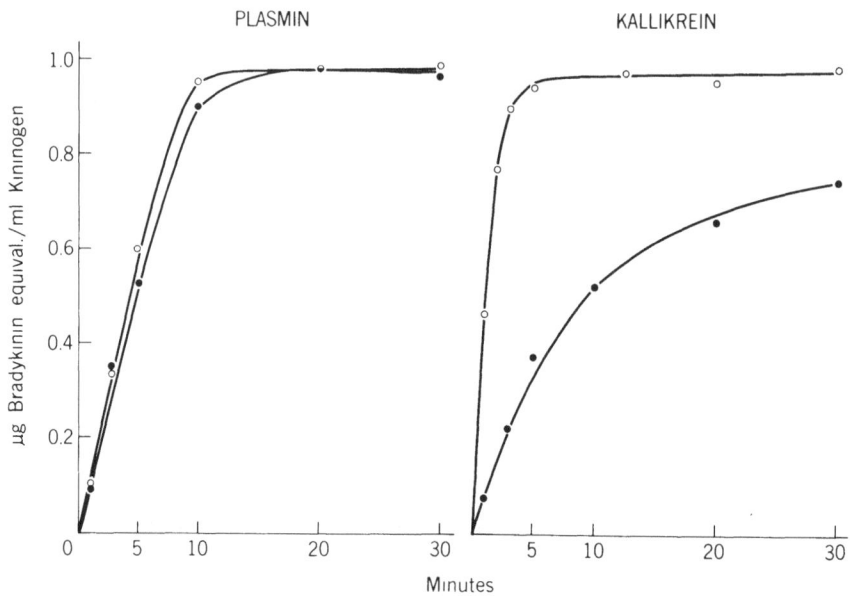

<u>Figure 4.</u>   Time course of the release of kinin from HMW-kininogen
            (open circles) and from LMW-kininogen (closed circles)
            by plasmin and by plasma kallikrein (see text).

      With both kallikrein and plasmin the amount of kinin generated
increased with increasing concentrations of kininogen, whereas the
rate of peptide formation was a function of enzyme concentration.

      As indicated in the introduction while there is no doubt
about the inhibition of plasmin and kallikrein by α_2-macroglobulin
and C1-inactivator there is some uncertainty about the effect of
α_1-antitrypsin and antithrombin III.   The two inhibitors eluted
together throughout anion exchange and molecular sieve chromatography and both adsorbed onto Concanavalin A-Sepharose.   Separation
could only be achieved by isoelectric focusing (pH 4.0-6.0) or by
affinity chromatography on heparin-Sepharose.   Even if the $Al(OH)_3$
adsorption suggested by Rosenberg and Damus (26) was used as the
initial step both inhibitors became adsorbed to the gel and were
separable only in the final step (Fig. 3).   As reported by
Heimburger <u>et al</u>. (29) trypsin is inhibited by both inhibitors,
but thrombin only by antithrombin III.   Antithrombin was found to
be a good inhibitor of both kallikrein and plasmin, particualrly
in the presence of small concentrations of heparin (Figs. 5 and 6).
Under the same conditions α_1-antitrypsin did not inhibit kallikrein and was a weak inhibitor of plasmin (Table 1).   In view of
the findings of Fritz <u>et al</u>. (17) the kallikrein was incubated

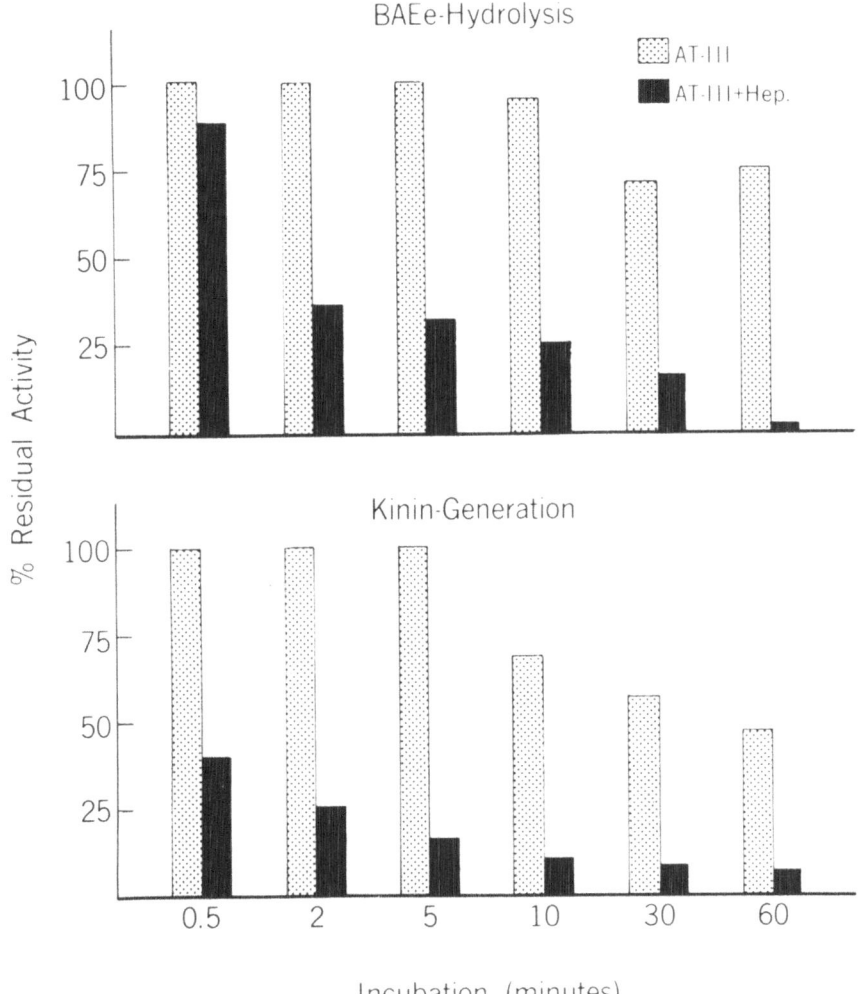

<u>Figure 5.</u> Inhibition of 0.1 ml plasmin (BAEe hydrolysing activity 215 mμmoles/min/ml) by 0.1 ml antithrombin III (12.5 μg) in the presence or absence of heparin (0.15 units). Inhibition of both arginine-esterase and kinin-generating activities are shown.

with the α_1-antitrypsin for 6 and for 24 hours at 37°. Under these extremely prolonged conditions inhibition of esterase activity was about 40% and 60% respectively. Kinin-generation was inhibited only 25% in 24 hours. Plasmin could not be tested

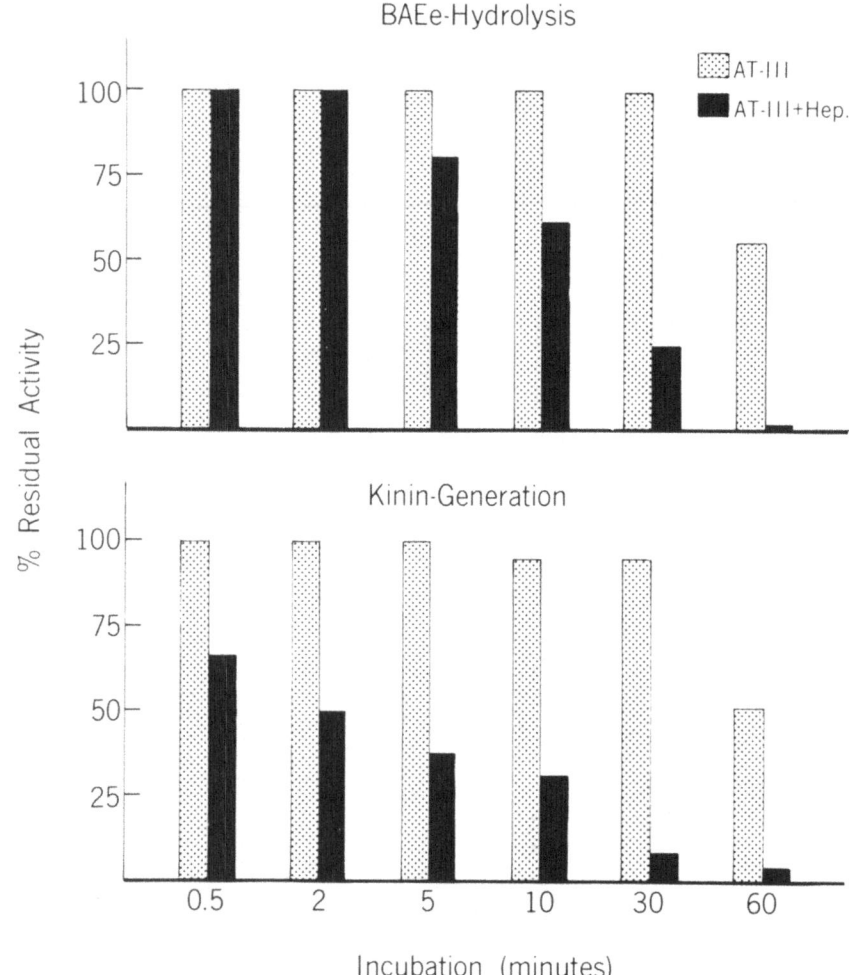

Figure 6.   Inhibition of plasma kallikrein (BAEe hydrolysing activity 207 mμmoles/min/ml) by antithrombin III. Conditions same as in Figure 5.

for a long period because the enzyme decays during incubation at 37°. To ascertain the data with α_1-antitrypsin shown in Table 1 are not due to trace contamination with antithrombin III, the α_1-antitrypsin was tested in the presence of heparin, but there was no enhancing effect. The α_1-antitrypsin used in the studies presented in Table 1 had a protein concentration of 13.0 μg by radial immunodiffusion (the concentration of antithrombin III 12.5 μg). Serial two-fold dilutions of the inhibitor were made and tested against trypsin. A twentieth-dilution of the inhibitor (0.65 μg) caused 100% inhibition of 1.0 μg of trypsin.

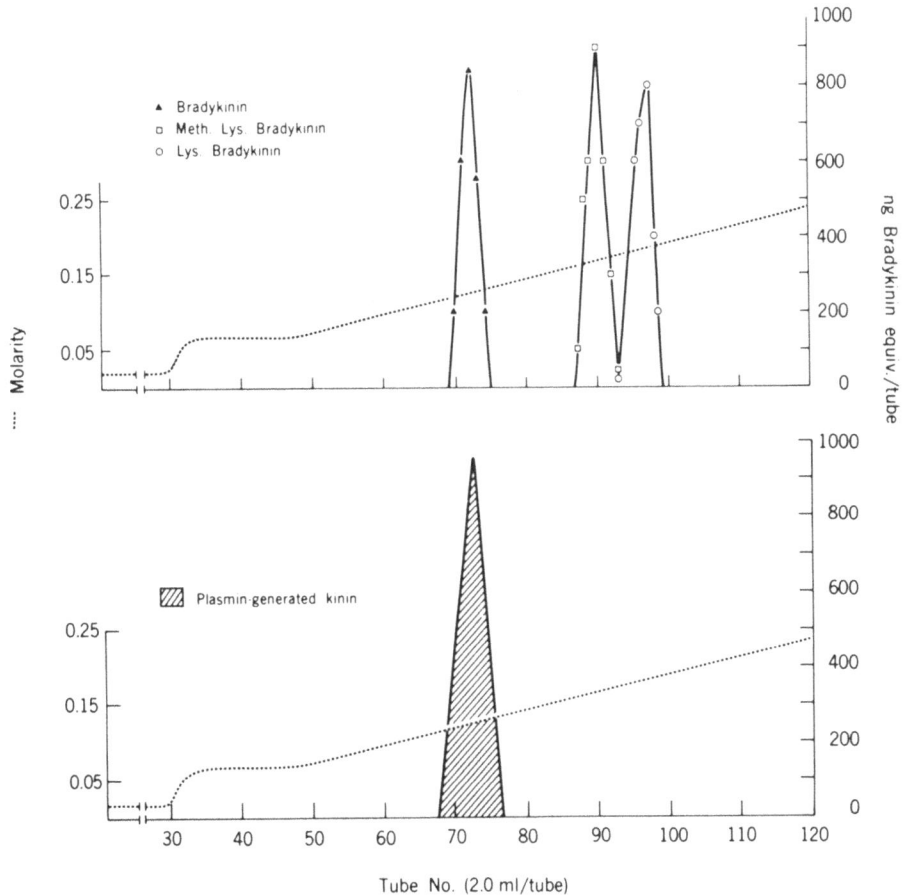

<u>Figure 7.</u> CM-cellulose chromatography of synthetic kinins and of
plasmin-generated kinin (see text).

This amount of trypsin had a BAEe-hydrolysing activity of 215
mμmoles/min/ml. More data are required to come to a more precise
understanding of the inhibition of the two kininogenases by the
two inhibitors. However, these preliminary data indicate that
<u>in vivo</u> probably only antithrombin plays any significant inhibitory
role.

In order to ascertain the nature of peptide cleaved by plasmin
HMW-kininogen and plasmin were dialysed for 4 hours against 0.02 M
ammonium formate adjusted to pH 7.4 with ammonium hydroxide. The
mixture was incubated at 37° for 20 minutes, the pH adjusted to
4.8 with formic acid and boiled for 10 minutes. After removal of
the protein precipitate, the supernatant was adjusted with distilled

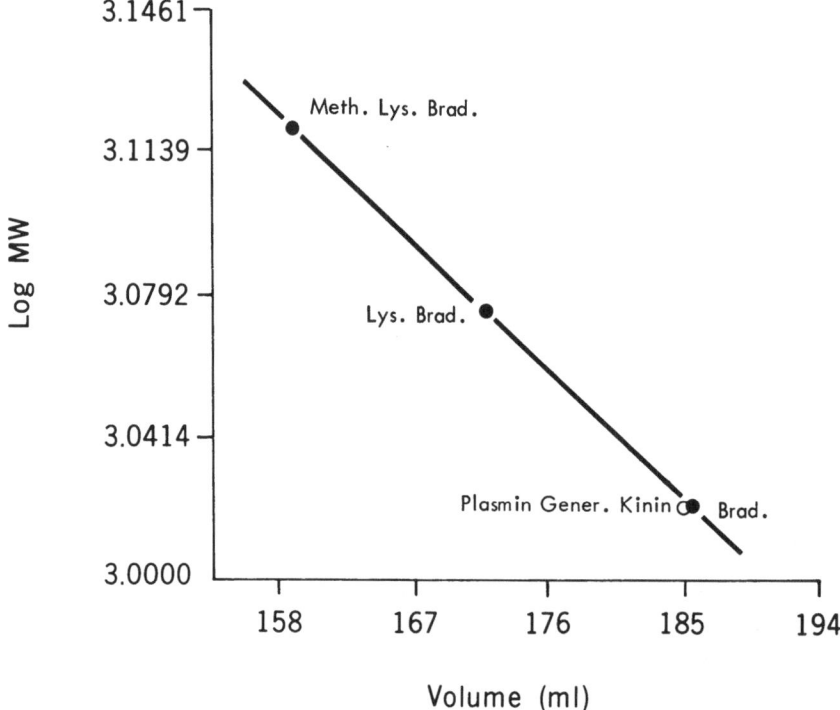

<u>Figure 8</u>.   Gel filtration of the plasmin-generated kinin on
             Sephadex G-15 (see text).

<u>TABLE 1</u>.   Inhibition of plasmin by α_1-antitrypsin

Activity	5	Incubation time (minutes)		
		10	30	60
		% Residual Activity		
BAEe-hydrolysis	0	8	29	62
Kinin-generation	0	0	13	40

0.1 ml plasmin (BAEe-hydrolysing activity 215 mμmoles/min/ml)
was incubated for ½-60 min. with 0.1 ml α_1-antitrypsin (13.0 μg)
at 37°. To this reaction mixture either BAEe or HMW-kininogen
was added and assayed as described under Materials and Methods.

water to the conductivity of 0.02 M ammonium formate-formic acid (pH 4.8) and applied to a 1.5 x 15 cm column of CM-cellulose equilibrated with 0.02 M formate buffer. After washing with the equilibrating buffer and with 0.08 M formate a linear gradient was applied between 0.08 and 0.3 M formate. Under similar conditions synthetic kinins eluted as described (21) and the peptide generated by plasmin eluted in the position of bradykinin (Fig.7). The pool containing the peptide was lyophilized, redissolved in 1.0 ml of distilled water and applied to two interconnected columns of Sephadex G-15 (1.6 x 100 cm). The gel was equilibrated with 0.2 M ammonium formate-formic acid, pH 4.0. Figure 8 shows the elution of the three synthetic kinins and that generated by plasmin. Amino acid analysis (30) confirmed the data obtained by CM-cellulose and Sephadex G-15 that the peptide generated by plasmin is bradykinin.

Concluding Remarks

Contrary to some earlier reports plasmin can generate kinin directly from kininogen, although it is known that it can activate prekallikrein indirectly by converting factor XII to prekallikrein activator. Whereas kallikrein cleaves kinin more readily from HMW-than from LMW-kininogen, plasmin forms kinin equally well from both substrates. Earlier reports notwithstanding, highly purified plasmin can liberate kinin from highly purified kininogens at a rapid rate. Both kallikrein and plasmin are readily inhibited by antithrombin III in the presence of heparin. Alpha$_1$-antitrypsin is a poor inhibitor of plasmin and its inhibition of kallikrein is negligible, since no inhibition was observed when incubated up to one hour; only after prolonged incubation. The peptide cleaved by plasmin from HMW-kininogen is the nonapeptide bradykinin.

References

1. Eisen, V. and Vogt, W.: Plasma kininogenases and their activators, In Handbook of Experimental Pharmacology, E.G. Erdos, ed., Springer, Berlin, (1970).

2. Wuepper, K.D.: Plasma prekallikrein: its characterization, mechanism of action and inherent deficiency in man, In Chemistry and Biology of the Kallikrein-Kinin System in Health and Disease, J.J. Pisano and K.F. Austen, eds., Fogarty Internat. Center Proc. No. 27, U.S. Gov. Printing Office, Washington, (1975).

3. Robbins, K.C. and Summaria, L.: Human plasminogen and plasmin, In Methods of Enzymology, E.G. Perlman and L. Lorand, eds., Academic Press, New York, (1970)

4. Lewis, G.P.: Formation of plasma kinins by plasmin. J. Physiol.
    140: 285, (1958).

5. Eisen, V.: Kinin formation and fibrinolysis in human plasma.
    J. Physiol. 166: 514, (1963).

6. Back, N. and Steger, R.: Activation of bovine bradykininogen
    by human plasma. Life Sci. 4: 153, (1965).

7. Hamberg, U.: Plasma protease and kinin release with special
    reference to plasmin. Ann. N.Y. Acad. Sci. 146: 517, (1968).

8. Gapanhuk, E. and Henriques, O.B.: Kinins released from horse
    heat-acid-denatured plasma by plasmin, plasma kallikrein,
    trypsin and bothrops kininogenase. Biochem. Pharmacol. 19:
    1091, (1970).

9. Bhoola, K.D., Calle, E.J.D. and Schachter, M.: The effect of
    bradykinin, serum kallikrein and other endogenous substances
    on capillary permeability in the guinea pig. J. Physiol.
    152, 75, (1960).

10. Vogt, W.: Kinin formation by plasmin: an indirect process
    mediated by activation of kallikrein. J. Physiol. 170
    153, (1964).

11. Buluk, K. and Malofiejew, M.: Urokinase-induced activation of
    kallikreinogen and the release of plasma kinins in renal
    blood. Acta Med. Pol. 6: 405, (1965).

12. Haustein, K.O. and Marquardt, F.: Untersuchungen uber die
    Gerinnungsund Fibrinolysevorgange im menschlichen Blut.
    Acta Biol. Germ. 16: 658, (1966).

13. Kaplan, A.P. and Austen, K.F.: A prealbumin activator of pre-
    kallikrein. II. Derivation of activators of prekallikrein
    from active Hageman factor by digestion with plasmin. J. Exp.
    Med. 133: 696, (1971).

14. Burrowes, C.E., Movat, H.Z. and Soltay, M.J.: The kinin system
    of human plasma. IV. The action of plasmin. Proc. Soc. Exp.
    Biol. Med. 138: 959, (1971).

15. Harpel, P.C.: Circulating inhibitors of human plasma kallikrein,
    In Chemistry and Biology of the Kallikrein-Kinin System in
    Health and Disease, J.J. Pisano and K.F. Austen, eds., Fogarty
    Internat. Center Proc. No. 27, U.S. Gov. Printing Office,
    Washington, (1975).

16. Harpel, P.C. and Cooper, N.R.: Studies on human plasma C1-
     inactivator-enzyme interactions. I. Mechanisms of inter-
     action with C1s, plasmin, and trypsin. J. Clin. Invest. 55:
     593, (1975).

17. Firtz, H., Wunderer, G., Kummer, K., Heimburger, N. and Werle,
     E.: α1-antitrypsin und C1-Inaktivator: Progressiv-Inhibitoren
     fur Serum-kallikrein von Mensch und Schwein. Hoppe- Seyler's
     Z. Physiol. Chem. 353: 906, (1972).

18. McConnell, D.J.: Inhibitors of kallikrein in human plasma.
     J. Clin. Invest. 51: 1611,(1972).

19. Highsmith, R.F. and Rosenberg, R.D.: The inhibition of
     human plasmin by human antithrombin-heparin cofactor.
     J. Biol. Chem. 249: 4335, (1974).

20. Habal, F.M., Movat, H.Z. and Burrowes, C.E.: Isolation of
     two functionally different kininogens from human plasma:
     separation from proteinase inhibitors and interaction with
     plasma kallikrein. Biochem. Pharmacol. 23; 2291, (1974).

21. Habermann, E. and Blennemann, G.: Uber Substrate und Reaktions-
     produkte der kininbildenden Enzyme Trypsin, Serum- und
     Pankreaskallikrein sowie von Crotalusgift. Naunyn-Schmiede-
     bergs Arch. Path. Pharm. 249: 357, (1964).

22. Ozge-Anwar, A.H., Movat, H.Z. and Scott, J.G.: The kinin
     system of human plasma. IV. The interrelationship between
     the contact phase of blood coagulation and the plasma kinin
     system in man. Thromb. Diath. Haemorrh. 27: 141, (1972).

23. Deutsch, D.G. and Mertz, E.T.: Plasminogen: purification from
     human plasma by affinity chromatography. Science 170:
     1095, (1970).

24. Burrowes, C.E., Movat, H.Z. and Soltay, M.J.: The role of
     plasmin in the activation of the kinin system. In Vaso-
     peptides, Chemistry, Pharmacology, and Pathophysiology,
     N.Back and F. Sicuteri, eds., Plenum Press, New York (1972).

25. Habal, F.M. and Movat, H.Z.: Some physicochemical and functio-
     nal differences between low and high molecular weight kinino-
     gens of human plasma, In Chemistry and Biology of the
     Kallikrein-Kinin System in Health and Disease, J.J. Pisano
     and K.F. Austen, eds., Fogarty Internat. Center Proc. No. 27,
     U.S.Gov. Printing Office, Washington (1975).

26.   Rosenberg, R.D. and Damus, P.S.: The purification and mecha-
      nism of action of human antithrombin-heparin cofactor. J.
      Biol. Chem. 248: 6490, (1973).

27.   Damus, P.S. and Wallace, G.A.: Purification of canine anti-
      thrombin III-heparin cofactor using affinity chromatography.
      Biochem. Biophys. Res. Comm. 61: 1147, (1974).

28.   Movat, H.Z., Poon, M.-C. and Takeuchi, Y.: The kinin system
      of human plasma. I. Isolation of a low molecular weight
      activator of prekallikrein. Int. Arch. Allergy 40: 89, (1971).

29.   Heimburger, N., Haupt, H. and Schwick, H.G.: Proteinase
      inhibitors of human plasma, In Proc. Internat. Res. Conf. on.
      Proteinase Inhibitors, H. Firtz and H. Tschesche, eds.,
      Walter de Gruyter, Berlin,(1971).

30.   Blackburn, S.: Amino Acid Determination, M. Decker, New York,
      (1968).

Acknowledgements

The authors wish to thank Dr. D.M. Wrobel and Mrs. I. Macdonald of the Canadian Red Cross for generous supplies of blood
and plasma. The skillful technical and secretarial assistance
of Mrs. Otti Freitag, Mrs. Anneliese Carré and Ms. Marica
Michael are gratefully acknowledged.

POTENT KININASES OBTAINED FROM MUSHROOMS

H. Moriya, K. Kizuki, Y. Hojima & C. Moriwaki

Lab. of Physiol. Chem., Science Univ. of Tokyo

Shinjuku-ku, Tokyo 162, Japan

In order to elucidate physiological functions or pathological meanings of the kallikrein-kinin system in the body, it might be an advantageous and important idea as one of the effective methods for approaching to find something strong and specific substance in the kinin system, for instance, to find specific kallikrein inhibitor, strong anti-kinin substance and potent kininase which would be sometimes developed to useful medicines for some diseases related to the kallikrein-kinin system.

The present paper deals with the potent kininases in mushrooms. As shown on Table 1, 2 kinds of Japanese mushrooms, "Shimeji (Tricholoma conglobatum) and Tsukuritake (Psalliota hortensis)" contained strong kininase activity. Other Japanese mushrooms did not contain so much. Those contained in other vegetables and fruits were almost none or weak.

For the determination of kininase activity, the assay was done by measuring inactivated contraction of synthetic bradykinin (Bdk) using guinea-pig ileum in 10 ml bath at 30^0. In order to get quantitative values from the proportional range of the inactivated response, incubation period of Bdk and enzyme, the range of inactivation % and other experimental conditions were examined, then an assay system was finally decided to yield about 50% inactivation during 3-5 min. incubation and was employed through this experiment. Thus 1 kininase unit was expressed as 1 μg of Bdk inactivated per min.

Following the first extraction of homogeneized mushrooms with distilled water, ammonium sulfate fractionation, dialysis,

37

Table I. Contents of Kininase Activity in Various Plants

	Kininase U*/g		Kininase U*/g
White potato [1]	0.5 - 0.9	Shimeji	40 - 334
Sweet potato	0.6 - 2.1	(Tricholoma conglobatum)	
Young taros	0.2 - 0.3	Tsukuritake	31 - 115
		(Psalliota hortensis)	
Lily bulb	0.3 - 0.7	Enokitake	13 - 17
Radish	0.9 - 1.5	(Collybia velutipes)	
		Matsutake	12 - 13
Pumpkin	0.5 - 3.9	(Armillaria Matsutake)	
Cabbage	0.1 - 0.8	Shiitake	5.4 - 6.4
Tomato	0.0 - 0.1	(Cortinellus edodes)	
		Nameko	1.6 - 1.7
Spinach	0.0 - 0.1	(Pholiota Nameko)	
Apple	0.2 - 0.4		

* Kininase Unit = 1 µg bradykinin inactivated/min(30°, pH 7.4)

DEAE-sephadex A-50 chromatography, sephadex gel-filtration etc. were applied. Shimeji kininase was finally prepared to yield 10% and 320 times purification through this procedure. Another highly pure enzyme from another mushroom Tsukuritake was also prepared by means of almost the same procedures except the concentration of buffers for elution chromatographies.

Table II summarizes the specific activities of the kininase compared with ever known enzymes, all of which values were measured by the same method in our laboratory. As shown on the Table II, especially big value of Tsukuritake kininase was found.

In order to examine which position of peptide bonds of Bdk molecule to be hydrolysed by the enzymes, techniques of detection of dancylated peptide which gives beautiful fluorescence on thin-layer chromatography was applied. This technique was originally developed by Gray and Hartley (3), then modified by Nakajima, Horishima Univ.

In Fig. 1., (A) shows the fluorescence of dancyl-Bdk and (B) shows one of fragments giving fluorescence after incubation of dancyl-Bdk and Shimeji kininase, and this fluorescence must be due to amino-terminal fluorescence of dancyl-Bdk itself. Other

Table II   Comparison of Activities of the Kininases from
Mushrooms and Other Plants

Enzymes	Kininase activity (U/mg)	
	Active form	Inactive form
Kininases from		
Tric. cong. (shimeji)	471*	
Psal. hort. (tsukuritake)	2284*	
Ficin	8.3	0.13
Ficin A[2)]	180	
B	7.5	
C	5.6	
D	0.3	
Bromelain	3.3	0.18
Papain	456	6.02
Kininase from potato	5.0*	

* Kininase U/E_{280}

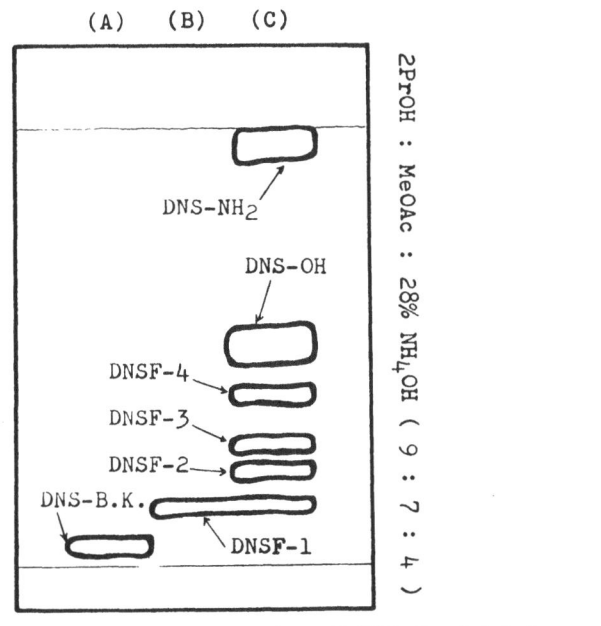

Fig. 1.   Thin-Layer Chromatography of DNS-Bradykinin
and DNS-Fragments from Bradykinin on Silicagel H

A : DNS-Bradykinin
B : DNS-Bradykinin + Kininase from
    Mushroom(Tric.cong., shimeji)
C : B treated with DNS-Cl

fragments were modified once more with dancyl chloride, then
developed on (C) in Fig. 1. and their fluorescence were observed.
There were 4 detectable fragments and 2 more upper spots (C)
giving fluorescence coming from reagent itself. Then amino-terminal
and composition of amino acids of each fragments were determined.
On the other hand the same experiment in the case of dancyl-Bdk
incubated with α-chymotrypsin was made sure in which the products
can be expected, and compared in the case of incubated with the
kininase. As shown on Table III, fragments-1, -2, -3, and -4,
N-terminal and amino acids compositions were determined, thus the
positions of Bdk molecule to be hydrolysed by this Shimeji kininase
were speculated and concluded (Fig. 2.). Just the same experiment
with another kininase of Tsukuritake was performed and the position
hydrolysed was determined.

Table III.   Amino Acid Analysis of the Fragments from DNS-Bdk

Fragment	N-terminal Amino Acids	Composed Amino Acids
DNSF-1	Arg	Arg , Pro , Gly
DNSF-2	Phe	Phe , Ser , Pro , Arg
DNSF-3	Phe	Phe , Arg
DNSF-4	Phe	Phe , Ser , Pro

Bradykinin : Arg-Pro-Pro-Gly-Phe-Ser-Pro-Phe-Arg

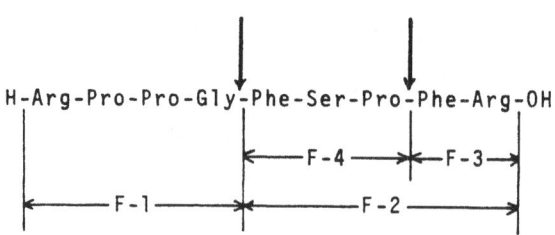

Fig. 2.   Sites of Action of Kininase from Mushroom
Tricholoma conglobatum (Shimeji)

Table IV.   Sites of Action of Some Kininases

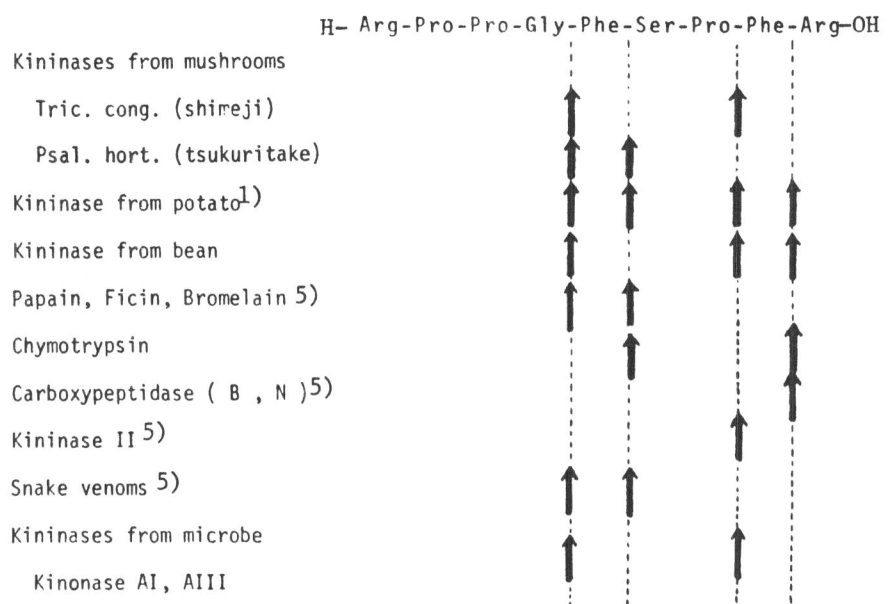

H– Arg-Pro-Pro-Gly-Phe-Ser-Pro-Phe-Arg–OH

Kininases from mushrooms

   Tric. cong. (shimeji)

   Psal. hort. (tsukuritake)

Kininase from potato[1]

Kininase from bean

Papain, Ficin, Bromelain [5]

Chymotrypsin

Carboxypeptidase (B , N)[5]

Kininase II [5]

Snake venoms [5]

Kininases from microbe

   Kinonase AI, AIII

The behaviours of two kininases against synthetic peptides substrates and the effect of various enzyme inhibitors on our both kininases were preliminarily tested. The details on these matters and other properties will be published in the future.

Table IV summarizes the positions of Bdk molecule hydrolysed by ever known proteinases. Kininases from potato and bean were also prepared in our laboratory and tested by the same experiment; however, the authors were afraid each of them was not homogenous, maybe mixture of some proteinases, giving the wide actions shown on Table IV. Papain, ficin, bromelain, chymotrypsin, carboxy-peptidase B, -N and kininase II in plasma cleaved the positions indicated (5). Kininases AI and AIII from microbe were the enzymes newly prepared from some kind of bacterial cultured fluid by Nakamura, Hiroshima Univ. and the position of Bdk hydrolysed by these enzymes was coincident with our Shimeji kininase.

REFERENCES

1. Y. Hojima, M. Tanaka, H. Moriya & C. Moriwaki, Japanese J.
   Allergology, 20, 755; 763 (1971).

2. M. Sugiura, M. Sasaki & C. Moriwaki, Folia Pharmacol. Japan.,
   69, 409 (1973).

3. W.R. Gray & B. S. Hartley, Biochem. J., 89, 379 (1963).

4. T. Nakajima, Metabolism and Disease, 6, 663 (1969).

5. E.G. Erdos & H.Y.T. Yang, "Handbuch der experimentellen
   Pharmakologie, vol. XXV Bradykinin, Kallidin and Kallikrein",
   p. 295, ed. by E. G. Erdos. Berlin-Heidelberg-New York:
   Springer-Verlag 1970.

CONFORMATION OF BRADYKININ IN RELATION TO SOLVENT ENVIRONMENT

D.I. Marlborough*, J.W. Ryan* and A.M. Felix**

*Papanicolaou Cancer Research Institute , P.O. Box 23-6188, Miami, Florida   33123 and **Hoffmann-La Roche Inc., Nutley, New Jersey   07110

For a small peptide, bradykinin has an unusually large percentage of proline residues in its primary structure. The occurrence of proline in a peptide chain tends to restrict the conformational flexibility of the peptide (1). Bradykinin would therefore be expected to show some degree of ordered structure in solution. Early optical rotatory dispersion (ORD) and circular dichroism (CD) results (2,3), however, suggested that the structure was freely flexible in aqueous solution. Later CD measurements on bradykinin and some of its homologs in aqueous and non-aqueous solvents (4) were interpreted as showing partial intramolecular hydrogen-bonding. An 8 → 6 hydrogen-bond across proline[7] was postulated for bradykinin in aqueous solution, while additional 9 → 7 and 4 → 2 hydrogen-bonds across phenylalanine[8] and proline[3] respectively were postulated in dioxane solution. The model on which Cann's conclusions are based is an intramolecularly hydrogen-bonded proline derivative in non-aqueous solvents. In non-aqueous solvents the possibility of other intramolecular interactions and solvent interaction with the peptide is minimized. It seems likely therefore, that the model for bradykinin in aqueous solution would be complicated by the possible interactions described above.

The pharmacological actions produced by hormones such as bradykinin are thought to be mediated through interaction with a receptor molecule as the first step in a chain of cellular processes leading to the hormonal response (5). A priori, the hormone "receptor-site" must be of such ionic and spatial character

that it will readily and specifically interact with the functional
groups on the hormone. Following this argument at least part of
the hormone must be in a definite orientation for interaction with
the receptor-site. Thus a knowledge of peptide conformation
appears to be essential to understand the peptide-receptor interaction. Intuitively it seems likely that the conformation of the
peptide is dictated by energetic preferences of the peptide-
receptor complex, particularly for peptides of the size of bradykinin. There is ample evidence of conformational changes when
peptides interact with proteins in solution (6). Thus the confor-
mative responses of peptide hormones such as bradykinin to environments which simulate possible properties of the receptor proteins
in hydrophobicity and nucleophilicity may well improve understanding
of the mechanism of action of these peptide hormones.

Based on the rationale given in the previous paragraph, the
CD spectra of bradykinin and some of its biologically active
analogs have been studied in a variety of solvent conditions. The
studies described here have attempted to give some basis for
relating conformational adaptation to pharmacological behavior.

EXPERIMENTAL SECTION

Bradykinin, obtained from BACHEM Inc., was shown to be electro-
phoretically and chromatographically homogeneous. L-3,4-dehydro-
lyl[3]-bradykinin, L-glutamyl[1]-kallidin and L-glutamyl[1]- L-3,4-
dehydroprolyl[3]-kallidin were prepared by solid-phase synthesis and
purified by gel filtration and preparative electrophoresis as
described by Felix, et al. (7). Each analog was shown to be homogeneous by tlc, paper electrophoresis and amino acid analysis.

Solutions were made up with distilled water passed through an
ion-exchange resin, and concentrations were estimated from dry
weights of the peptides. The urea used was analytical reagent
grade obtained from MALLINCKRODT and recrystallized from boiling
water prior to use. 2,2,2-trifluoroethanol (TFE) was obtained
from MATHESON, COLEMAN and BELL, and redistilled prior to use.

The CD spectra were measured on a JASCO ORD-UV/5 spectropolarimeter at ambient temperatures. The instrument was calibrated with
d-10 camphorsulfonic acid (C = 0.14% in water) in accordance with
the published data of Krueger and Pshigoda (8). Prior to measuring all spectra, the aqueous solutions were passed through a
Millipore filter and the non-aqueous solutions filtered through
glass wool.

RESULTS AND DISCUSSION

Bradykinin in aqueous solution has a CD spectrum with a trough
at 234-5nm (molar ellipticity - 500°) and a peak at 222-3nm (molar
ellipticity, + 600°). In solutions of increasing urea concentration, the trough shifted to 236-7nm and the molar ellipticity
changed to -320°. The peak shifted to 223-4nm and the molar
ellipticity increased in magnitude to +750°. These results are
shown in figure 1 as a titration of $[\theta]_{230}$ against urea concentration. However, in TFE the trough was blue-shifted to 227nm and
the negative magnitude of the ellipticity increased. The titration of $[\theta]_{230}$ against TFE concentration in water is also shown
in figure 1. TFE, a known order-promoting medium, has a significant effect on the CD of bradykinin relative to the effect of the
order-disrupting agent urea. The CD data suggest that in aqueous
solution bradykinin has little secondary structure to be disrupted
but adopts a less flexible conformation in the non-interacting
environment of TFE.

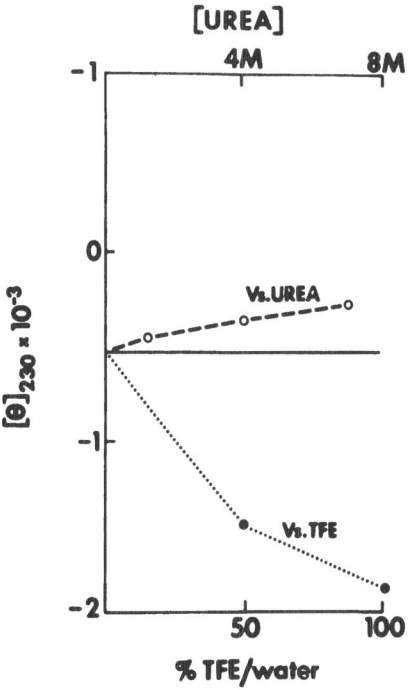

Figure 1. Optical titration of molar ellipticities at 230 nm for
bradykinin against urea and TFE/water.

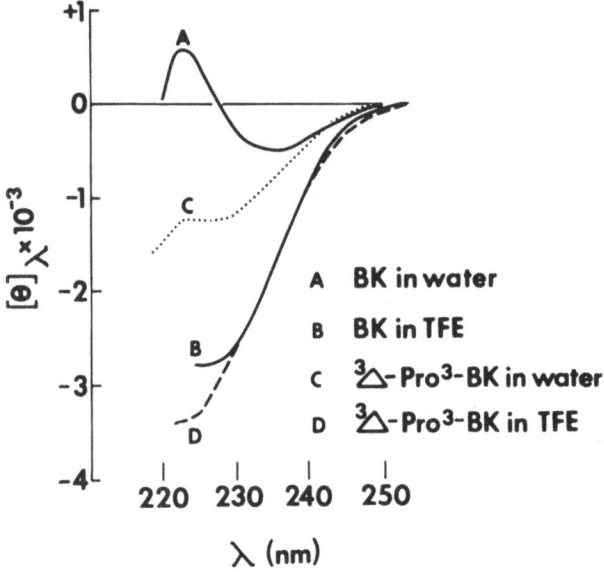

Figure 2. Circular dichroism spectra for bradykinin (BK) and
L-3,4-dehydroprolyl[3]-bradykinin ($^3_\Delta$-Pro[3]-BK) in TFE and water.

     The CD spectrum of L-3,4-dehydroprolyl[3]-bradykinin in water
is intermediate between that of bradykinin in water and bradykinin
in TFE. The CD of L-3,4-dehydroprolyl[3]-bradykinin in TFE is,
however, much closer to that of bradykinin in TFE (figure 2). The
CD spectrum of L-glutamyl[1]-kallidin in water superimposes that of
bradykinin in water within experimental error. Also the CD spectrum of L-glutamyl[1]-L-3,4-dehydroprolyl[3]-kallidin in water is
very close to that of L-3,4-dehydroprolyl[3]-bradykinin in water.
In TFE the CD spectra of bradykinin and L-glutamyl[1]-L-3,4-
dehydroprolyl[3]-kallidin are close to each other in profile (figure
3). The similarity of the CD spectra of the 1-L-glutamyl homologs
of bradykinin and L-3,4-dehydroprolyl[3]-bradykinin to bradykinin
and L-3,4-dehydroprolyl[3]-bradykinin, respectively, suggests that
extension from the α-amino terminal has little effect on conformation, even though a side-chain of opposite polarity to arginine
has been introduced. The orientation of the peptide bond around
the proline[3] in bradykinin, and its analogs, appears, from the
CD data, to strongly influence the overall conformation.

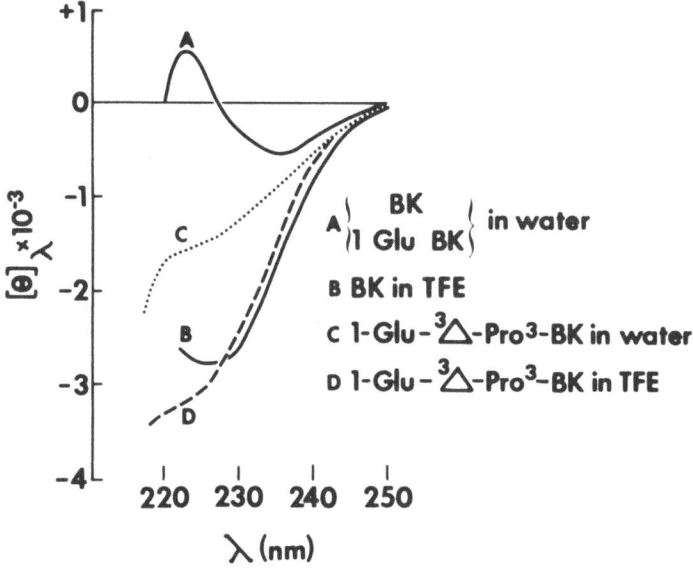

Figure 3. Circular dichroism spectra of bradykinin (BK), L-glutamyl[1]-kallidin (1-Glu BK) and L-glutamyl[1]-L-3,4-dehydroprolyl[3]-kallidin (1-Glu-3Δ-Pro[3]-BK) in water and TFE.

Figure 4 shows the change of the molar ellipticities at 230nm for bradykinin, L-3,4-dehydroprolyl[3]-bradykinin and L-glutamyl[1]-L-3,4-dehydroprolyl[3]-kallidin with a change of solvent from water to TFE. The graph in figure 4 demonstrates that, despite the differences in molar ellipticities for the three peptides in aqueous solution, the molar ellipticities are equivalent in TFE.

The influence of hydrophobic environment on the conformation of bradykinin is additionally illustrated by the effect of the detergent sodium dodecyl sulfate (SDS) on the CD spectrum of bradykinin (figure 5). The CD profile for bradykinin in 0.1% SDS is similar to that for bradykinin in TFE, suggesting similar conformations in the two media. Reynolds and Tanford (9) have suggested that protein-SDS complexes may be good models for polypeptides which are not easily dissociated from membrane lipids, and probably associated with the lipid through primarily hydrophobic forces. If the interactions of the membrane proteins with lipids parallel that of SDS then an extended ordered polypeptide chain can be postulated which is associated with the hydrophobic regions of the bimolecular leaflet. Applying the above reasoning to the interaction of bradykinin with SDS it can be postulated that an ordered

extended chain conformation could be adopted by bradykinin in
hydrophobic environments such as those associated with membrane
lipids.

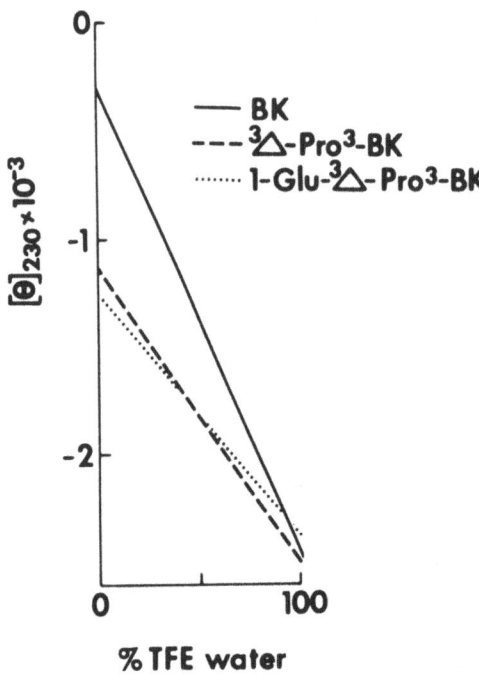

Figure 4.   Titration of molar ellipticities at 230 nm against TFE/
water for bradykinin (BK), L-3,4-dehydroprolyl[3]-bradykinin ([3]$_\Delta$-
Pro[3]-BK), and L-glutamyl[1]-L-3,4-dehydroprolyl[3]-kallidin (1-Glu-[3]$_\Delta$-
Pro[3]-BK).

The analogs described in this paper have pharmacological
activities like those of bradykinin (7), yet their conformations
as measured by CD are similar in hydrophobic rather than aqueous
environments.   Therefore it seems possible that the pharmacological
actions are expressed in a hydrophobic environment.

The change in aqueous CD spectra on going from bradykinin to
L-3,4-dehydroprolyl[3]-bradykinin is similar to the spectroscopic
change observed by Madison and Schellman (10) for N-acetyl-L-
proline-N,N'-dimethylamide.   Madison and Schellman found with
this proline compound that a low magnitude CD trough at 224 nm in
cyclohexane (attributed to a cis-configuration) increases in
negative magnitude and blue-shifts to 197 nm in water (attributed
to a trans configuration).   If the N-terminal fragment of brady-

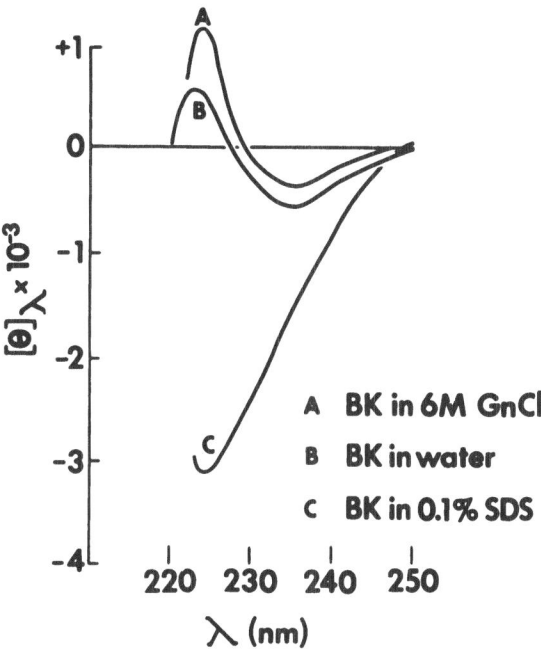

Figure 5. Circular dichroism spectra of bradykinin in (A) 6 molar guanidine hydrochloride (B) water and (C) 0.1% sodium dodecyl sulfate.

kinin, arginyl-prolyl-prolyl-glycine, is placed in a trans peptide configuration around prolyl[2]-proline[3] like that of poly-L-proline II (figure 6), the guanidino-group of the arginine side-chain adopts a position proximate to the proline[3] ring. Such a position could be marginally stabilized by attraction between the electrophilic guanidino-group and the π-orbitals of the olefinic bond in L-3,4-dehydroproline. The interaction between the guanidino group and dehydroproline is similar to one described by Sugihara, et al. (11) for interactions between cyclic peptides and benzene, where there is an attraction between the electron-rich benzene plane and the partial positive charge on the nitrogens of the peptide groups. Any reinforcement of this conformation around arginyl[1]-prolyl[2]-proline[3] such as might occur in a hydrophobic medium would result in a very specific orientation of these groups. Whether this specific orientation of residues in bradykinin is an essential requisite for the binding of bradykinin to its receptor site remains to be determined.

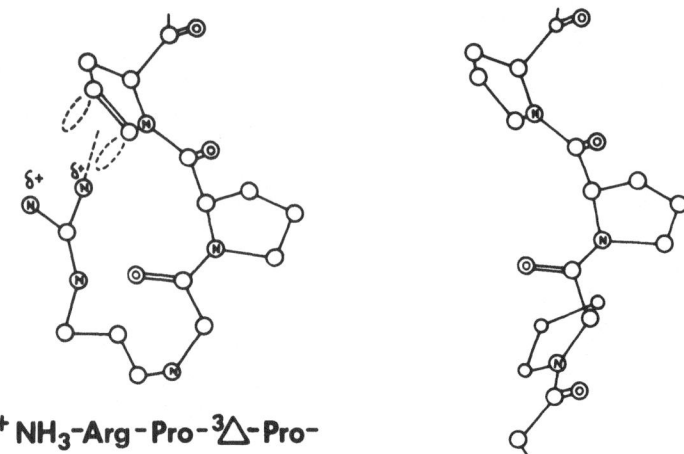

Figure 6. Molecular models for poly-L-proline II and the proposed conformation of the arginyl-prolyl-3,4-dehydroprolyl terminal of L-3,4-dehydroprolyl[3]-bradykinin.

ACKOWLEDGEMENT

The authors would like to thank Dr. K. Wellman of the Chemistry Department, University of Miami, Coral Gables, Florida for his generosity in allowing access to the JASCO spectropolarimeter. This work was supported in part by a NIH General Research Support Grant 5-S01-RR05690-05.

REFERENCES

1.   C.M. Venkatachalam and G.N. Ramachandran, Ann. Rev. Biochem. 38, 45-82 (1969).

2.   A. Bodanszky, M. Bodanszky, E.J. Jorpes, V. Mutt and M.A. Ondetti, Experientia 26, 948-950 (1970).

3.   A. H. Brady, J.W. Ryan and J.M. Stewart, Biochem. J. 121, 179-184 (1971).

4.   J.R. Cann, J.M. Stewart and G.R. Matsueda, Biochemistry 12, 3780-3788 (1973).

5.   M.A. Devynck, M.-G Pernollet, P.Meyer, S. Fermandjian, P. Fromageot and F.M. Bumpus, Nature 249 67-69 (1974).

6.   Cf. J. Rudinger in, "Proceedings of 3rd International Sympos- ium on Endrocrinology; London", Heinemann, London 1971.

7.   A.M. Felix, M.H. Jimenez, R. Vergona and M.R. Cohen, Int. J. Peptide Protein Res. 5, 201-206 (1973).

8.   W.C. Krueger and L.M. Pshigoda, Anal. Chem. 43, 675 (1971).

9.   J.A. Reynolds and C. Tanford, J. Biol. Chem. 245, 5161-5165 (1970).

10.   V. Madison and J. Schellman, Biopolymers 9, 65-94 (1970).

11.   T. Sugihara, Y. Imanishi and T. Higushimura, Biopolymers 14, 733-747 (1975).

PERMEABILITY FACTOR AND SURFACE ESTERASE

Brenda Mason

The Lister Institute of Preventive Medicine, Chelsea

Bridge Road, London SW1W 8RH, England

Both vascular permeability factor and surface factor (SF), which have been implicated in the activation of the kinin-releasing system in plasma, are activated when plasma is exposed to glass (1, 2). SF is adsorbed by the glass and, as a consequence, permeability-increasing activity is generated in solution (3).

Prekininogenase activator (PKA) is present in activated human and guinea-pig plasma at a dilution that contains strong permeability-increasing activity (4, 5), an observation confirmed on a range of dilutions by Oh-Ishi and Webster (6) with purified prekallikrein as a substrate.

However, since unadsorbed SF in solution might account for the PKA activity, an attempt was made to remove all the SF from dilute plasma in order to re-examine the product for permeability-increasing activity and PKA. Preliminary tests on human plasma indicated that PKA activity was retained when all the SF was adsorbed (7). This study demonstrates that a similar separation can be achieved with dilute guinea-pig plasma, and that treatment of the adsorbed surface factor with an esterase inhibitor has an effect on its capacity to generate permeability-increasing activity in plasma.

Two hundred ml of guinea-pig plasma diluted 1/100 in 0.15 M phosphate saline, pH 7.5, were added to 100 ml of dry glass ballotini, and adsorbed by rotation for 10-15 min. at 20 C. At each stage, samples were taken of the adsorbed plasma, which were set aside in chilled silicone tubes, and of the coated ballotini, which were washed ten times with phosphate saline.

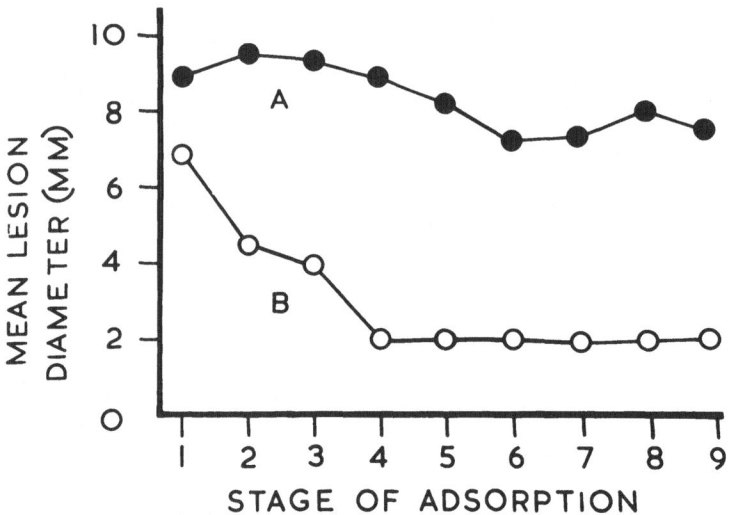

Fig. 1. The separation of permeability-increasing activity (A)
and surface factor (B) in a volume of dilute guinea-pig by
repeated adsorptions with glass ballotini at 20 C.
A = The permeability-increasing activity of 0.1 ml samples of the
1/100 guinea-pig plasma taken at every adsorption. B = The
activity of surface factor adsorbed to the lots of glass ballotini
as indicated by the permeability-increasing activity that washed
samples of the ballotini subsequently generated in 1/100 Hageman
trait plasma after rotation for 10 min. at 20 C.

The vascular permeability-increasing activity in 0.1 ml
injections, assayed in guinea-pigs having circulating pontamine
blue (8), was generated by the first contact with ballotini.
Although the initial strength declined to some degree, possibly
due to the fading of kinin and kininogenase activity (5), the major
permeability activity of the adsorbed plasma was substantially
retained throughout the process (Fig. 1, A). The final product
that was adsorbed nine times contained PKA, because in 4 min. at
29 C it released kinin from intact plasma but not from heated
plasma.

Since guinea-pig plasma generates permeability-increasing
activity in Hageman trait plasma, the SF borne on the ballotini
was also measured. The well-washed samples of ballotini were
rotated in the ratio of one volume of ballotini to two volumes of
1/100 Hageman trait plasma for 10 min. at 20 C, and 0.1 ml of the
activated plasma was injected intradermally.

The SF was taken up in successively decreasing quantities by
the ballotini during the first four adsorptions (Fig. 1, B), and

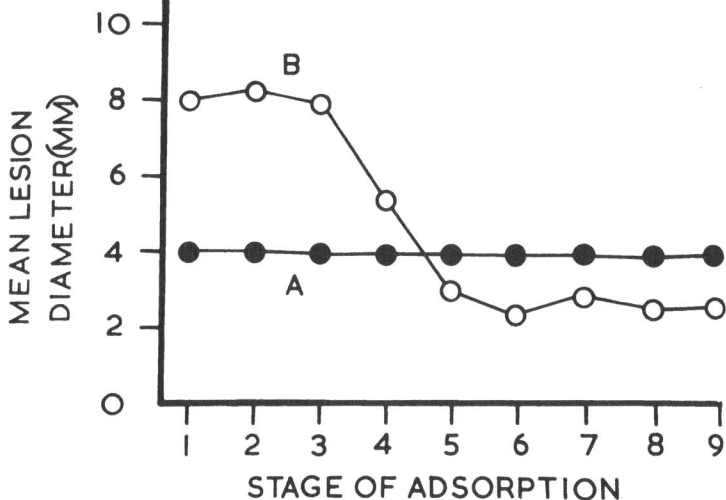

Fig. 2.   The separation of unactivated permeability-increasing
activity (A) and surface factor (B) in a volume of dilute guinea-
pig plasma by repeated adsorptions with glass ballotini at 3 C.
A = The permeability-increasing activity of 0.1 ml samples of the
1/100 guinea-pig plasma taken at every adsorption.   B = The
activity of surface factor adsorbed to the lots of glass ballotini
as indicated by the permeability-increasing activity that washed
samples of the ballotini subsequently generated in 1/100 Hageman
trait plasma after rotation for 10 min. at 20 C.

none at subsequent adsorptions.   Therefore, the final product,
adsorbed dilute plasma, was free of SF though it contained permeability-increasing activity and PKA.

Further evidence distinguishing SF from the major permeability
factor was provided by the results of cold adsorption.   A volume
of 1/100 guinea-pig plasma was adsorbed with nine quantities of
ballotini at 3 C.   Samples of the plasma at each stage were set
aside in chilled silicone tubes, and samples of the ballotini were
washed ten times with phosphate saline at 3 C before testing against
1/100 Hageman trait plasma at 20 C.   The results are illustrated
in Figure 2.   Cold adsorbed dilute plasma had no detectable
permeability-increasing activity at any stage of the procedure,
though all the SF was adsorbed during the first five adsorptions.
The final product, which was free of SF, had no PKA activity, and
permeability-increasing activity was not generated in it by clean
glass at 20 C (Fig. 3, B).   But exposure to well-washed ballotini,
prepared by coating in 1/100 intact guinea-pig plasma, stimulated
the production of permeability-increasing activity in the cold

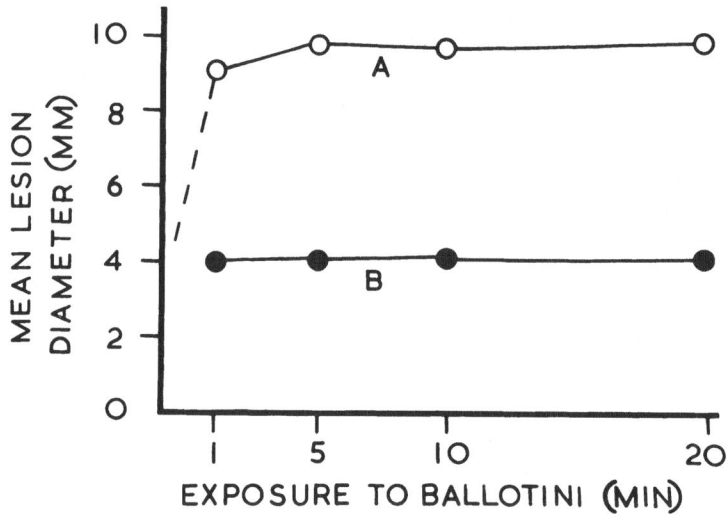

Fig. 3.   The time course of permeability-increasing activity
of 1/100 guinea-pig plasma that was previously adsorbed at 3 C
with glass ballotini.   Activity of 0.1 ml samples of this dilute
plasma when continuously rotated at 20 C with ballotini coated in
1/100 intact guinea-pig plasma (A), and with uncoated ballotini (B).

adsorbed plasma dilution (Fig. 3, A), and on the removal of the
ballotini the plasma had the ability to activate prekininogenase.
These two activities were not diminished by subsequent rotation
with clean glass.

The results indicate that the PKA of dilute guinea-pig plasma
dilutions is not unadsorbed SF, and provide further support for the
correlation of permeability-increasing activity with PKA activity.

As the technique of cold adsorption appears to yield a preparation that has permeability-increasing activity in an unactivated
form, which is activable by SF on glass, the effects of di iso
propylphosphofluoridate (DFP) were tested on the glass borne SF.
Sets of ballotini were coated with SF from graded dilutions of
intact guinea-pig plasma by rotating for 10 min. at 20 C.   They
were then washed ten times in phosphate saline.   Since there was
a linear relation between the log dilution of the intact coating
plasma and the mean lesion diameter induced by the cold adsorbed
plasma dilution when reacted with these graded amounts of SF, a
measurement could be made of the degree of inhibition of the SF
activity.   Each set of coated ballotini was treated by rotating
in test solutions for 3 hr at 37 C followed by 18 hr at 3C.   Set A
was rotated in 0.01 M DFP in Tris HCl buffer, set B was rotated in

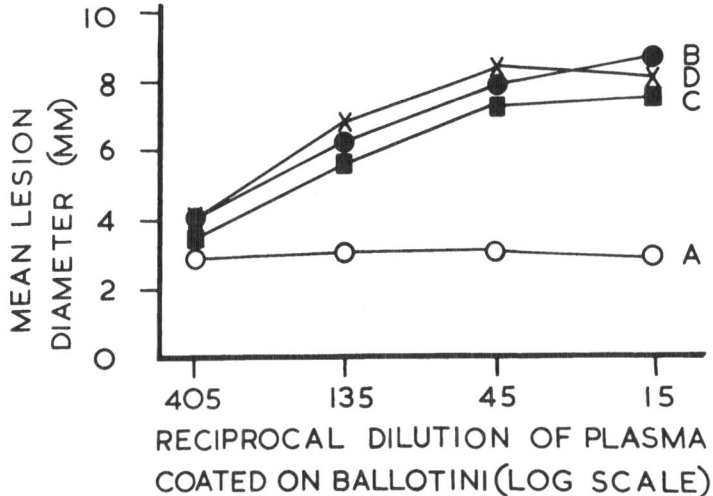

Fig. 4.   The effect of pretreatment with DFP and TAMe followed
by washing, on the ability of surface factor borne on the glass
ballotini to activate permeability-increasing activity in 1/100
guinea-pig plasma that was previously adsorbed at 3 C.   The permeability-increasing activity of 0.1 ml 1/100 cold adsorbed guinea-pig
plasma rotated for 5 min at 20 C with coated ballotini pretreated
with DFP(A), with DFP and TAMe (B), with TAMe (C) and with buffer
solution only (D).

a mixture of 0.01 M DFP and 0.05 M tosyl arginine methyl ester
(TAMe), set C was rotated in 0.05 M TAMe, and set D was rotated in
buffer only.   All specimens of ballotini were then washed ten times
in phosphate saline and tested against unactivated cold adsorbed
plasma in the ratio of one volume of ballotini to two volumes of
plasma.   Rotations were for 5 min at 20 C and 0.1 ml injections
were made of the activated plasma.

The results, depicted in Figure 4, indicate that the DFP pretreatment inhibits the activity of SF more than 27 fold in its
capacity to generate permeability-increasing activity in the cold
adsorbed plasma when exposed for 5 min.   The finding that TAMe
protected the SF from inhibition is evidence that the generation
of permeability-increasing activity by surface material is dependent
upon the presence of an active esterase adsorbed from plasma.
Since kallikrein is adsorbed to glass from plasma there is the
possibility that it is responsible for this esterase activity.

REFERENCES

1.   Mackay, M.E., Miles, A.A., Schachter, M. and Wilhelm, D.L.
     (1953) Susceptibility of the guinea-pig to pharmacological
     factors from its own serum. Nature, Lond., 172, 714.

2.   Margolis, J. (1957) Plasma pain-producing substance and blood
     clotting. Nature, Lond., 180, 1464.

3.   Margolis, J. (1958) Activation of a permeability factor in
     plasma by contact with glass. Nature, Lond., 181, 635.

4.   Mason, B. and Miles, A.A. (1962) Globulin permeability factors
     without kininogenase activity. Nature, Lond., 196, 587.

5.   Mason, B. (1972) The profile of vascular permeability factors
     in dilute guinea-pig plasma. Br. J. exp. Path., 53, 597.

6.   Oh-Ishi, S. and Webster, M.E. (1975) Vascular permeability
     factors (PF/Nat and PF/Dil) - their relationship to Hageman
     factor and the kallikrein-kinin system. Biochem. Pharmac.,
     24, 591.

7.   Mason, B. (1975) The relation between surface factor and
     permeability factor. Life Sci., 16, 781.

8.   Wilhelm, D.L., Mill, P.J., Sparrow, E.M., Mackay, M.E. and
     Miles, A.A. (1958) Enzyme-like globulins from serum reproducing
     the vascular phenomena of inflammation. IV. Activable perme-
     ability factor and its inhibitor in the serum of the rat and
     the rabbit. Br. J. exp. Path., 39, 228.

THE REGULATION OF KALLIKREIN SECRETION FROM ISOLATED SUBMANDIBULAR

GLAND SLICES BY NEUROTRANSMITTERS, CYCLIC NUCLEOTIDES AND CALCIUM

K. D. Bhoola, P.F. Heap and M.J.C. Lemon

Departments of Pharmacology and Anatomy

The Medical School, University of Bristol, Bristol BS8 ITD

Evidence suggests that neurotransmitters interact with specific receptors on the plasma membrane of cells which results in the formation within the cell of a chemical messenger. Enzyme secretion in exocrine glands is considered to be controlled by the chemical messengers, adenosine 3'5' monophosphate (cyclic AMP), guanosine 3'5' cyclic monophosphate (cyclic GMP) and calcium. This second messenger concept was examined using isolated guinea-pig submandibular gland slices, incubated in modified Krebs-Ringer at 37°C and gassed with a mixture of 95% O_2-5% CO_2 (Fig. 1). The secretion of kallikrein into the incubation medium together with the morphological changes which accompany the secretory process were determined in response to noradrenaline, acetylcholine, dibutyryl cyclic AMP and dibutyryl cyclic GMP.

Noradrenaline activates adenylate cyclase and raises the intracellular levels of cyclic AMP in the submandibular gland of the guinea-pig (Lemon & Bhoola, 1975; Bhoola & Lemon, 1975). The relative role of α- and β- adrenoceptors in mediating kallikrein secretion was investigated. Phenylphrine (α and partial β agonist) was marginally more effective than isoprenaline (β and partial α agonist) at the incubation time of 15 min, but neither was as potent as noradrenaline (Fig. 2). Both propranolol (β antagonist) and phentolamine (α antagonist) were required to fully inhibit the noradrenaline response (Table 1). The release of kallikrein evoked by noradrenaline was accompanied by depletion of secretory granules and vacuolation in the acinar cells (Plate 1 and 2), with no apparent changes in the striated duct cells. Although dibutyryl cyclic AMP stimulated kallikrein secretion and produced similar morphological events, they were not as pronounced

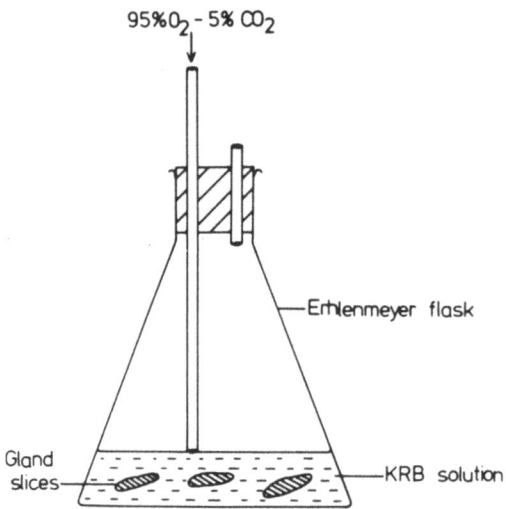

Fig. 1   Diagrammatic representation of the incubation of isolated
         submandibular gland slices in a modified Krebs-Ringer solu-
         tion. The buffer solution contained NaCl 121 mM, KCl 14.3
         or 5.0 mM, NaHCO$_2$ 25.2 mM, CaCl$_2$ 2.6 mM, MgSO$_4$ 1.2 mM,
         glucose 5.6 mM and β-hydroxybutyric acid 6.1 mM.

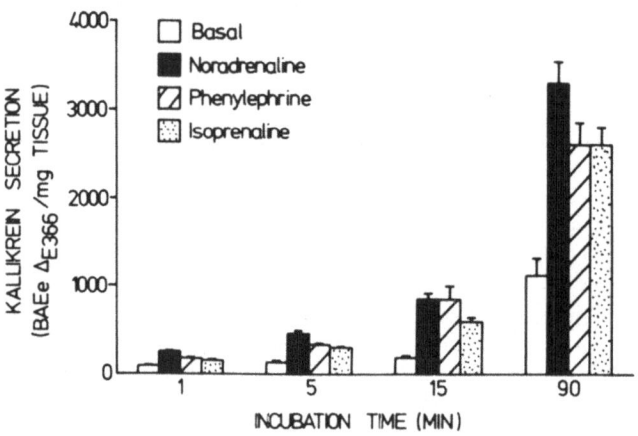

Fig. 2   Comparison of the kallikrein releasing potency of
         phenylephrine, noradrenaline and isoprenaline. Kallikrein
         (BAEe Δ_{E366}/mg tissue) secreted from the gland slices into
         the medium. The concentration of each drug was 400μM.
         Bar shows 1 S.E. of mean, n = 3.

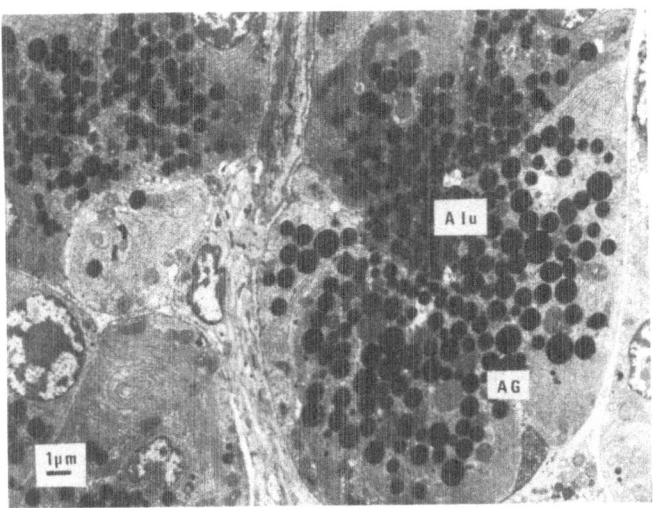

Plate 1 Ultrastructural appearance of isolated submandibular
        gland slices incubated in vitro in Krebs-Ringer solution.
        The morphological architecture of the control slices is
        apparently intact after incubation for 90 min. The
        acinar cells are packed with secretory granules (AG) and
        the acinar lumen (Alu) is small and not distended.

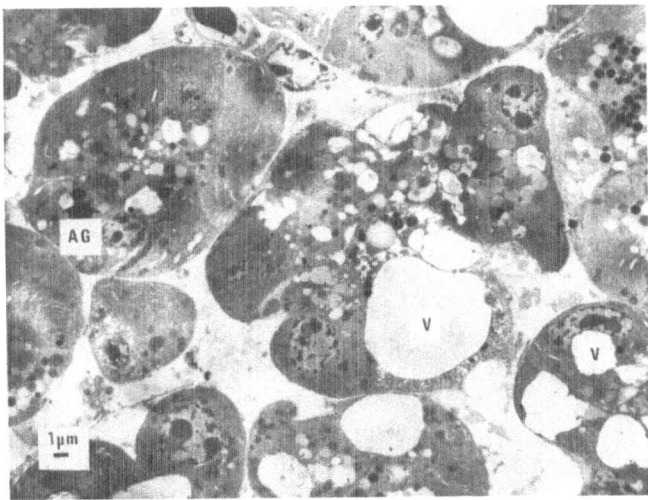

Plate 2 Five structural changes in the isolated gland slices
        induced by noradrenaline. Many of the acinar cells show
        a marked loss of secretory granules (AG) and considerable
        vacuolation (V).

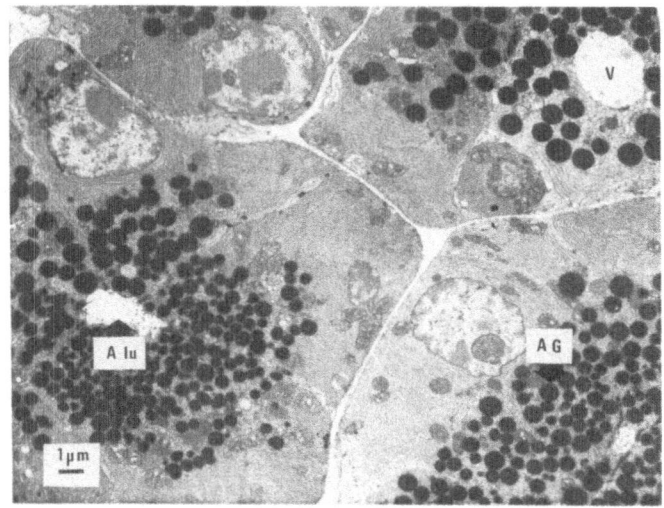

Plate 3   Five structural changes in the isolated gland slices
           evoked by acetylcholine. The depletion of secretory
           granules by (AG) and vacuole formation (V) in the acinar
           cells is much less in magnitude than that observed with
           noradrenaline. Alu = acinar cell lumen.

Table 1   Inhibition of noradrenaline stimulated kallikrein secre-
           tion by adrenoceptor antagonists. Gland slices were
           incubated with the antagonists for 15 min, and after the
           addition of noradrenaline for a further 15 min period.
           Values represent kallikrein activity expressed as BAEe
           E366/mg tissue, ± S.E. of mean, n= 6.

	KALLIKREIN ~ BAEe Δ_{366}U/mg TISSUE	
	CONTROL	NORADRENALINE 0·4 mM
BASAL	77·8 ± 15·0	–
NORADRENALINE 0·4mM	400·0 ± 46·9	400·0 ± 46·9
PROPRANOLOL 4·0mM	107·8 ± 14·0	269·0 ± 45·9
PHENTOLAMINE 4·0mM	84·3 ± 10·9	279·4 ± 57·0
PROPRANOLOL 4·0mM PHENTOLAMINE 4·0mM	71·3 ± 5·0	119·3 ± 20·6

Table 2   Inhibition of acetylcholine stimulated kallikrein secretion by atropine. Gland slices were incubated for 2 min, and after the addition of acetylcholine for a further 15 min period. Values represent kallikrein activity expressed as BAEe Δ_{E366}/mg tissue, ± S.E. of mean, n = 6.

| | KALLIKREIN—BAEeΔ_{366}U/mg TISSUE | |
	CONTROL	ACETYLCHOLINE 4 mM
BASAL	137·5 ± 22·2	-
ACETYLCHOLINE 4·0mM	361·0± 53·1	361·0 ± 53·1
ATROPINE 0·04mM	129·0	131·0
ATROPINE 0·4 mM	133·2 ± 14·5	129·8 ± 27·8
ATROPINE 4·0 mM	84·8 ± 20·8	90·0 ± 21·1

Table 3   Effect of calcium on kallikrein release stimulated by acetylcholine, noradrenaline, isoprenaline, dibutyryl cyclic AMP and dibutyryl cyclic GMP. Gland slices incubated with different concentrations of calcium. Values represent kallikrein activity expressed as BAEe Δ_{E366}/mg tissue, ± S.E. of mean, n = 6 - 8.

| | KALLIKREIN—BAEe Δ_{366}—U/mg TISSUE | | | |
| | CALCIUM— FREE 1mM EGTA | CALCIUM (mM) | | |
		2·6	5	10
BASAL (15 MIN)	88·1± 12·6	162·4 ± 23·8	191·4 ± 32·3	262·8± 65·8
ACETYLCHOLINE 4mM	127·9± 15·8	417·0± 45·9	638·9± 73·9	769·0± 96·3
NORADRENALINE 4 mM	257·8± 21·5	610·2±77·8	541·7±68·5	682·7±49·4
ISOPRENALINE 4mM	192·2± 20·5	469·1±66·3	468·2± 51·2	438·6± 46·7
BASAL (30 MIN)	157·4± 24·6	258·2± 43·1	201·4± 47·0	416·0±120·9
dcAMP 40 mM	212·9±17·1	314·0± 30·9	350·7±39·3	467·0±73·8
dcGMP 40 mM	151·0± 11·2	312·0± 47·0	241·3±32·0	425·3±78·8

as those observed with noradrenaline.

Significant secretion of kallikrein was obtained with acetylcholine which was completely blocked by atropine (Table 2). Kallikrein secretion stimulated by acetylcholine was associated with depletion of granules and vacuolation in acinar cells which were not as marked as those observed with noradrenaline (Plate 3). Since acetylcholine does not activate adenylate cyclase nor does it raise cyclic AMP levels in the submandibualr gland (Lemon * Bhoola, 1975; Bhoola & Lemon, 1975), it is considered that the secretory effects of acetylcholine may be mediated by cyclic GMP. Dibutyryl cyclic GMP produced a transient stimulation of kallikrein release.

Incubation of the gland slices in calcium-free Krebs-Ringer solution containing 1 mM EGTA markedly reduced the secretory response to acetylcholine but to a lesser extent that of noradrenaline and isoprenaline (Table 3). Incubation in medium containing 5 and 10 mM calcium significantly increased the secretion of kallikrein to only acetylcholine.

Our results support the view that noradrenaline, acetylcholine and cyclic nucleotides stimulate kallikrein secretion from isolated guinea-pig submandibular gland slices with varying degrees of efficacy. The secretion of kallikrein was accompanied by depletion of secretory granules and vacuolation in the acinar cells with no obvious morphological changes in the granule populations of the intercalated and junctional duct cells.

We are particularly grateful to Mrs. Lindsey Smith and Mr. P. Summers for very able technical assistance. We thank the Medical Research Council for financial support.

REFERENCES

Bhoola, K.D. & Lemon, M.J.C. (1975). J. Physiol. (Lond) 245, 121-122P.

Lemon, M.J.C. & Bhoola, K.D. (1975). Biochem. Biophys. Acta. 385, 101-113.

A SENSITIVE KININ LIBERATING ASSAY FOR KININOGENASE IN RAT URINE, ISOLATED GLOMERULI AND TUBULES OF RAT KIDNEY

K. Mann*, R. Geiger**, and E. Werle**

*I. Med. Klinik, **Institut für Klinische Chemie und

Klinische Biochemie der Universität Munchen

8000 Munich, Germany

There are several hints, that the kallikrein-kinin-system of the kidney is involved in physiological regulation mechanisms and in pathological processes (1, 2, 3, 4, 5, 6, 7). A prerequisite to evaluate the significance of the system, is the possibility of measuring kallikrein activities in tissues, where it is formed, excreted and inactivated. Recently Nustad and Pierce (8) showed, that the rat kidney synthesizes four kallikreins, which are re- leased unchanged into urine. But the localisation of kallikreins in the nephron is not known. Moreover, there is no specific rat-urine kallikrein assay available, which is sensitive enough to measure enzyme activities in isolated structures of the kidney. This report will be focused on these points.

First of all we developed a reliable rat-uterus-test, which allows measurement of bradykinin equivalents from 0.4 ng to 4 ng. Figure 1 shows a typical recording. Dose differences of 0.13 ng can be measured between 0.91 to 1.43 ng. The measurement is the diastolic tone between two contraction waves (see Fig. 2). The inter-assay variation coefficient of the method is about 3%.

Substrate was prepared in a modification of the method, suggested by Habal, Movat (9, 10), Spragg and Austen (11). An activation of kallikrein in plasma was suppressed very well, when we used Hexadimethrine, SBTI, Na_2EDTA and dialysed against a 0.05 M Tris-HCl-buffer pH 7.4, which contained 10^{-3} M DFP. Human HMW-kininogen was eluted from QAE-Sephadex A 50 in the 0.4 M NaCl fractions as shown in Figure 3.

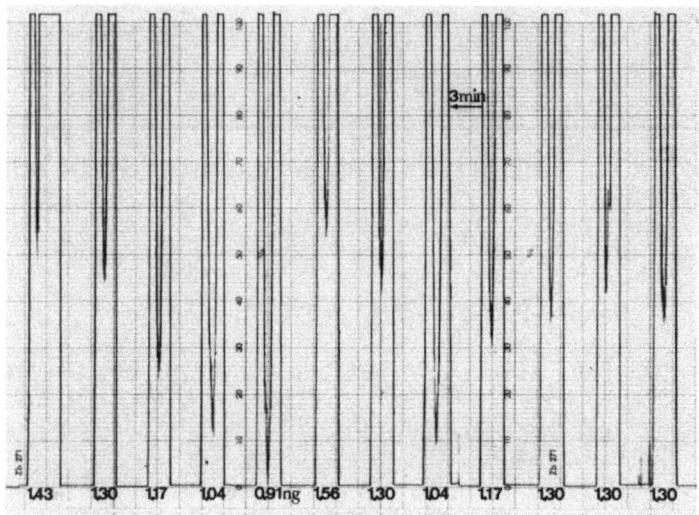

Fig. 1. Rat uterus test. Measurement of bradykinin standard
solution containing from 0.91 to 1.43 ng.

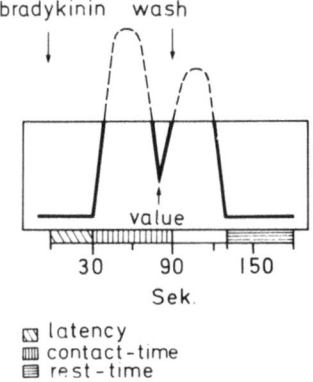

Fig. 2. Scheme of kinin measurement.

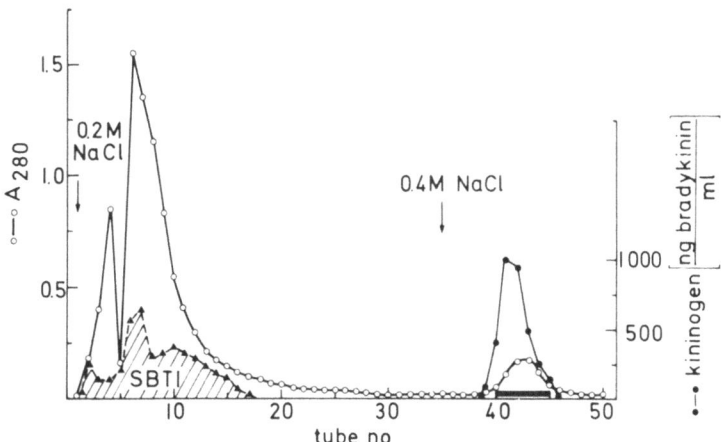

Fig. 3. Chromatography of 100 ml human plasma, containing
500 mg Na$_2$EDTA, 100 mg Hexadimethrine, 30 mg SBTI and 10^{-3} M DFP
at room temperature on a column of QAE-Sephadex A 50, equilibrated
with 0.06 M Phosphate-buffer pH 7.4 at a flow rate of 420 ml/h,
containing 10^{-3} M DFP. Substrate eluted with 0.4 M NaCl. Kininogen
content is expressed as ng/ml of bradykinin equivalents. SBTI
eluted with 0.2 M NaCl.

SBTI was eluted completely in the 0.2 NaCl fractions. After
dialysing kininogen-containing fractions against distilled water
containing 500 mg/l Na$_2$EDTA and 10^{-3} M DFP the lyophilized substrate
was sufficiently purified for a sensitive assay. Hog pancreas and
rat urine kallikreins released about 250 ng bradykinin/mg protein.
The total yield from 100 ml plasma was about 18 ug bradykinin-
equivalents. So called "spontaneous kinin forming activity" is
about 2% of the total kinin formation of enzymes tested. Kalli-
krein-inhibitors as α-2-macroglobulin, C̄-1-inactivator and α-1-
antitrypsin could not be detected in double diffusion tests.

Kininase activity in the substrate was completely inhibited
over a period of 24 hours by 4 x 10^{-3} M Na$_2$EDTA and 10^{-2} M 8-hy-
droxyquinoline (Fig. 4).

In the final assay the kininogenase activity of pooled dialysed rat-urine was determined by incubating 0.1 - 1.0 µl urine
with 800 ng/ml bradykinin equivalents of substrate in a total
volume of 250 µl 0.15 M Tris-HCl-buffer pH 8.6, containing 4 x 10^{-3}M
Na$_2$EDTA and 10^{-2}M 8-hydroxyquinoline for 4 hours at 37° C. Under
these conditions maximal velocity of the reaction was observed as
Fig. 5 demonstrates. The reaction was stopped by adding 50 µl

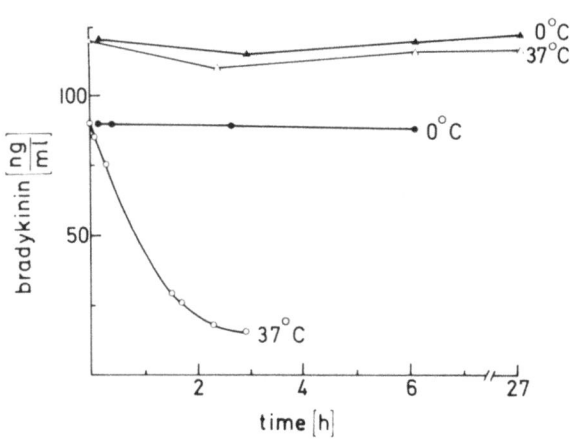

Fig. 4. Pattern of kininase inhibition in substrate with
4 x 10⁻³M Na₂EDTA and 10⁻²M 8-hydroxyquinoline.

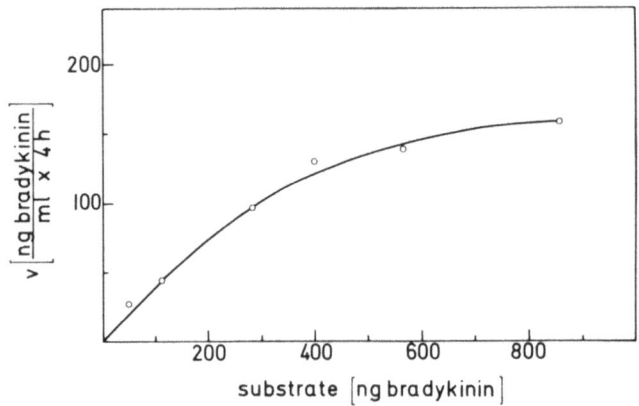

Fig. 5. Velocity of formation of kinin at constant kallikrein concentration with increasing concentrations of semi-
purified human kallikrein substrate.

Trasylol (500 KIU) and boiling for 10 min. No more than 15% of the
substrate was consumed.

Figure 6 shows that the kinin formation was directly proportional to the amount of urine used. Optimal kinin formation
was observed at pH 8.6 (see Fig. 7), at 37° C (see Fig. 8), and

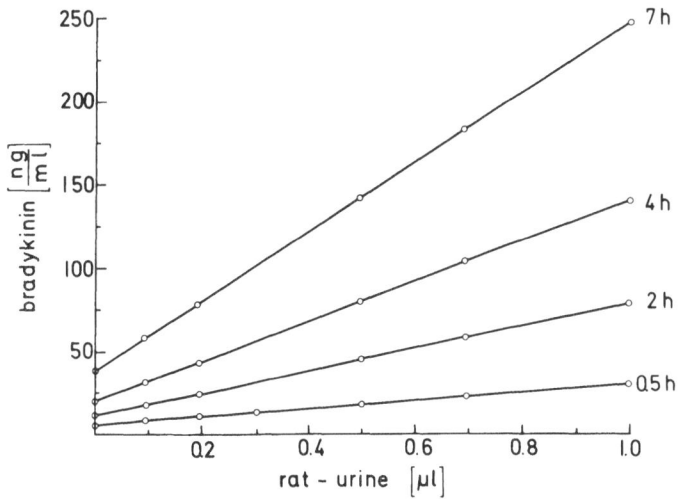

Fig. 6. Dependence of kinin-releasing activity on added urine
(kallikrein) and incubation time. Conditions: 800 ng/ml substrate,
incubation at 37ºC with 0.15 M Tris-HCl-buffer pH 8.6 containing
Na$_2$EDTA and 8-hydroxyquinoline, incubation volume 250 µl; the
reaction was stopped by 50 µl Trasylol (500 KIU) and 10 minutes
boiling.

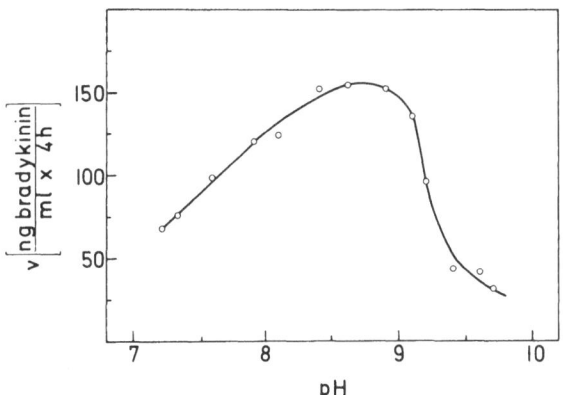

Fig. 7. pH-activity curve for rat urine. Conditions: 800 ng/
ml substrate, 1 µl dialysed pooled rat urine. Incubation time
4 h at 37º C; 0.15 M Tris-HCl-buffer containing Na$_2$EDTA and
8-hydroxyquinoline; incubation volume 250 µl. The reaction was
stopped by 50 µl Trasylol (500 TIU) and 10 minutes boiling.

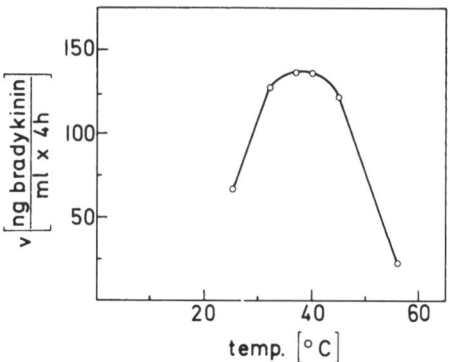

Fig. 8. Temp. activity curve for rat urine. Conditions:
800 ng/ml substrate, pH 8.6, 0.15 M Tris-HCl-buffer containing
4×10^{-3}M Na$_2$EDTA, and 10^{-2}M 8-hydroxyquinoline, 1 µl dialysed
pooled rat urine, incubation time 4 hours, other conditions were
as described before.

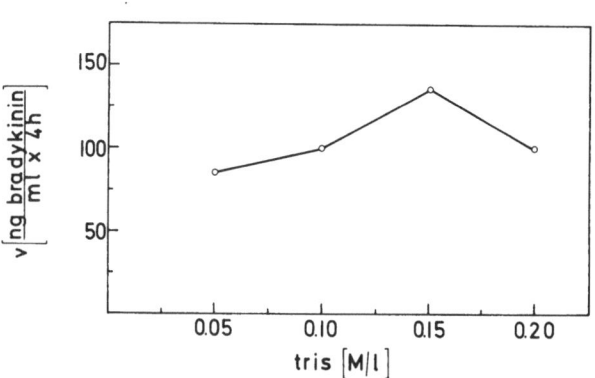

Fig. 9. ion-strength activity curve for rat urine. Conditions:
800 ng/ml substrate, 1 µl dialysed pooled rat urine. Incubation
time 4 hours at 37^0 in 250 µl Tris-HCl-buffer containing Na$_2$EDTA
4×10^{-3}M and 10^{-2}M 8-hydroxyquinoline. The reaction was stopped
by 50 µl Trasylol (500 KIU) and 10 minutes boiling.

at 0.15 M Tris-HCl-buffer ion strength (see Fig. 9). The assay
can also be used for measurement of human urine kallikrein.

Isolation of glomerula was done by microdissection. Tubules
were isolated after "Dissociative" treatment with collagenase,
according to Guder (12).

During incubating the same amount of substrate with different
amounts of glomerula (Fig. 10), the specific activity in all
samples was nearly the same. Enzyme activity of 50 glomerula was
the lowest measureable.

In contrast, after incubating increasing amounts of homogenized
tubular cell supernatants, no linearity could be observed (Fig. 11).
Preliminary results show a hyperbolic decrease in the specific
activity kinin formation, as enzyme concentrations increased. For
homogenisation and incubation we used the same Tris-HCl-buffer,
which inhibited completely kininase activity of glomerula and
tubules.

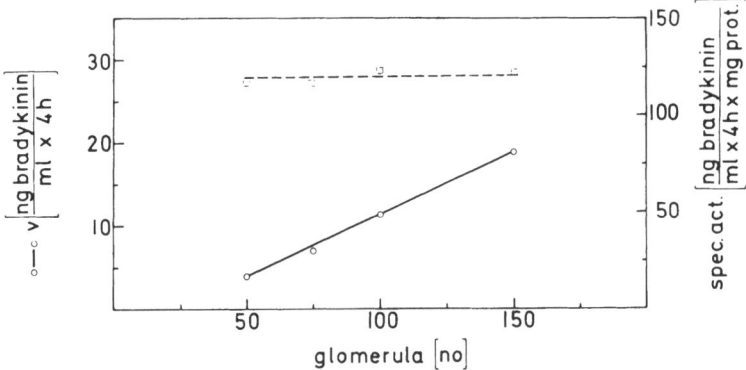

Fig. 10. Effect of the number of glomerula on kinin
formation. Glomerula were homogenized by ultrasonic treatment in
120 µl incubation buffer containing 0.5% deoxycholic acid. 50 µl
of supernatant were incubated under conditions described. 50 µl
were used for protein determination after Folin-method.

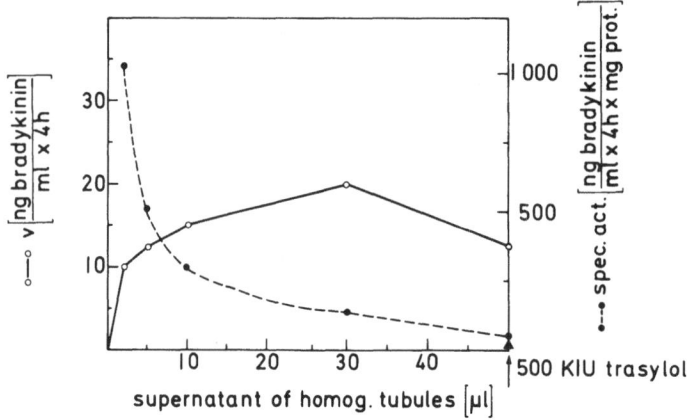

Fig. 11. Effect of the amount of supernatant of homogenized
tubular cells. 40 mg of tubule-cell sediment was mixed with 400 μl
incubation buffer, containing 0.5% deoxycholic acid. After homo-
genization of the sediment in a hand homogenizator increasing
amounts of the supernatant were incubated under conditions
described. Protein determination was carried out in the corresponding volume.

We considered the possibility that there could be a kallikrein inhibitor in our tubular preparation. Indeed, after gel-
filtration on G-100 Sephadex we found fractions which strongly
inhibited the kinogenase activity of the rat urine. Further
investigations are in progress.

The identification of kallikrein and kinins was done indirectly. Trasylol inhibited kinin formation to about 95% in
urine, glomerula and tubules. Chymotrypsin and carboxypeptides
B destroyed the uterus-contracting material, whereas trypsin did
not. All samples had no effect on the blood pressure of Pentolinium-
treated rats, even after application of substrate treated with high
doses of urine, glomerula and tubules. Renin and angiotensin
were not detectable.

There were several hints of a tubular localization of renal
kininogenases (6,13,14,15,16). It is now evident that renal
kallikreins are located in glomerula as well as in tubules. We
are planning micropuncture studies to find out the exact local
distribution and function of kallikrein in the rat nephron.

REFERENCES

1. Adetuyibi, A., and Mills, J.H. (1972) Lancet 2, 203

2. Geller, R.G., Margolius, H.S., Pisano, J.H., and Keiser, H.R. (1972) Circ. Res. 31, 857

3. Croxatto, H.R., and San Martin, M. (1970) Experientia (Basel) 26, 1216

4. Marin-Grez, M., Cottone, P., and Carretero, O.A. (1972) Amer. J. Physiol. 223, 794

5. Carretero, O.A., and Oza, N.B. (1973) Proc. of a Int. workshop conference Los Angeles, International congress series No. 302

6. Scili, A.G., Carretero, O.A., Hampton, A., and Oza, N.B. (1975) Fed. Proc. 37, 378

7. Frey, E., Kraut, H., and Werle, E. (1968) Ferdinand Enke Verlag, Stuttgart

8. Nustad, K., Vaaje, K., and Pierce, J.V. (1975) Br. J. Pharmac. 53, 229

9. Habal, F.M., and Movat, H.Z. (1972) Res. Comm. in Chem. Pathol. and Pharmacol. 4, 477

10. Habal, F.M., Movat, H.Z., and Burrowes, C.E. (1974) Biochem. Pharmacol. 23, 2291

11. Spragg, J., and Austen, K.F. (1974) Biochem. Pharmacol. 23, 781

12. Guder, W., Wiesner, W., Stukowski, B., and Wieland, O. (1971) Hoppe-Seyler's Z. Physiol. Chemie 352, 1319

13. Werle, E., and Vogel, R. (1960) Archs. int. Pharmacodyn. The. 126, 171

14. Nustad, K. (1970) Br. J. Pharmac. 39, 87

15. Nustad, K., and Rubin, J. (1970) Br. J. Pharmac. 40, 326

16. Schachter, M., and Barton, S. (1974) Conference on Chemistry and biology of the kallikrein-kinin system in health and disease. Okt. 20-23

(This research was supported by Sonderforschungsbereich 51 Munich)

INHIBITORS OF KININ-FORMING ENZYMES

Setsuro Fujii

Professor of Department of Enzyme Physiology
Institute for Enzyme Research, School of Medicine
Tokushima University, Tokushima, Japan

The typical trypsin-like protease in animals were plasmin, kallikrein, thrombin, factor X, XI, XII, cathepsin B, plasminogen tissue activator and urokinase, and so on. Among them plasmin and kallikrein have kinin-forming activity. A synthetic reversible inhibitor of plasmin, and anticoagulant factor of blood, has been extensively studied. The first effective fibrinolytic inhibitor, ε-aminocaproic acid (εACA) was discovered by Okamoto, et al. in 1958 (1). This discovery was followed several years later in 1964 by an announcement of two additional inhibitors which were shown to possess greater potency; trans-4-aminomethyl-cyclohexanecarboxylic acid (trans-AMCHA [2]) and p-aminomethyl-benzoic acid (3).

Baumgarten,et al. in 1969 reported several new fibrinolytic inhibitors and the most outstanding representative of them was 4-aminomethylbicycle [2,2,2]-octane-1-carboxylic acid (4).

It was reported by us (5) in 1963 that ε-ACA and trans-AMCHA inhibited fibrinolytic activity of human plasmin, and did not suppress acetone-activated human kallikrein and thrombin. Plasmin does catalyse not only fibrinolysis, but also caseinolysis, esterolysis and kinin formation. Fibrinolysis was inhibited by ε-ACA and trans-AMCHA, while caseinolysis, esterolysis and kinin formation were not affected by these inhibitors. Later on there have been published several reports on the inhibitory action of these compounds, suggesting that they eliminated the activation of plasminogen to plasmin but little affected plasmin activity. In 1968, Abiko,et al. (6) investigated the interaction between plasminogen and trans-AMCHA using ultracentrifugation and gel

TABLE I   Inhibitory effects of various compounds on trypsin-like enzyme (50% inhibitory concentration).

The abbreviations used are: α_2-MG, $\alpha_2$macroglobline; TAME, Tosyl-arginine methyl ester; AGLME, Acetyl-glycyl-lysyl methyl ester; ATEE, Acetyl-tyrosine ethyl ester.

Enzyme	Substrate	Compound (M)			
		DV-1006	FOY	Leupeptine	Trasylol*
Trypsin	TAME	3.1×10^{-5}	9.4×10^{-6}	1.1×10^{-4}	0.2
Plasmin	TAME	1.0×10^{-5}	3.0×10^{-5}	9.0×10^{-5}	2.7
Plasmin + α_2	TAME		8.6×10^{-5}	7.6×10^{-5}	>500
$C1\bar{r}$	AGLME		7.0×10^{-5}	2.3×10^{-4}	
$C1\bar{s}$	ATEE	$>2 \times 10^{-4}$	5.2×10^{-4}	6.0×10^{-5}	>500
Plasma-kallikrein	TAME	1.3×10^{-4}	4.1×10^{-5}	2.0×10^{-5}	>10
Pancreatic-kallikrein	TAME		1.3×10^{-3}		8
Thrombin	TAME	9.0×10^{-4}	1.1×10^{-4}	$>10^{-3}$	>500

*; KIU

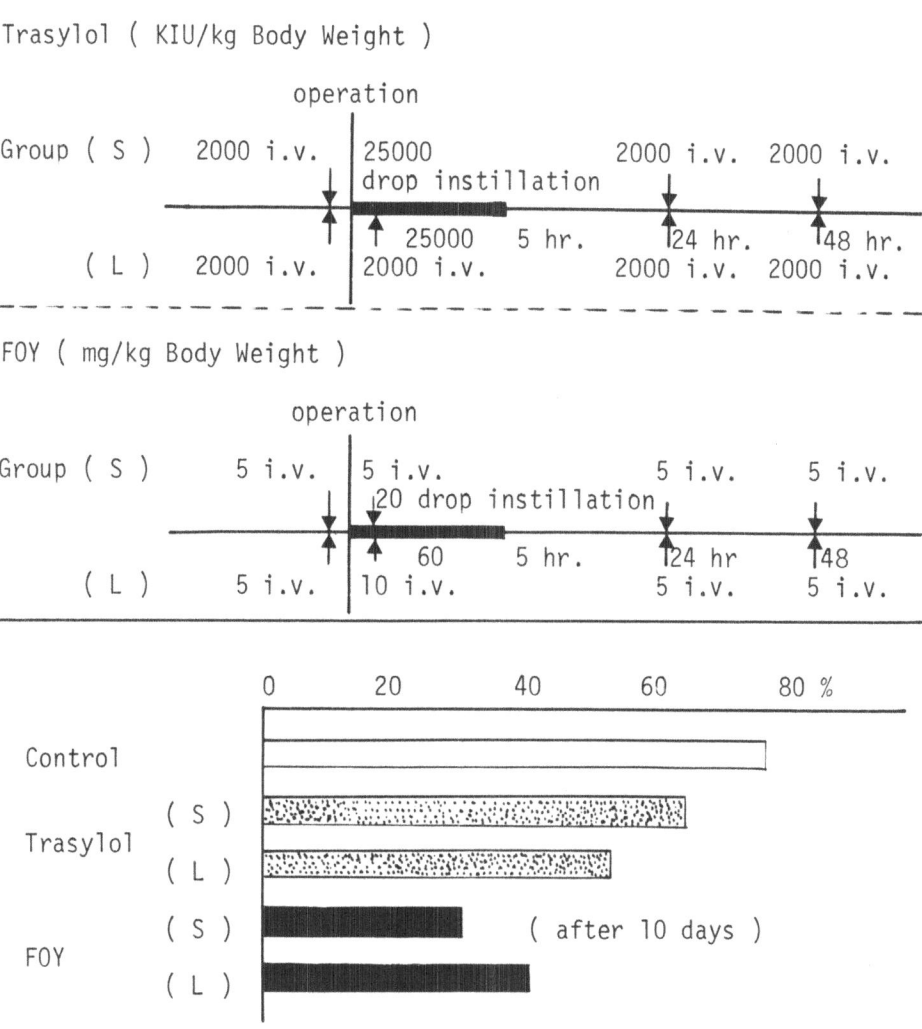

Fig. 1 Effects of FOY and Trasylol on mortality in dogs with experimental pancreatitis

filtration techniques, and concluded that these compounds inhibited the activation of plasminogen through the formation of a
stoichiometric equilibrium complex with plasminogen, accompanying
a conformational change of plasminogen molecule and did not inhibit caseinolysis and esterolysis of plasmin as we described previously.

The various derivatives of benzoyl and phenyl esters of ε-ACA,
trans-AMCHA and ε-guanidinocaproic acid were synthesized as reversible inhibitor of kinin-forming activity of human plasmin and
acetone-activated kallikrein in blood (7).

Finally, 4'-(2""-carboxyl)ethylphenyl-4-aminoethyl-cyclo-
hexane-carboxylate (DV 1006) and p-carboethoxyphenyl εguanidino-
caproate (FOY) were chosen as the most potent inhibitors of plasmin
and kallikrein. These inhibitors suppress fibrinolysis and caseinolysis of plasmin, and esterolysis of kallikrein. The 50% inhibitory dose of DV 1006 was 2×10^{-4} M for kinin-forming activity of
plasmin and 1×10^{-4} M for that of kallikrein from kininogen II, and
those of FOY were 1×10^{-3} M and 5×10^{-5} M, respectively. The effects
of DV 1006, FOY, leupeptin and trasylol on the trypsin-like enzymes
are shown in Table 1. DV 1006, FOY and leupeptin have almost the
similar inhibitory effect on these proteases and no effect on
chymotrypsin. FOY and leupeptin inhibit Cl esterase, and Leupeptin
has no effect on thrombin.

It is well known that in blood active plasmin combines with
α_2-macroglobulin. This complex still has a little plasmin activity (8). Trasylol inhibits active plasmin but does not affect
plasmin activity of the complex, while FOY eliminates the enzymatic activity of free and combined plasmin with α_2-macro-
globulin.

As shown by Haines and Lepow (9), Cl esterase hydrolyses
acetyl tyrosine ethylester, which is representative substrate of
chymotrypsin, preferentially to tosylarginine methylester. The
inhibitory effect of p-aminophenyl-β-phenyl propionate on chymotrypsin was reported to us and 50% inhibitory dose of this compound was about 6×10^{-5} M, but Cl esterase activity was not
affected by the chymotrypsin inhibitor (10).

It has been reported that trasylol exerts a favorable therapeutic effect on pancreatitis in clinical trial. Subsequently,
the effects of FOY and trasylol were examined on the experimental
pancreatitis of dogs induced by Elliot's method. In the upper
part of Fig. 1 the time sequence of experiment was presented.
Trasylol and FOY were administered into animals intravenously
before and after operation. The results were demonstrated in the
lower part of the figure and the mortality of dogs treated with
trasylol and FOY was diminished less than that of control.

REFERENCES

1. Okamoto A., et al Keio J. Med. 8: 211 (1959).
2. Dubber, A.H.C., McNicol, G.P., Douglas, A.S., Melander, B.
   Lancet 11: 1317 (1964); Dubber, A.H.C., McNicol, G.P.,
   Douglas, A.S., Haemat, J. 11: 237 (1965); Melander, B.,
   Granstrand, G.B., Hanshoff, G., Acta Pharmacol. 22: 340 (1965).
3. Markwardt E.F., Haustein, K.O., Klocking, H.P. Arch. int
   Pharmacodyn 152: 233 (1964).
4. Baumgarten, W., Priester, L.L., Stiller, D.W., Duncan, A.E.W.,
   Ciminera, J.L., Loeffler, L.J. Throm. Diabetes Haemorrh.,
   22:263 (1969).
5. Muramatsu, M., Onishi, T., Fujii, S. Proceedings of Symposium
   on Chemical Physiology and Pathology, 3: 142 (1963);
   Muramatsu, M., Onishi, T., Sato, T., Makino, S., Hayakumo, Y.,
   Kitajima, K., Fujii, S. Proceedings of Symposium on Chemical
   Physiology and Pathology, 3: 142 (1963).
6. Iwamoto, M., Abiko, Y., Shimizu, M. J. Biochem., 64: 759
   (1968); Iwamoto M., Abiko, Y. J. Biochem., 65: 821 (1969);
   Abiko, Y., Iwamoto, M., Tomikawa, M. Biochim. Biophys. Acta
   242: 203 (1971).
7. Muramatsu, M., Fujii, S. Biochim. Biophys. Acta 242: 203,
   (1971); Muramatsu, M., Fujii, S. Biochim Biophys. Acta
   268: 221 (1972).
8. Hamberg, V., Stelwage, P., Ervast, H. Eur. J. Biochem. 40
   439 (1973).
9. Haines,A.L., Lepow, I.H. J. Immunol. 99: 456 (1964).
10. Muramatsu, M., Shiraishi, S., Fujii, S. Biochim. Biophys.
    Acta 285: 224 (1972).

MECHANISM OF THE SIALAGOGIC EFFECT INDUCED BY BRADYKININ IN DOGS: POSSIBLE MEDIATION BY ENDOGENOUS PROSTAGLANDIN*

Corrado, A.P., Grellet, M.

Departments of Pharmacology and Surgery, Faculty of

Medicine of Ribeirao Preto, USP, Sao Paulo, Brazil

The increase of the dog submaxillary gland secretion induced by bradykinin (3 µg/kg) by intracarotideal route is low, short-lasting and tachyphylatic. It is unaffected by hexamethonium (2 mg/kg, i.v.) and is still present in chronically denervated glands. The effect is abolished by atropine (1 mg/kg, i.v.), morphine (10 µg/kg, i.v.) or following the ganglionic block by depolarization induced by nicotine (1 mg) by intracarotideal route.

A possible adrenergic mediation of bradykinin effect was excluded, since: a) the polypeptide does not increase the secretion when injected into the artery leading towards the superior cervical ganglion; b) isoproterenol, but not bradykinin, elicits secretion in the atropinized animals; c) even though bradykinin release catecholamines from the adrenal gland, there is no secretion in the right submandibular gland when the injection is made on the left side. The last observation also makes improbable the participation of the central nervous system in bradykinin effects.

Our results indicate that bradykinin interacts with receptors sensitive to blockade by morphine which are probably located in the postsynaptic membrane of cells of the parasympathetic ganglion of the submaxillary gland. The mechanism of action of McN-A-343 and pilocarpine resembles that of bradykinin; they differ in their

---

* This work was partially supported by a Research Grant from "Fundacao de Amparo a Pesquisa do Estado de Sao Paulo (FAPESP)".

susceptibility to blockade by indomethacin. This nonsteroidal anti-inflammatory agent was more specific in blocking bradykinin and the sialagogic effect induced by chorda stimulation. The correlation of these results with the finding that Prostaglandin $PGF_{2\alpha}$ is very potent sialagogic agent in the dog (Hahn and Patil, 1972, 1974; Corrado, 1974), suggests that the effect of the polypeptide could be mediated by endogenous prostaglandins which probably have an important role in salivary secretion physiology.

INTRODUCTION

A relationship has been found between salivary secretion and functional vasodilation with the release of a hypotensive substance which is not acethylcholine (Feldberg and Guimaraes, 1935; Hilton and Lewis, 1955a, a,b). According to Hilton and Lewis (1955 a,b) the functional vasodilation of the cat's submandibulary gland was due to a bradykinin-like substance produced in the intersticial space by the action on plasma proteins of an enzyme released by the physiologically activated gland.

Bradykinin and Kallidin (Werle and Lorenz, 1966) as well as other hypotensive peptides such as physalaemin and eledoisin (Bertaccini and Caro, 1965; Emmelin and Lenninger, 1967) have been found to increase salivary secretion in the dog. Physalaemin and eledoisin are effective in doses ranging from 10^{-9} to 10^{-8} g/kg and seem to act directly on the effector cells. On the other hand, not much is known about the potency and mechanism of action of bradykinin. In the present paper we compared the action of the polypeptide with the effects of other well known sialagogic agents and with the electrical stimulation of the chorda tympani.

METHODS

Mongrel dogs of either sex, weighing 9 to 15 kg were anesthetized with sodium pentobarbital (30 mg/kg intravenously). After surgical exposure, the submaxillary ducts were cannulated, at the chorda-ligual triangle, using a polyethylene tubing (PE 50); the lingual nerve was cut below and above the emergence of chorda tympani which was kept under mineral oil at 39ºC and stimulated with stainless steel electrodes. The drops of saliva secreted were recorded using a Palmer photoelectric drop-timer. The impulses thus generated were converted through a control unit to a Thorp impulse-counter, and cumulatively recorded on a smoked drum.

In all experiments the trachea, the right femoral artery and the left femoral vein were cannulated for respiration and arterial blood pressure recording and for intravenous drug administration, respectively. The lingual artery was cannulated for injection of sialagogic drugs.

Secretory stimuli. The secretory responses of the dogs were
obtained by means of two kinds of stimuli: 1) physical - a Grass
model S_4 square-wave stimulator was used to stimulate the chorda
tympani at a frequency of 50 c/sec., 2 ms duration, 1, 5 V, during
30 sec.; 2) chemical- the following sialagogic drugs were used:
bradykinin*, acethycholine chloride, nicotine, pilocarpine nitrate,
physalaemin*, isoprenaline hydrochloride, McN-A-343* (4-chlorphenyl-
carbomoyloxy-2-butynyltrimethylammonium chloride) and prostaglandin
$F_{2\alpha}$*.

When the drugs were injected directly toward the sub-mandibular
gland, the external carotid artery was clamped immediately below
the emergence of the lingual artery. On the contrary, when they
were injected in a reverse direction, in order to reach the internal
carotid, ascending pharynx, occipital and other arterial branches
in the vicinity of the common carotid bifurcation, clamping of
the external carotid immediately above the emergence of the lingual
artery was carried out. In this way, it was possible to investigate
the role played by the central nervous system, superior cervical
ganglion or release of biogenic amines, as possible mediators of
the sialagogic effect of bradykinin. Salivary secretion was recorded on a smoked drum for 15 min after drug injections. The
polypeptides freed from their preserving solvent by previous eva-
poration were dissolved in saline which in control experiments did
not elicit flow of saliva. The total volume injected via the
lingual artery never exceeded 0.4 ml; 0.2 ml corresponding to the
drug and 0.2 ml to washing of the catheters with saline.

RESULTS

1. Cardiovascular and respiratory effects: The intra-
arterial administration of 1-5 µg/kg of bradykinin caused, apnea,
bradycardia and arterial hypotension when the external carotid
artery above the emergence of the lingual artery was temporarily
occluded. If the occlusion was performed below this artery we
observed the appearance of hyperpnea and a sialagogic effect
(Fig. 1).

2. Sialagogic effect: Was always observed with a dose of
3 µg/kg of bradykinin; the response was reproducible for the first
four injections with tachyphylaxis occuring thereafter (Fig. 2).

---

* McN-A343, physalaemin, prostaglandin $F_{2\alpha}$ and bradykinin were kindly
supplied by Dr. A. P. Rozskowsky (McNeil Lab. Philadelphia, USA), Dr.
G. Bertaccini (Lab. Farmitalia, Parma, Iyaly), Dr. C. Taaues (UpJohn
Lab., Sao Paulo, Brazil)and S. Bricarello (Sandoz Lab., Sao Paulo,
Brazil).

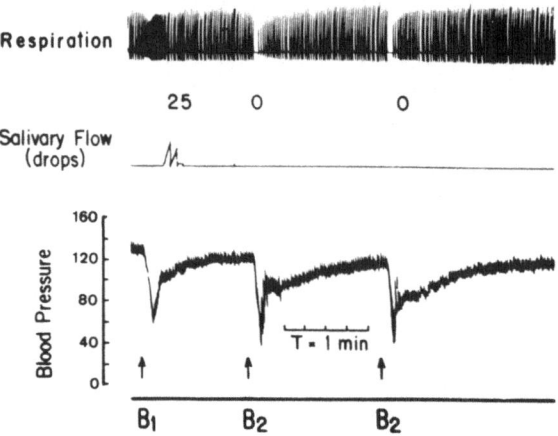

Figure 1. Dog 10kg, anesthetized with pentobarbital sodium (30 mg/kg, i.v.). Respiratory, sialagogic, and circulatory effects of bradykinin (3μg/kg) injected via lingual artery during temporary carotid occlusion below (B_1) and above (B_2) the emergence of the lingual artery. Note the absence of salivation and the presence of apnea and bradycardia at B_2. The number above the tracing of salivary flow indicates the total amount of drops of saliva.

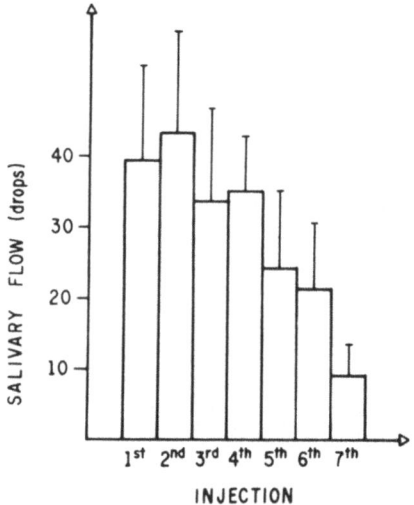

Figure 2. Salivatory response induced by successive intracarotid injection of 3.0 μg/kg of synthetic bradykinin. Each point represents the mean of 10 experiments. The vertical bars are the standard error of the mean. The polypeptide was injected through the lingual artery during carotid occlusion below the lingual emergence.

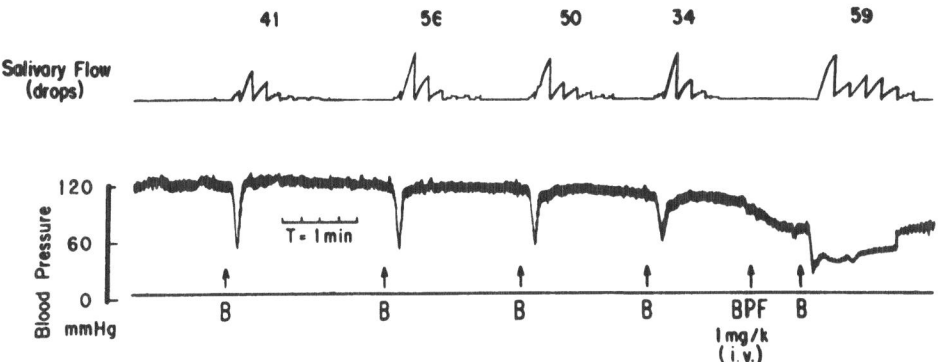

Figure 3. Records of salivary secretion and arterial blood pressure of an 11 kg dog anesthetized as described in Figure 1. Note the potentiation induced by Bradykinin Potentiating Factor - BPF (1 mg/kg, i.v.) of sialagogic and hypotensive effects caused by 3 µg/kg of bradykinin (B) injected via lingual artery as indicated in Figure 2.

Table I. Effects of atropine (1 mg/kg, i.v.) on the salivary flow induced by different stimuli in five dogs

Secretory Stimulus	Before	After
Bradykinin (3 µg/kg)	43.2 + 17.1*	0
Physalaemin (100 µg/kg)	11.0 + 2.0	10.6 + 1.7
Acetylcholine (4 µg/kg)	40.4 + 12.5	0
Isoprenaline (2 µg/kg)	21.3 + 2.0	20.0 + 1.5
McN-A-343 (3 µg/kg)	60.6 + 12.7	0
Chorda ⎡-30 sec	37.8 + 11.8	0
Stimulation ⎢-15 min	49.6 + 14.5	0
15 V-50 c/s ⎣-Total	87.4 + 25.9	0
Nicotine (10 µg/kg)	14.2 + 3.2	0
Pilocarpine (1 µg/kg)	156.6 + 26.3	0

* All numbers indicate the mean ± S.E. of drops of saliva. All sialagogic drugs were injected via lingual artery during carotid occlusion below the lingual emergence.

3. <u>Interference caused by drugs on the salivatory secretion</u>
<u>induced by bradykinin, cholinergic agents and chorda stimulation</u>:

a) <u>Bradykinin potentiating factor</u> (<u>BPF</u> - Ferreira, 1964;
Ferreira and Rocha e Silva, 1965). We have investigated the effect
of BPF (1 mg/kg, i.v.) given after the 4th injection of bradykinin.
Fig. 3 illustratesone of such experiments in which instead of
observing the expected fall of salivary flow, BPF strikingly enhanced bradykinin effects. Note also the potentiation of systemic
hypotension induced by the polypeptide.

b) - <u>Atropine</u>. When injected intravenously at a dose of 1
mg/kg in 5 animals, atropine completely inhibited the sialagogic
effects due to bradykinin, nicotine, stimulus of chorda tympani
and to muscarinic agents such as acetylcholine, McN-A-343 and pilocarpine. Physalaemine and isoprenaline were not affected by atropine
(Table 1).

c)- <u>Hexamethonium followed by morphine</u>. Hexamethonium (1
mg/kg, i.v.) which completely blocked the arterial hypertension
due to nicotine (1 mg i.a.), did not interfere or, in some cases,
facilitated the sialagogic effects due to bradykinin, McN-A-343
and pilocarpine (Table II). The ganglioplegic agent decreased the
salivation resulting from the stimulus of the chorda tympani
during the 30-second period following its application, the inverse
being observed with the salivary flow registered during the 15
minutes period after interruption of the stimulus (Table II). In
the same animals, morphine (10 µg/kg, i.v.) was shown to reduce
markedly the effect of bradykinin, McN-A-343 and pilocarpine but
not the action of nicotine. Salivary flow induced by the stimulus
of the chorda tympani was also blocked by morphine; the inhibitory
action of the opiate was most pronounced on the salivation recorded
during the 15 minutes following the end of the electric stimulation
(Table II).

d) - <u>Morphine followed by hexamethonium</u>. Morphine at a dose
(10 µg/kg, i.v.) sufficient to block the non-nicotinic ganglionic
receptors (Trendelenburg, 1959) markedly inhibited the sialagogic
effect of bradykinin and moderately inhibited that of muscarinic
agents such as McN-A-343 and pilocarpine. The effect of nicotine
was facilitated by the opiate. The salivary secretion induced by
the stimulus of the chorda was blocked more intensely during the
15 minutes following the end of the stimulus (Table wII). Hexamethonium (1 mg/kg, i.v.) on the other hand, facilitates the
sialagogic effect of bradykinin, McN-A-343 and pilocarpine and
inhibited that of nicotine as well as that obtained during the
30 second period of chorda tympani stimulation (Table III).

Table II. Comparison of effects of hexamethonium followed by morphine on the salivary flow induced by different stimuli

Secretory Stimulus		Before	After	
			HEXAMETHONIUM (1 mg/kg, i.v.)	MORPHINE (10 µg/kg, i.v.)
Bradykinin (3 µg/kg)		18.0 ± 5.7*	24.3 ± 6.1	7.6 ± 1.5
Acetylcholine (4 µg/kg)		41.1 ± 9.1	27.1 ± 4.4	14.6 ± 5.5
McN-A-343 (3 µg/kg)		30.0 ± 6.2	37.8 ± 7.3	13.8 ± 3.4
Chorda	-30 sec	13.3 ± 2.2	8.1 ± 2.3	6.6 ± 1.8
Stimulation	-15 min	20.0 ± 1.3	31.3 ± 2.4	10.8 ± 2.4
15 V-50 c/s	-Total	33.3 ± 5.1	39.5 ± 4.3	17.5 ± 3.9
Nicotine (10 µg/kg)		10.3 ± 3.9	4.8 ± 1.1	6.8 ± 1.3
Pilocarpine (1 µg/kg)		74.0 ± 11.0	81.8 ± 12.7	37.1 ± 8.1

*Numbers indicated drops of saliva (Mean ± S.E. of six animals) caused by sialagogic drugs injected as indicated in Table I.

Table III. Effects of morphine followed by hexamethonium on the salivary flow induced by different stimuli

Secretory Stimulus		Before	After	
			MORPHINE (10 µg/kg, i.v.)	HEXAMETHONIUM (1 mg/kg, i.v.)
Bradykinin (3 µg/kg)		40.0 ± 12.7[*]	10.3 ± 4.3	13.1 ± 5.5
Acetylcholine (4 µg/kg)		57.5 ± 13.3	44.8 ± 13.8	37.6 ± 11.9
McN-A-343 (3 µg/kg)		65.8 ± 16.0	40.3 ± 16.1	50.5 ± 22.4
Chorda	−30 sec	36.8 ± 2.6	31.3 ± 3.7	7.0 ± 1.8
Stimulation	−15 min	85.8 ± 11.9	52.1 ± 11.3	52.0 ± 10.5
15 V−50 c/s	−Total	122.6 ± 14.0	83.5 ± 13.2	59.0 ± 1.3
Nicotine (10 µg/kg)		9.6 ± 1.3	12.0 ± 2.2	4.8 ± 0.7
Pilocarpine (1 µg/kg)		131.1 ± 31.7	109.1 ± 28.4	134.1 ± 33.1

[*]Numbers indicate drops of saliva (Mean ± S.E. of six animals) caused by chorda stimulation and sialagogic drugs injected as indicated in Table I.

Table IV. Effects of indomethacin (100 µg/kg, i.v.) on the salivary flow induced by secretory stimuli

Secretory Stimulus		Before	After
Bradykinin (3 µg/kg)		20.2 $\pm$ 3.4[*]	4.0 $\pm$ 0.7
Acetylcholine (4 µg/kg)		29.2 $\pm$ 5.7	25.0 $\pm$ 6.0
McN-A-343 (3 µg/kg)		43.0 $\pm$ 9.0	56.2 $\pm$ 14.8
Chorda	-30 seg	24.0 $\pm$ 5.7	17.2 $\pm$ 4.9
Stimulation	-15 min	52.2 $\pm$ 18.9	29.2 $\pm$ 9.3
15 V-50 c/s	-Total	76.2 $\pm$ 22.4	46.5 $\pm$ 13.6
Nicotine (10 µg/kg)		11.0 $\pm$ 1.0	14.0 $\pm$ 1.9
Prostaglandin $F_{2\alpha}$ (5 ng/kg)		95.0 $\pm$ 15.0	72.0 $\pm$ 10.5

[*] Numbers indicate drops of saliva (Mean $\pm$ S.E. of four animals) caused by chorda stimulation and sialagogic drugs injected as indicate in Table I.

e) - <u>Nicotine</u>. When injected through the lingual artery
in small doses (10 g/kg) the alkaloid produced only moderate salivation (Tables I, II, III, IV). At doses of 1 mg, besides a more
pronounced sialagogic effect, a temporary block of salivation after
stimulation of the chorda or elicited by bradykinin was observed
(Fig. 4). However, successive injections of high doses (1, 3, 5
mg or more) of nicotine reversed the blockade of the effect of
bradykinin while salivary flow due to chorda stimulation remained
blocked only during 30 second period of electrical stimulation
(Fig. 4).

f) - <u>Indomethacin</u>. Given in a dose of 100 µg/kg by lingual
artery in 5 animals, this anti-inflammatory agent almost completely
blocked the sialagogic effect of bradykinin and decreased the salivation induced by chorda tympani stimulation; the actions of
McN-A-343 and nicotine were, on the other hand, facilitated.
The effect of prostaglandin $F_{2\alpha}$ is slightly decreased (Table IV).

DISCUSSION

The potentiation of the sialagogic effect of bradykinin
induced by BPF (Fig. 3), suggests the presence of kininases in the
glandular parenchyma, in accordance with the inactivation of vasoactive polypeptides directly applied to this tissue (Nobilli, 1965).
However, the possibility that BPF produces this potentiation partly
through the inhibition of plasma kininases, eventually accumulated
in the extracellular space of the edematous gland, cannot be discarded. Edema could occur as a result of successive injections of
bradykinin, which is known to enhance vascular permeability.

Contrary to other pharmacologically active polypeptides, such
as physalaemin and eledoisin, which act "directly" on the effectors
of the salivary secretion (Bertaccini and Caro, 1965; Emmelin and
Lenninger, 1967) the sialagogic effect of bradykinin is completely
blocked by the previous intravenous injection of atropine, suggesting an "indirect" mechanism of action which would involve nervous
structures and/or the liberation of chemical mediators directly
from their stores.

The participation of the central nervous system, of the
superior cervical ganglion or release of endogenous catecholamines
was ruled out since no salivation was observed in the heterolateral
control duct and in the duct under observation, following the
occlusion of the external carotid above the emergence of the lingual artery. In this case, the respiratory and hemodynamic effects
which accompany the sialagogic effect were greatly increased (Fig.
1) corroborating the results of Riccioppo Neto and col. (1970,
1974). The persistence of the sialagogic effect of isoproterenol

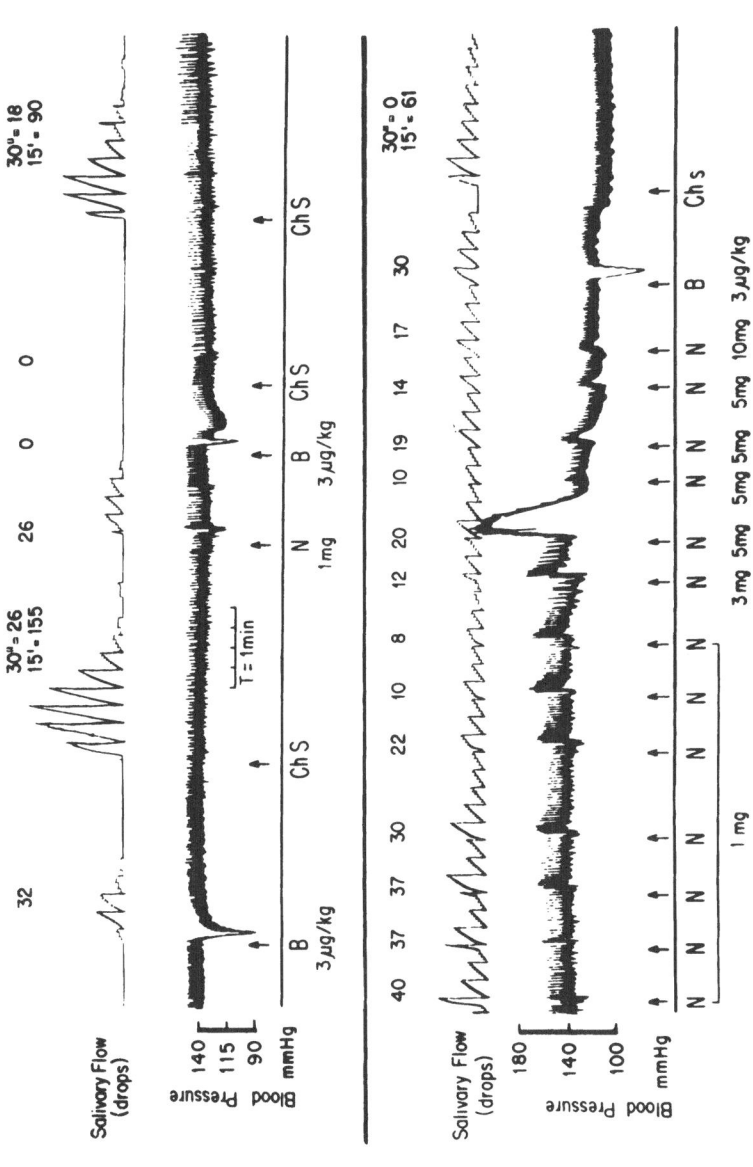

Figure 4. Effects caused by depolarizing and competitive phases of the ganglionic blockade induced by nicotine (N) on the salivary flow elicited by bradykinin (B) and chorda tympani stimulation (Chs). Dog 12 kg under sodium pentobarbital anesthesia (30 mg/kg, i.v.). Note the absence of salivation during the depolarizing phase of the ganglionic blockade by nicotine and the reappearance of saliva after repeated applications of the alkaloid (no depolarizing or competitive phase). All drugs were injected bia lingual artery as indicated in Figure 2.

in atropinized animals provides one more piece of evidence against
the participation of the sympathetic system in the action of
bradykinin since, according to Emmelin and Lenninger (1967), in
the submandibular gland of the dog only sympathetic β-receptors
are present.

That hexamethonium facilitates, instead of blocks, the
sialagogic effect of bradykinin suggests that this effect involves
postganglionic nervous structure or that bradykinin acts on ganglionic sites not susceptible to blockade by hexamethonium i.e.,
on non-nicotinic receptors, as demonstrated in the superior cervical ganglion of the cat (Lewis and Reit, 1965, 1966; Trendelenburg,
1966). An analogous facilitation was also observed with pilocarpine and McN-A-343, known to exert a stimulatory action on the
non-nicotinic receptors of the sympathetic ganglion (Roszkowski,
1961; Trendelenburg, 1966). Thus, it could be suggested that these
agents exert their sialagogic effect, at least in part, through
activation of non-nicotinic receptors, probably present in the
submandibular ganglion.

A special comment must be made regarding the effect of hexamethonium on the salivary flow elicited by stimulus of the chorda
tympani. Contrary to what was expected, in almost all cases a
facilitation of total flow was observed, the increase being
mainly due to the flow recorded after 30 seconds of stimulus application. Admitting the existence of ganglionic non-nicotinic receptors, such results suggest that the salivary flow observed
during the 30 seconds stimulus, results from the activation of
the nicotinic receptors, whereas the delayed flow is due to non-
nicotinic receptor stimulation. This suggestion is reinforced by
the fact that high-frequency stimulation (50 c/s), as employed in
our experiments, has been reported to activate non-nicotinic ganglionic receptors (Eccles and Libet, 1961; Takeshige and Volle,
1952). The participation of non-nicotinic receptors could also
play a role in the salivary flow induced by acetylcholine. In
fact, morphine, which is considered a typical non-nicotinic blocking
agent in sympathetic and parasympathetic ganglia (Trendelenburg,
1959), partially blocked the salivary flow induced by acetylcholine,
suggesting the probable existence of both nicotinic and non-nicotinic
receptors in the submandibular ganglion. In contrast, Alonso de La
Sierra (1962) reported no significant changes in salivary flow of
cats following McN-A-343 and pilocarpine, in the presence of
effective doses of intravenously injected morphine (1 mg/kg). This
discrepancy could be due to differences in animal species as well
as routes of administration. Although the present results do not
completely rule out a "direct" action of McN-A-343 on effector
cells, as proposed by Alonso de La Sierra (1962), they nevertheless
strongly suggest a preferential action of McN-A-343 on the maxillary
ganglion. Our results with pilocarpine suggest a predominant

peripheral action, in agreement with Alonso de La Sierra (1962).

The fact that morphine mainly blocked the delayed salivary flow after electrical stimulation of chorda tympani, in contrast to hexamethonium, agrees with the former suggestion on the role of non-nicotinic receptors in this phenomenon.

The inhibition of sialagogic effect of bradykinin during the depolarized state period induced by nicotine, as well as the recovery of the sialagogic action during the non-depolarizing blockade phase, reinforces the hypothesis of a ganglionic action of the polypeptide.

The fact that bradykinin was able to induce salivation in animals with cronically decentralized glands suggests that preganglionic nerve endings are not involved in the sialagogic action of the polypeptide.

Indomethacin has been reported to inhibit the synthesis of prostaglandin (Vane, 1971; Ferreira, et al.,1971). In addition, prostaglandin $F_{2\alpha}$ has been shown to be a very potent sialagogic agent in the dog, a prolonged salivatory response being induced by only 5 ng/kg of this substance, in agreement with Hahn and Patil (1972, 1974) and Corrado (1974). Therefore, the specific antagonism by indomethacin of the sialagogic effect of bradykinin, as shown by present results, suggests that the effect of the polypeptide could be mediated by endogenous prostaglandins. Taking into account the potent sialagogic action of prostaglandin $F_{2\alpha}$ and the blockade induced by indomethacin on the low frequency chorda stimulation (A.P. Corrado & R.T.N. Ribeiro, unpublished) it can be suggested the participation of prostaglandins as the mediators of the physiological neurotransmission of the submandibular gland. The inhibition of prostaglandin action by atropine and its potentiation by neostigmine (Hahn & Patil, 1972; Corrado, 1974) indicate that following the nervous impulse there is a mobilization of prostaglandins which in turn release acetylcholine.

REFERENCES

Alonso de La Sierra, B.G. (1962) Action of some ganglion-stimulating substances on the secretion of saliva from the submandibular gland. Brit. J. Pharmacol. 18, 501.

Bertaccini, G. and Caro, G. de (1965) The effect of physalaemin and related polypeptides on salivary secretion. J. Physiol. 181, 68.

Corrado, A.P. (1974) Mecanismo da acao sialagoga da prostaglandina $F_{2\alpha}$ em caes. Ciencia e Cultura 26 (Supl.), 521.

Eccles, R.M. and Libet, T. (1961) Origin and blockade of the synaptic responses of curarized sympathetic ganglia. J. Physiol. 157, 484.

Emmelin, N. and Lenninger, S. (1967) The "direct" effect of phy-
    salaemin on salivary gland cells. Brit. J. Pharmacol. Chemother.
    $\underline{30}$, 676.
Feldberg, W. and Guimaraes, J.A. (1935) Some observations on sali-
    vary secretion. J. Physiol. $\underline{85}$, 15.
Ferreira, S.H. (1964) A bradykinin-potentiating factor (BPF) present
    in the venom of Bothrops jararaca. Thesis, Faculty of Medicine
    of Ribeirao Preto, USP, Brazil.
Ferreira, S.H. and Rocha e Silva, M. (1965) A Bradykinin-potentiating
    factor (BPF) present in the venom of Bothrops jararaca. Brit.
    J. Pharmacol. $\underline{24}$, 1963.
Ferreira, S.H., Moncada, S. and Vane, J.R. (1971) Indomethacin and
    aspirin abolish prostaglandin release from the spleen. Nature
    New Biol. $\underline{231}$, 237.
Hahn, R.A. and Patil, P.N. (1972) Salivation induced by prostaglandin
    $F_{2\alpha}$ and modification of the response by atropine and physos-
    tigmine. Brit. J. Pharmacol. $\underline{44}$, 527.
Hahn, R.A. and Patil, P.N.·(1974) Further observations on the inter-
    action of prostaglandin F_{2x} with cholinergic mechanisms in
    canine salivary glands. Eur. J. Pharmacol. $\underline{25}$, 279.
Hilton, S.M. and Lewis, G.P. (1955a) The cause of the vasodilatation
    accompanying activity in the submandibular salivary gland.
    J. Physiol. $\underline{128}$, 235.
Hilton, S.M. and Lewis, G.P. (1965b) The mechanism of the functional
    hyperaemia in the submandibular salivary gland. J. Physiol.
    $\underline{129}$, 253.
Lewis, G.P. (1962) Bradykinin-biochemistry, pharmacology and its
    physiological role in controlling local blood flow. Lectures
    on the Scientific Basis of Medicine $\underline{14}$, 242.
Lewis, G.P. and Reit, E. (1965) The action of angiotensin and
    bradykinin on the superior cervical ganglion of the cat. J.
    Physiol. (London) $\underline{179}$, 538.
Lewis, G.P. and Reit, E. (1966) Further studies on the actions of
    peptides on the superior cervical ganglion and suprarenal
    medulla. Brit. J. Pharmacol. 26, 444.
Nobilli, M.B. (1965) Sulla inativazione della eledoisina e della
    physalaemina da parte del sangue totale e di omogenati
    tessuatali di alcuni vertebrati. Arch. int. Pharmacodyn.
    $\underline{158}$, 187.
Riccioppo Neto, F., Reis, D.S. and Corrado, A.P. (1970) Stimulation
    of paravascular intracraneal receptors by bradykinin and
    kallidin. In: Bradykinin and Related Kinins: Cardiovascular,
    Biochemical and Neural Actions, Edit. Sicuteri, F., Rocha e
    Silva, M. and Back, N., pg. 547, Plenum Press, New York.
Riccioppo Neto, F., Corrado, A.P. and Rocha E Silva, M. (1974)
    Apnea, bradycardia, hypotension and muscular induced by
    intracarotid injection of bradykinin. J. Pharmacol. Exp.
    Ther. $\underline{190}$, 316.

Roszkowski, A.P. (1961) An unusual type of sympathetic ganglionic
    stimulant. J. Pharmacol. exp. Ther. 132, 156.
Takashige, C. and Volle, R.L. (1962) Bimodal response of sympathetic
    ganglia to acetylcholine following eserine or repetitive pre-
    ganglionic stimulation. J. Pharmacol. 138, 66.
Trendelenburg, U. (1959) Non-nicotine ganglion-stimulating sub-
    stances. Fed. Proc. 18, 1001.
Trendelenburg, U. (1966) Receptores muscarinicos del ganglio
    cervical superior del gato. Acta Physiol. Latino Amer. 36, 297.
Vane, J.R. (1971) Inhibition of prostaglandin synthesis as a
    mechanism of action for aspirin-like drugs. Nature New Biol.
    231, 232.
Werle, E. and Lorenz, W. (1966) Speicheldrüsensekretion nach
    Pilocarpin, Histamin und Kininen. Arch int. Pharmacodyn.
    161, 477.

KININS AND INFLAMMATION: CHANGES INDUCED ON THE LEVELS OF CYCLIC NUCLEOTIDES

Bertelli, A., Caciagli, F., Schinetti, M.L.

Institute of Pharmacology

University of Pisa, Pisa

Cyclic nucleotides have an important role in the regulation of several biological phenomena, as shown by many experimental results (1, 2).

The relations between 3'5' AMP and 3'5' GMP proved to be particularly important.

Changes in their tissue concentrations seem to affect some hormonal actions, or tissue reactions to different stimuli (3, 4).

The inhibiting effect of cAMP administration on bronchial spasm reaction, induced by chemical mediators such as serotonin, histamin or bradykinin was previously pointed out by us; on the contrary, the same bronchospastic reactions were increased after 3'5'GMP administration (5, 6, 7).

Observations of a number of experimental inflammatory reactions also showed how these cyclic nucleotides have a role in regulating several biological reactions (8, 9).

The observations showed that external cAMP administration inhibited carrageenin-induced rat's paw edema and the increase in permeability induced by serotonin, histamin or bradykinin (10).

The inflammatory reaction by PGs was also reduced by cAMP, but increased, by cGMP administration. In these communications we expose the results of research carried out by us to analyse (11) the effects of cyclic nucleotides, such as 3'5'AMP and 3'5'GMP, on other

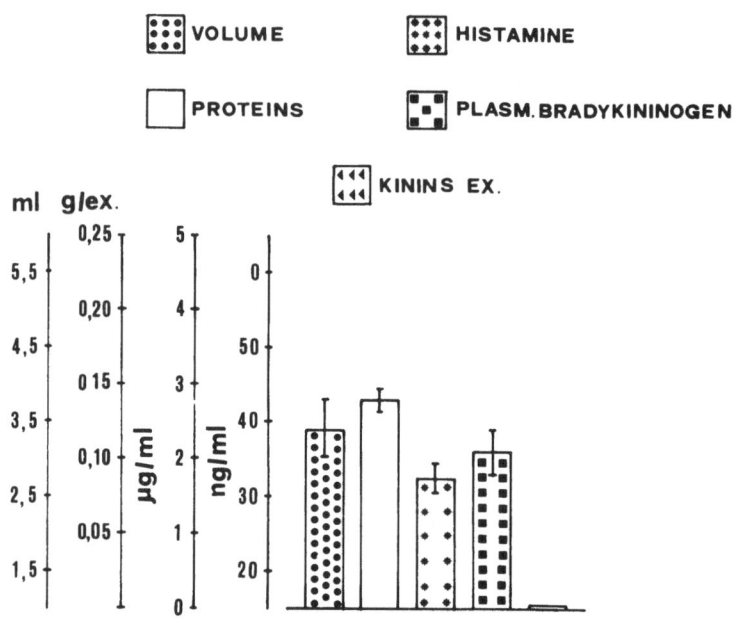

Fig. 1. Evaluation of exudate volume, protein content, histamine concentration and plasmatic kininogen variations in 2% acetic acid induced pleuritis in rats.

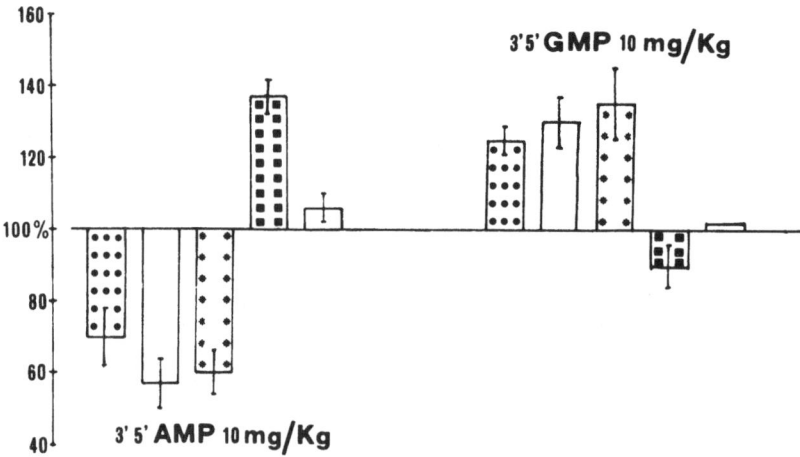

Fig. 2. Modification induced by 3'5'AMP and 3'5'GMP administration on some biochemical variables of 2% acetic acid induced pleuritis. For symbols references, see Fig. 1.

experimental models of phlogosis are investigated to obtain further information on their role in inflammatory processes. Acetic acid-induced pleuritis seemed a suitable model for investigating the relation between intensity of stimulation and phlogistic reaction (12) like pyrophosphate pleurisy.

The intensity of the reaction actually proved to be related to the concentration of intra-pleurically injected acetic acid. Moreover, the temporal behavior of the reaction with respect to exudate volume and protein content can be followed with this method.

The biochemical analysis of exudate as for its histamine and bradykinin content, as well as plasmatic bradykininogen levels can be carried out in such a model (Fig. 1).

In this situation, as well as in those previously studied by us, the administration of cAMP has an inhibiting effect on the phlogosis; the exudate volume, the concentration of its chemical components, in particular histamine and bradykinin are decreased.

The phlogistic reaction is increased by cGMP (thus behaving in opposite way with respect to cAMP); this had been also seen in some broncho-pneumonic spastic reactions (Fig. 2) (7, 13).

In other experiences endogenous 3'5'AMP and 3'5'GMP were dosed in the pleuric exudate in the acetic acid induced pleuritis; this seemed to better signify the importance of the role of these nucleotides in the inflammatory reaction. After a prepurification proposed by Mao and Guidotti (14), the method of evaluation was the protein binding assay of Gilman for 3'5'AMP (15) and radio-immunoassay method of Steiner for 3'5'GMP (16).

The tables we reproduce show a clear decrease in 3'5'AMP, an increase of 3'5'GMP in the exudate obtained after the stimulation by acetic acid. The concentrations are 1%, 2%, 5% and 10% (Fig. 3).

Both changes show a relation to the intensity of the phlogistic stimulation: an increase in the acetic acid concentration (and, consequently, in the phlogistic reaction induced by this substance) is related to a decrease in cAMP and, on the contrary, to a relative increase in cGMP.

These results suggest that the inflammatory reaction may develop if the intracellular concentration of cAMP decrease, while those of cGMP increase (as we already suggested a few years ago).

Other experimental models were investigated to control whether the same changes in cyclic nucleotides could be found in phlogistic reactions.

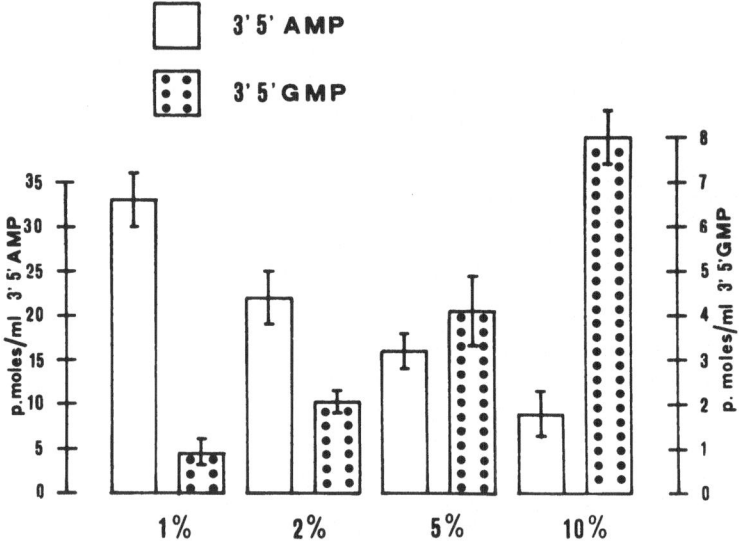

Fig. 3. Levels of 3'5'AMP and 3'5'GMP in acetic acid induced
pleuritis in rats. The concentration's variations are proportional
to phlogistic stimulus intensity.

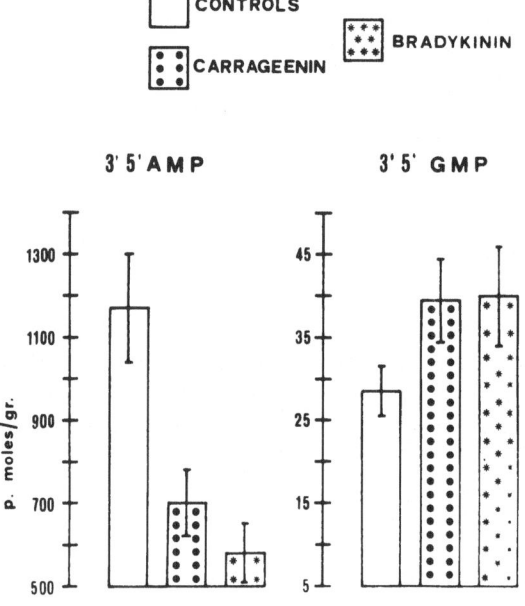

Fig. 4. 3'5'AMP and 3'5'GMP concentration's changes in rat's paw
edema induced by 1% carrageenin and bradykinin (10 μg in 0.1 ml).

In other words, we wish to see whether the same changes in cyclic nucleotides we observe in acetic acid-induced pleuritis appear in the carrageenin or bradykinin induced rat's paw edema.

Moreover, we want to see whether these changes in rat's paw also show a relation between intensity of stimulation and changes in nucleotides concentrations ratios.

The results of these experiments show a decrease in endogenous cAMP, and increase in cGMP in the tissues of rat's paw injected with carrageenin, or even bradykinin (Fig. 4).

Our results therefore confirm the importance of the role of cAMP and cGMP, as well as the importance of their concentrations ratios, in conditioning the intensity and time course of the inflammatory reaction.

Other models, besides these, have been used to classify the behavior of the cyclic nucleotides in inflammatory reaction.

Recent findings for instance indicate that changes similar to those we have described intervene in 3'5'AMP concentrations of bronchial tissue in the broncho-spastic reaction induced by immunological reaction (17).

We conclude that inflammatory reactions result from an imbalance between the concentration of tissue cAMP and cGMP (18).

This finding is of importance not only for a better understanding of the phenomena which regulate the inflammatory reaction, but also for the more profitable study of pharmacological means which may deal with such processes.

ACKNOWLEDGEMENT

The authors thank Mr. Sauro Pellegrini for his invaluable cooperation during the experimental work.

REFERENCES

1. Sutherland, E.W., Rall, T.W., Pharmacol. Rev., 18; 145, 1960.

2. Rasmussen, H., Pechet, M., Fast, D., J. Clin. Invest. 47; 1853 1968.

3. Levine, R.A., Vogel, J.H., J. Pharmacol. 151; 262, 1966.

4. Abe, J., Morimoto, S., Yamamoto, K., Meda, J., Jap. J. Pharmacol. 18; 271, 1968.

5. Bertelli, A., Bianchi, C., Beani, L., J. Pharm. Pharmacol.
    25; 60, 1973.

6. Bertelli, A., Bianchi, C., Beani, L., Experientia 29; 300,
    1973.

7. Bertelli, A., Caciagli, F., Pellegrini, S., In Press.

8. Fleischer, N., Donald, R.H., Butcher, R.W., Am. J. Physiol.
    217; 1287, 1969

9. Bowers, C.Y., Lee, K.L., Shally, A.V., Endocrinology 82; 75,
    1968.

10. Ichikawa, A., Nagasaki, M., Umezu, K., Hayashi, H., Tomita, K.,
    Biochem. Pharmacol. 21; 2015, 1972.

11. Bertelli, A., Caciagli, F., Schinetti, M.L., In Press

12. Willoughby, D.A., Dunn, C.J., Yamamoto, S., Capasso, R.,
    Deporter, D.A., Giroud, J.P., Agents and Actions, 5; 35, 1975.

13. Caciagli, F., Bertelli, A., In Press

14. Mao, A., Guidotti, Anal. Biochem. 31; 618, 1974.

15. Gilman, F., Biochem. Biophys. Acta 18; 530, 1972.

16. Steiner, A., et al., Anal. Biochem. 3, 1974.

17. Gillespie, E., Valentine, M.D., Lichtenstein, L.M., J. All.
    Clin. Immunol. 53; 27, 1974.

18. Goldberg, N.D., Haddox, M.K., Estensen, R., Withe, J.G.,
    Lopez, C., Hadden, J.W., Cyclic AMP, Cell Growth and the
    Immune Response, Ed. W. Braun, L.M. Lichtenstein C. Parker,
    Springer Verlag, Berlin 1974, pg. 247.

AN IMPROVED PREPARATION FOR DETERMINATION OF BRADYKININ

H. Edery and Z. Abraham

Israel Institute for Biological Research, Tel Aviv

University-Medical School, Ness Ziona, Israel

Presently the most sensitive methods for determination of kinins in general and bradykinin in particular include assays on smooth muscle preparations. A variety of organs have been suggested but the most commonly used are the guinea pig ileum and rat uterus. The sensitivity of these preparations towards bradykinin greatly increased after exposure to proteolytic enzymes including chymotrypsin (Edery & Grunfeld, 1969). In addition, the sensitizing action of chymotrypsin has been found to be a useful and simple mean to identify bradykinin (Edery, 1967). Kinins elicit contraction of cat isolated intestine (Schachter, 1956; Erspamer & Erspamer, 1962) and it has been reported that the jejunum showed particular sensitivity to bradykinin (Ferreira & Vane, 1967). It was then considered of interest to see if the spontaneous sensitivity of this preparation could be increased even more when subjected to chymotrypsin.

METHODS

Cats of either sex (3 to 5 kg body weight) were sacrificed by intravenous injection of an overdose of chloroform or sodium pentobarbital. To obtain a piece of jejunum laparotomy was performed. In the cat there is no clear anatomically visible separation between duodenum and jejunum (Reighard & Jennings, 1957). Therefore, to avoid the duodenum and insure that the piece taken was indeed of jejunum, the rostral cut was made at least 16 cm from the pylorus. The piece of jejunum excised was freed of adjacent mesentery and the lumen rinsed with warm Krebs solution. Strips 4-6 mm wide and 5 cm long were then cut parallel to the mesenteric edge. A single strip was (a) mounted into a 10 ml

organ-bath and fitted with an isotonic lever or (b) superfused at a
rate of 2 ml/min while contractions were recorded with a B-myograph
(E & M Instrument Co.). In all experiments the nutrient fluid was
Krebs solution at 35°C (Ferreira & Vane, 1967) and bubbled with a
mixture of 95% O_2 + 5% CO_2.

Drugs

The drugs used were: bradykinin (Sandoz), acetylcholine chloride (Light), 5-hydroxytryptamine creatinine sulphate (Sigma), doses refer to the base, and alpha-chymotrypsin (Nutritional Biochem.).
Drugs were dissolved in the nutrient fluid and strength of solutions was so adjusted that no more than 0.5 ml was either introduced into the organ-bath or injected into the superfusion fluid.

RESULTS

Cat isolated jejunum strip contracted when 5 to 50 ng bradykinin, 10 to 20 ng acetylcholine or 0.5 to 2 µg 5-hydroxytryptamine
were introduced into the organ-bath.

After application of 1 mg chymotrypsin the response to bradykinin was potentiated. In addition, immediately after the exposure
to chymotrypsin, the preparation became sensitized to the kinin.
These effects are illustrated in Fig. 1.

The degree of sensitization varied from preparation to preparation but in all cases the threshold dose was raised to such an
extent that contractions could be elicited by concentrations of
bradykinin ranging from 100 to 300 pg/ml. Moreover the height of
responses to supraliminal doses of bradykinin was increased two to
three fold. In no case was there sensitization to acetylcholine
or to 5-hydroxytryptamine and in some experiments, responses to
these agonists diminished following exposure to chymotrypsin.

Cat jejunum strip contracted after injection of 5 to 20 ng of
bradykinin or acetylcholine into the fluid superfusing the preparation. Chymotrypsin (1 mg) sensitized the tissue to bradykinin
but in a different manner than when the strip was kept in an
organ-bath. Sensitivity was increased only after delay. This is
shown in Fig. 2. Moreover, in most cases maximal sensitization
was attained after applying two or three doses of chymotrypsin.

Use has been made of sensitized preparations, either kept in
an organ-bath or superfused, to determine bradykinin-like material
in extracts of dog blood samples obtained before, during and after
the appearance of "dumping syndrome". This was induced by administration of 150 ml of 50% glucose through a permanent catheter
fixed in the duodenum. The severity of the syndrome as well as

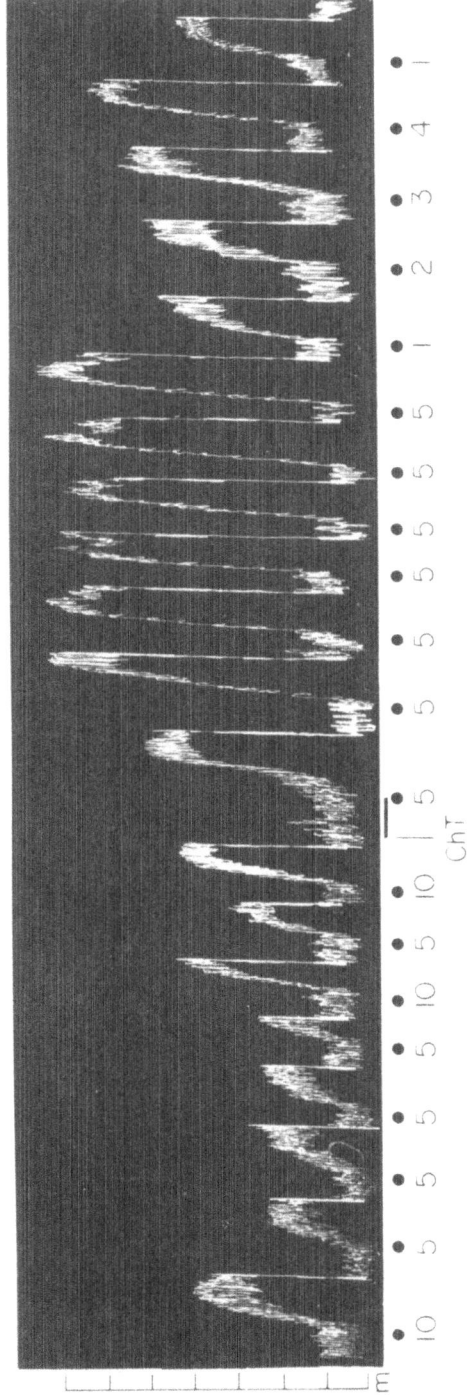

Fig. 1. Cat isolated jejunum strip suspended in 10 ml Krebs solution at 35°C. Contractions elicited by bradykinin (numbers indicate doses in ng introduced into the bath; contact time 1.5 min at 5 min intervals; preparation being washed at least twice after each contraction).

Note that chymotrypsin (ChT, 1 mg; horizontal bar indicates that the preparation was not washed after addition of the enzyme) potentiated the response to bradykinin and subsequently the preparation became sensitized to the peptide.

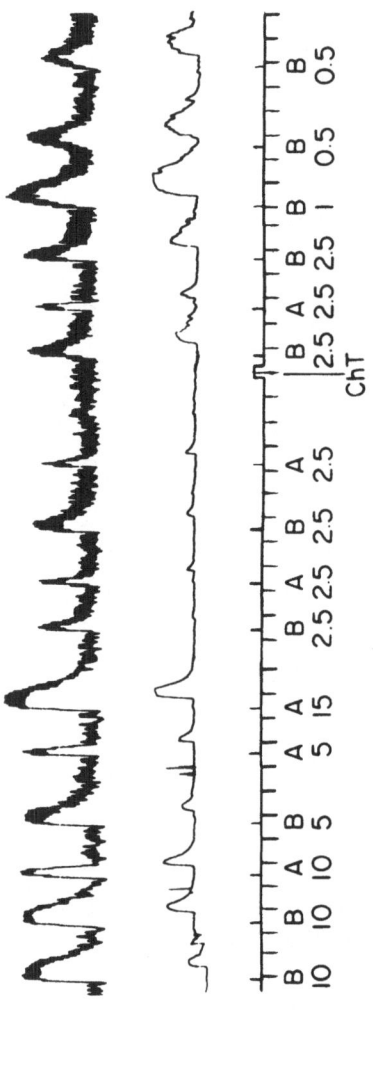

Fig. 2.   Twin preparations of cat isolated jejunum superfused with Krebs solution (2 ml/min), time marker, 60 sec. Contractions induced by injection (upward stroke) into the perfusion fluid of bradykinin (B) or acetylcholine (A), (numbers refer to ng).

Note the delayed sensitization to bradykinin which developed after injection of 1 mg of chymotrypsin (ChT).

blood kinin activity were diminished by previous administration of 20 ml ethanol. Full details of these experiments will be reported separately.

COMMENT

The present work showed that by treating cat isolated jejunum with chymotrypsin, the preparation became sensitized to bradykinin, thus allowing to detect minute amounts of the peptide. The time course of sensitization differed according to the experimental conditions. During superfusion only a minimal amount of chymotrypsin might have been retained by the tissue owing to the short contact time. Consequently a relatively long lapse had to pass until bradykinin receptors could be uncovered by the enzyme as this has been postulated to be the likely mechanism of sensitization by proteolytic enzymes (Edery & Grunfeld, 1969). Likewise, the failure of chymotrypsin to induce sensitization of jejunum strip after injection into superfusing blood (Ferreira & Rocha e Silva, 1969) might also have been due to the fact that minimal amounts, if any, could have been taken up by the tissue. It would thus appear that in order to increase sensitivity to bradykinin when using superfused preparations, it might be advisable either to inject up to three doses of chymotrypsin, or beforehand to incubate the preparation with the enzyme for a short period.

SUMMARY

The cat isolated jejunum kept either in an organ-bath or under superfusion can be rendered extremely sensitive to bradykinin after exposure to chymotrypsin. Treated preparations responded to as little as 100 pg/ml of the peptide.

Use has been made of sensitized preparations to determine bradykinin-like material of dog blood extracts obtained in experimental "dumping syndrome".

REFERENCES

Edery, H. (1967). Nature, 217, 70.

Edery, H. & Grunfeld, Y. (1969). Br. J. Pharmacol., 35 , 51-61.

Erspamer, V. & Erspamer, G.F. (1962). Br. J. Pharmacol., 19, 337-354.

Ferreira, S. & Vane, J.R. (1967). Br. J. Pharmacol., 29, 367-377.

Reighard, J. & Jennings, H.S. (1957). Anatomy of the cat. 4th ed., H. Holt & Co. New York p. 236.

Schachter, M. (1956). Br. J. Pharmacol., 11, 111-118.

EFFECT OF ISOPROTERENOL ON THE KALLIKREIN CONTENT OF THE SUBMANDIBULAR GLAND OF RATS

Namir S. Lauar, O.L. Catanzaro*, R.B. Rossoni and
W. T. Beraldo

Departments of Physiology-Biophysics and Morphology
ICB, UFMG, Belo Horizonte, Brazil

Selye et al. (1961) and Brown-Grant (1961) demonstrated that isoproterenol (IPR) elicited enlargement of submandibular and parotid gland in rats and mice. Barka (1965) verified that the drug stimulates DNA synthesis and mitotic activity in these organs. IPR, as a sialagogue, causes a depletion of secretory material in the salivary glands followed by a period of resynthesis of proteins (Byrt, 1966; Schirley and Mills, 1971).

Since an increase in the kallikrein content in the rat sub-mandibular gland during postnatal development was observed by Beraldo,et al (1972) it was decided to investigate the influence of IPR on the kallikrein content of the gland in young and adult rats during chronic treatment with the drug. This effect of the IPR was correlated with the structure of the gland.

MATERIAL AND METHODS

Used were 5, 15, 56 and 84 day old rats (Holtzman) injected intraperitonealy with IPR (1.6 mg/100g) twice a day for 6 days. Groups of 5 to 9 male animals were used. They were sacrificed 20 hours after the last injection of the drug. The submandibular glands were excised and homogenized in saline. The homogenate was centrifuged at 20.000 r.p.m. for 1 hour at 4°C and supernatant used for protein determination (Lowry et al 1951). Kallikrein bioassay was performed according to Beraldo et al (1972).

---

* From the CONICET, Argentina, and visiting professor of the CNPq, Brazil.

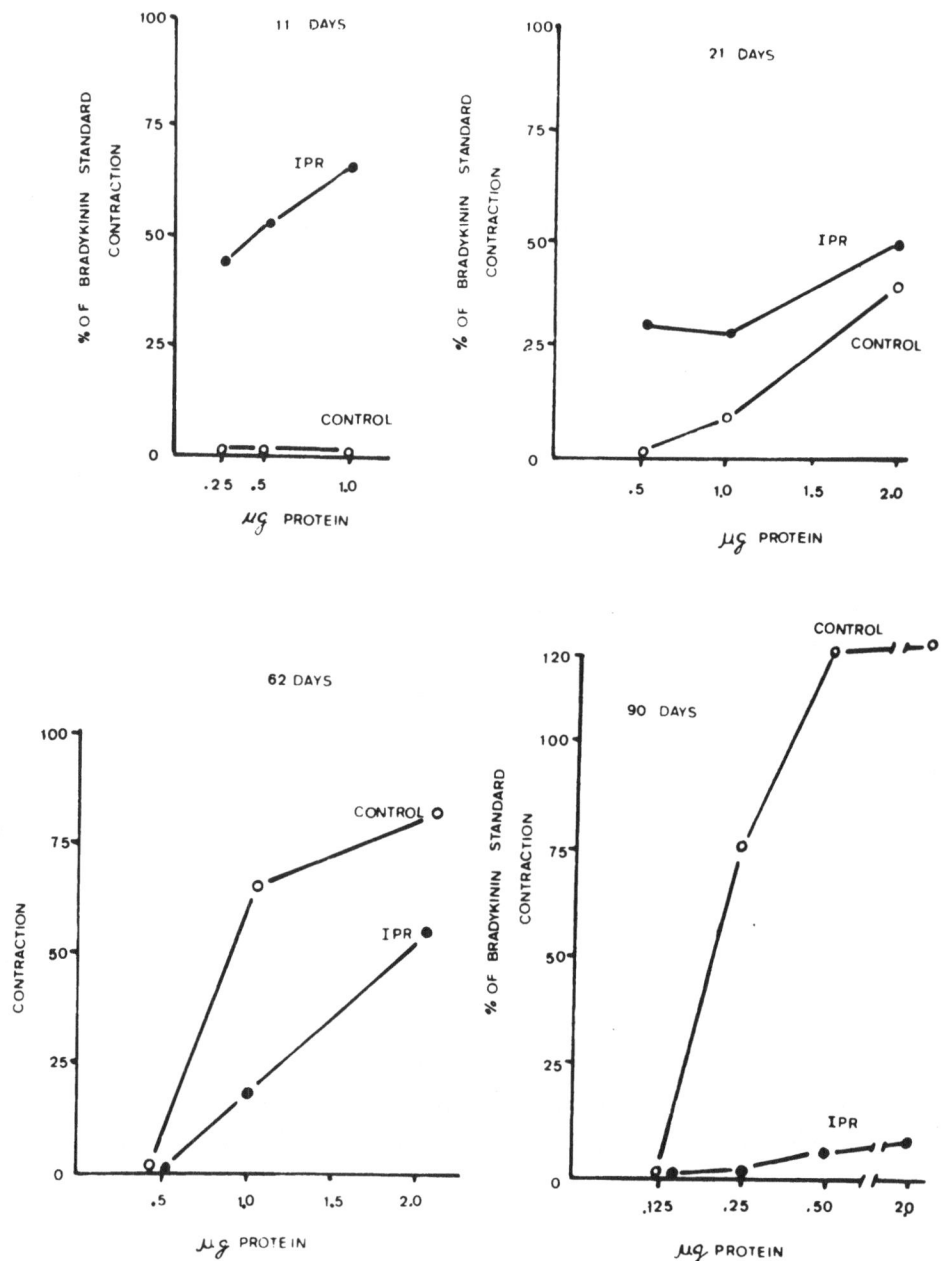

Fig. 1. Kallikrein content of submandibular gland of rats from 11, 21, 62, and 90 days old. Each point represents the mean of 8 to 12 glands.

For the histological studies glandular fragments of the control and IPR treated animals were fixed in Helly fluid and embedded in paraffin. Sections were cut at 6 μm stained with periodic-Schiff (PAS) and haematoxylin.

RESULTS

When 0.2 to 0.5 μg protein of submandibular gland of 11 day old rats were added to the organ bath containing rat uterus, the preparation did not respond at all. However, if the same amount of gland protein from a rat of the same age, previously injected with IPR, were added to the bath the muscle contracted. Whereas gland protein of 21 day old rats both IPR treated and control showed kallikrein activity, quite different results were obtained when the submandibular gland extract protein of adult rats (62 and 90 day old rats) were assayed for kallikrein content. IPR, instead of increasing the kallikrein of the gland, produced a decrease as shown in Figure 1.

Figure 2 summarizes the results of the effect of IPR on the kallikrein content of the submandibular gland at different ages. The drug showed a striking effect on young rats, but its effectiveness progressively decreased with the age of the animals. On the 62 and 90 day old rats, the gland of controls presented greater amounts of kallikrein as compared to the IPR treated ones.

Marked histological differences occurred between the submandibular glands of the control and IPR treated rats (Fig. 3 and 4). The gland of the control 11 day old rats showed inter and intralobular ducts and terminal tubules with PAS-positive acinar cells budding off from them. The gland of the 11 day old rats injected with IPR did not present terminal tubules but well developed acini dominated the picture. The acini showed a great amount of secretory granules intensely stained with PAS but in many acini they were slightly stained or unstained. In the submandibular gland of the control 21 day old rats, acini and terminal tubules surrounded by acinar cells were the most evident structures. At the same age, the IPR treated rats showed the gland predominantly occupied by large acini with a similar aspect to that of the injected 11 day old rats. No granulated ducts were developed in the submandibular gland of the control and treated 11 and 21 day old rats. In the submandibular gland of the control 62 day old rats, apart from the acini with PAS-positive granules and the ductal system, granulated ducts were already seen. In the IPR treated animals the most evident alteration was the enlargement of the acini. The granulated ducts showed a moderate degranulation. The submandibular gland of 90 day old control rats exhibited a structure similar to that described for the control 62 day old ones,

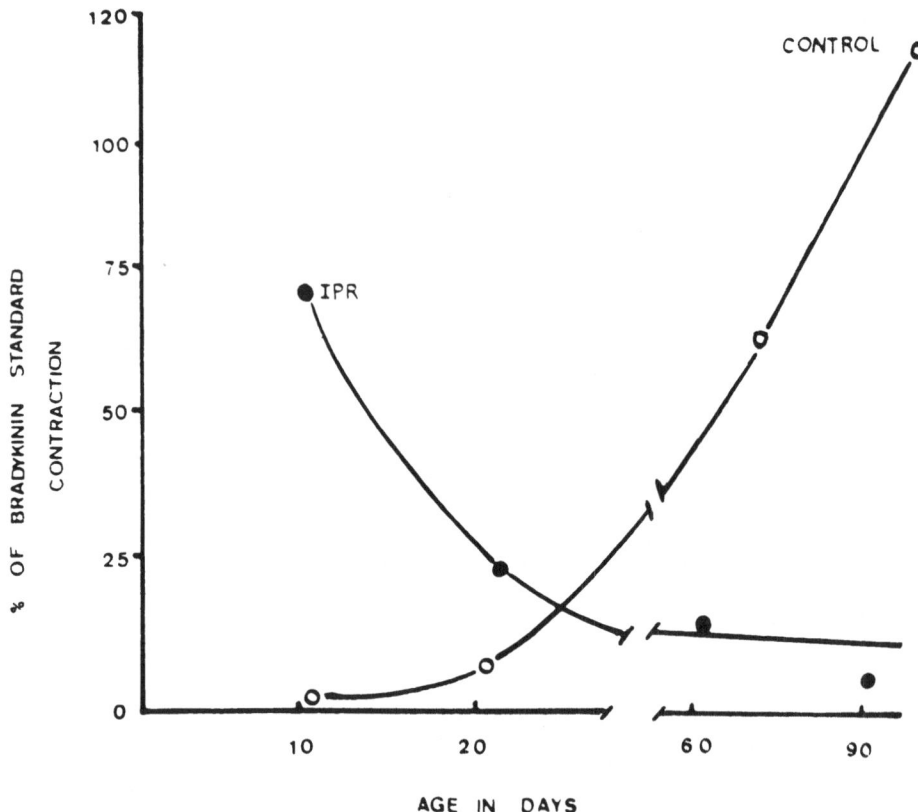

Fig. 2. Kallikrein content of submandibular gland of rats at different ages. These results were replotted from Fig. 1. The kallikrein activity contained in 1 μg of gland extract protein was
chosen.

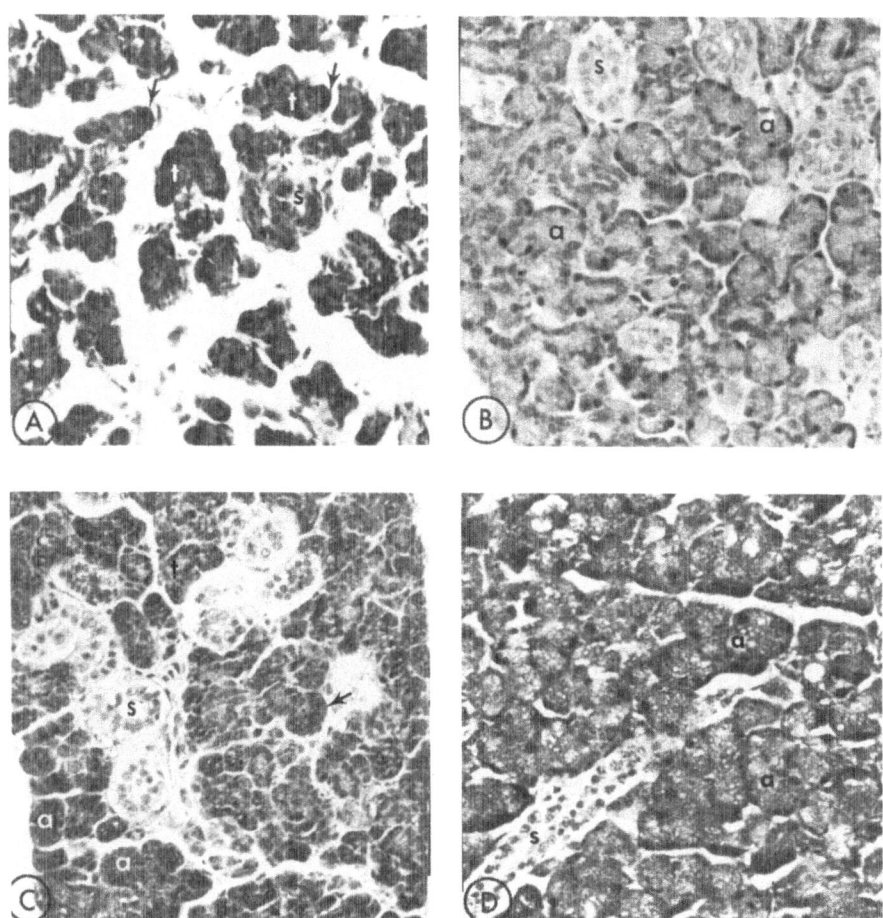

Fig. 3. Submandibular gland of rats. A, control 11 days old. B, IPR treated 11 days old. C, control 21 days old. D, IPR treated 21 days old. Arrows, budding cells; t, terminal tubules; a, acini; s, striated ducts. (275x)

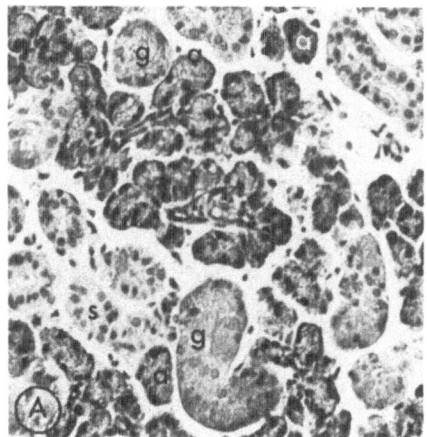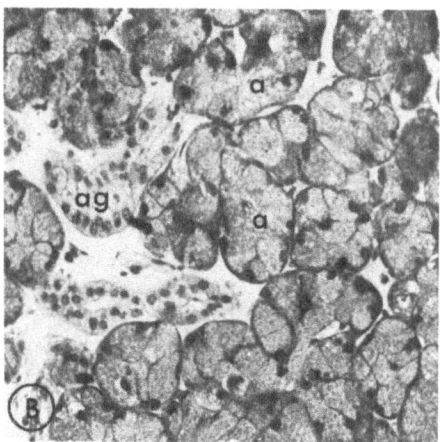

Fig. 4. Submandibular gland of rats. A, control 90 days old. B, IPR treated 90 days old. a, acini; s, striated ducts; g, granulated ducts; ag, atrophic granulate duct. (275x)

although the granulated ducts were more developed. In 90 day old IPR treated animals the gland showed hypertrophied acini with most of their granules slightly stained or unstained. The granulated ducts were atrophied and its granular content was decreased or absent.

DISCUSSION

Postnatal changes in number, size and degree of maturation of the acinar cells of salivary glands are regulated by the auto-nomic innervation (Hall et al., 1969; Schneyer, et al., 1969). A correlation between the postnatal differentiation of the acini and the kallikrein content of submandibular gland of the rat was already demonstrated (Beraldo et al., 1972). Our present results showed that the early appearance of well developed acini induced by IPR was closely associated with an increase in the kallikrein content of the gland in the 11 and 21 day old rats. In fact, hypertrophied acini were described in the submandibular gland of young and adult rats tréated with IPR and they would indicate a condition of marked functional engagement (Mira et al., 1971). The participation of the granulated ducts as sourcesof kallikrein in the 11 and 21 day old rats can be ruled out, since these structures are absent at this stage of development.

In the 62 and 90 day old IPR treated rats the histological
modifications of the granulated ducts, coinciding with the
decrease of kallikrein content of the gland may suggest that
these last structures are related to the production of kallikrein.
This hypothesis, however, cannot explain the decrease of kallikrein observed in the 21 day old IPR treated animals as compared
with the 11 day old IPR treated ones, since the submandibular
gland of these animals did not show granulated ducts.

It is interesting to point out that the kallikrein activity
was higher in the 11 day than in the 21, 62 and 90 day old IPR
treated rats. The increase of kallikrein content in the gland
of 11 and 21 day old rats could be due to the ineffectiveness of
the secretory mechanism to eliminate enzymes produced by the gland.
The progressive decrease in the kallikrein content in
the gland of 11 to 90 day old rats could be explained by the
functional maturation of the autonomic nervous system and the
mechanism of glandular secretion as a whole. Finally, it could
be suggested that the receptor sites in the acinar cell membrane
in the young animals are not completely prepared to receive the
drug and trigger the secretory mechanism. However, the receptors
are well differentiated to perform enlargement, increasing the
mitotic activity and enzyme content in the acinar cells.

SUMMARY

The influence of IPR on the kallikrein content of the submandibular gland of 11, 21, 62 and 90 day old rats was investigated.
The appearance of acini in IPR treated rats was associated with
an increase in the kallikrein content of the gland in 11 day old
rats. The decrease of kallikrein in the gland of 21 to 90 day
old animals was attributed to the maturation of the autonomic
nervous system and the mechanism of glandular secretion.

We wish to thank Mr. Rubens Miranda for the technical
assistance.

REFERENCES

Barka, T. Stimulation of DNA synthesis by isoproterenol in the
    salivary gland. Exp. Cell Res. 39, 355, 1965.

Beraldo, W.T., G. Siqueira, J.A.A. Rodrigues and C.R.S. Machado.
    Changes in kallikrein activity of rat submandibular gland
    during postnatal development. Adv. Exp. Med. Biol. 21, 239,
    1972.

Brown-Grant, K. Enlargement of the salivary gland in mice
    treated with isopropylnoradrenaline. Nature. 212, 1212, 1966.

Byrt, P., Secretion and synthesis of amylase in the rat parotid gland after isoprenaline., Nature. 212, 1212, 1966.

Hall, H.D. and C.A. Schneyer. Physiological activity and regulation of growth of developing parotid. Proc. Sox. Exp. Biol. Med. 131, 1288, 1969.

Lowry, O.H., N.J. Rosebrough, A.L. Farr and R.J. Randall. Protein measurement with the Folin phenol reagent. J. Biol. Chem. 193, 265, 1951.

Mira, E., G. Gerzeli, P. de Piceis Polver and I. Vidi. Histo-functional changes in isoproterenol enlarged submaxillary glands of adult male rats. Acta Anat. 80, 235, 1971.

Schirley, B.A. and K.S. Mills. Amylase changes accompanying stimulated salivary gland growth. Comp. gen. Pharmac. 2, 205, 1971.

Schneyer, C.A. and H.D. Hall. Growth pattern of postnatally developing rat parotid gland. Proc. Soc. Exp. Biol. Med. 130, 603, 1969.

Selye, H., R. Veilleux and M. Cantin. Excessive stimulation of salivary gland growth by isoproterenol. Science. 133, 44, 1961.

WHICH IS THE EFFECTIVE AGENT - BRADYKININ OR PROSTAGLANDINS - ON THE ISOLATED MAMMALIAN HEART (*)

M. Rocha e Silva, M. Morato (**), A.P. de Almeida
and A. Antonio

Department of Pharmacology, Faculty of Medicine, USP
Ribeirão Preto, São Paulo, Brazil

It is well known that bradykinin in minute doses increases perfusion flow and the height of the beats of the isolated mammalian heart (1). In Reston, Va., last October, the question was raised whether the effects of bradykinin (Bk) on the isolated mammalian heart perfused by the Langendorff technique, could be due to a release of prostaglandin (PGE_2), since the latter was able to produce a similar effect on the coronary perfusion flow and on the force of contraction. Such an indirect effect of Bk mediated by PGE_2 could be reasonable owing to the many reports establishing that Bk is able to stimulate synthesis of prostaglandins (2). On the other hand PGE, has been found to potentiate the effects of Bk in pain production (3), swelling of the rat's paw (4), increase in vascular permeability (5) and in the so-called pseudo-affective reaction to Bk when injected into the splenic artery (6). In a series of experiments on the isolated guinea pig heart (Langendorff's technique) the effects of Bk and PGE were compared and the results obtained fully demonstrated the impossibility of explaining by synthesis or release of PGE_2 the immediate effect of minute doses (0.001 to 0.01 μg) of Bk on the perfusion flow and height of contraction. In our experiments, PGE_2 acts in a quite different way in higher (0.1 to 1.0 μg) doses inducing an immediate reduction in the height of contraction and a rather delayed effect on the perfusion flow accompanied by sustained increase in height of contraction. The opposite possibility, namely that prostaglandin (PGE_2) may act by release of an endogenous mediator is more likely to explain the delayed

(*) Aided by Grants from CNPq and FAPESP
(**) Under a fellowship of CNPq

effect on coronary flow and height of contraction. A release of catecholamines by PGE_2 has been considered but excluded, since a β-sympatholytic agent (Inderal) which blocks the effect of epinephrine, did rather enhance (potentiate) the secondary effect of PGE_2. The alternative possibility of formation of Bk from endogenous sources of bradykininogen was considered as a likely by the fact that a bradykinin potentiating factor (BPF) definitely enhanced the secondary effects of PGE_2. Furthermore, Inderal which potentiated the secondary effect of PGE_2 also increased the primary effect of Bk alone or associated with BPF. If confirmed, the possibility that prostaglandins may release Bk from its precursor in tissue, would be a first instance in which prostaglandin may constitute a Bk-forming agent, that could explain part of the potentiating action of PGE, on several effects of Bk, as mentioned above. These results await further confirmation by experiments currently being carried out in our laboratory.

REFERENCES

1. Antonio, A. and Rocha e Silva, M. 1962, Circulation Res. 11, 910.

2. Vane, J.R. and Ferreira, S.H., 1975, In: Meet. on Chemistry and Biology of the Kallikrein-Kinin System in Health and Disease (Reston, Va.). In press.

3. Ferreira, S.H., Moncada, S. and Vane, J.R., 1974, Brit. J. Pharmacol. 50, 461P.

4. Thomas, G. and West, G.B., 1973, J. Pharm. Pharmacol. 25, 747.

5. Isoda, K., Tanaka, K. and Katori, M., 1975, In: Meet. on Chemistry and Biology of the Kallikrein-Kinin System in Health and Disease (Reston, Va., 1974). In press.

6. Ferreira, S.H., Moncada, S. and Vane, J.R., 1973, Brit. J. Pharmacol. 49, 86.

ISOLATION OF PROCINE URINARY KALLIKREIN

H. Tschesche[+], G. Mair[+], B. Förg-Brey[++], H. Fritz[++]

[+]Organisch-Chemisches Institut der Technischen Universität München,[++]Klinisch-Chemisches und Klinisch-Biochemisches Institut der Universität München
[+]8 München 2, Arcisstr. 21, [++]8 München 2, Nußbaumstr.20

Purification and characterization of urinary kallikrein was stimulated by its assumed significance for the renin-angiotensin system. It still remains to be clarified whether urinary kallikrein is identical with renal kallikrein and which relationships are between urinary and pancreatic kallikrein.

Fresh porcine urine was collected from urinary bladders after death of the animals. The urine was preserved from bacterial deterioration by addition of toluene and storage at 4° C. One liter urine contains about 60 U (BAEE/ADH-test) of active enzyme. The first purification step was fractionated acetone precipitation at 4° C (step 1). The second fraction with 50 - 75 % acetone contained almost the total BAEE-hydrolyzing activity. The precipitate was redissolved in deionized water, dialyzed against deionized water and concentrated by ultrafiltration using Amicon Hollow Fiber DC 2 with H1DP10 Diafibers. Further purification was achieved by Sephadex G-75 gel filtration in 0.05 M ammonium acetate, pH 6.8, saturated with chloroforme at 6° C (step 2). Inactive coloured material was separated from a single active fraction. This fraction was further purified by DEAE-Sephadex chromatography using a linear ammonium acetate gradient from 0.1 - 1.0 molar concentration, pH 6.8, Fig. 1 (step 3). The BAEE-hydrolyzing activity was resolved into two active peaks, A and B, the first one not completely separated from acidic, coloured material with high 280 nm absorbance. The specific activity from steps 1 to 3 was increased by a factor of 50 - 70.

Additional purification after step 2 can be achieved by affinity chromatography using bovine trypsin-kallikrein inhibitor (Kunitz)

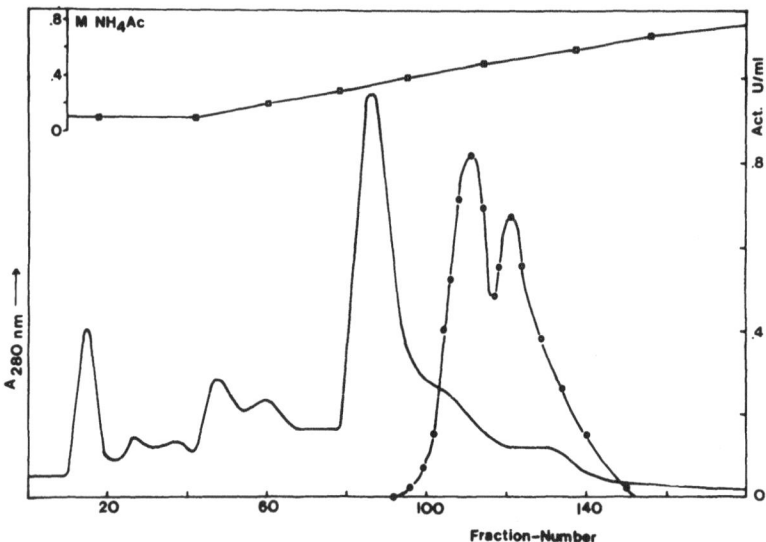

Fig. 1 Elution profile of crude porcine urinary kallikrein after
    DEAE-Sephadex A-50 chromatography. Column 4.2 x 30 cm, 0.1 M
    ammonium acetate, pH 6.8. Gradient from 0.1 - 1.0 M ammonium
    acetate: □ ── □. Flow rate 30 ml/h; 9 ml/fraction. Absorbance
    at 280 nm: ── . Esterolytic activity (BAEE/ADH): o ── o.

bound at pH 5.0 to BrCN-activated Sepharose. The active enzyme was
eluted from the affinity column by 0.5 M benzamidine/HCl in trie-
thanolamine/HCl, pH 6.5. However, the affinity of porcine urinary
kallikrein to the bovine trypsin-kallikrein inhibitor was very weak
when compared to the binding of the porcine pancreatic kallikrein.
There is a significant difference in the association constants between the two enzymes and the bovine inhibitor as is obvious from
their titration curves, Fig. 2.

    Both enzyme preparations from affinity chromatography and from
DEAE-Sephadex chromatography were subjected to isoelectric focussing
using polyacrylamide ampholyte slab gels, Fig. 3. Numerous bands
appeared in the acidic pH-range from pH 3 - 4 and 3.5 - 5, respectively.

    The Michaelis constant of enzyme from peak B (Fig. 1) was de-
termined to 125 μMol (0.1 M Tris/HCl, pH 7.8).

    The amino acid composition of the porcine urinary enzyme puri-
fied by affinity chromatography closely resembles that of porcine
pancreatic kallikrein. Preliminary data from a 16-h hydrolysate indicate the composition given in the Table.

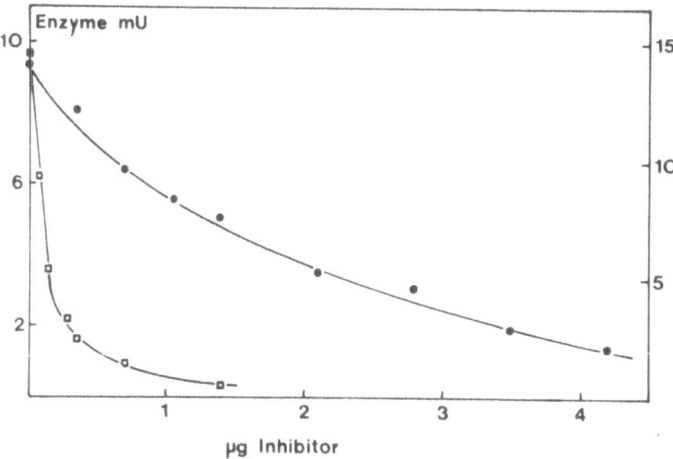

Fig. 2 Titration of porcine urinary kallikrein (●, left ordinate)
and pancreatic kallikrein (□, right ordinate) with trypsin-
kallikrein inhibitor (Kunitz).

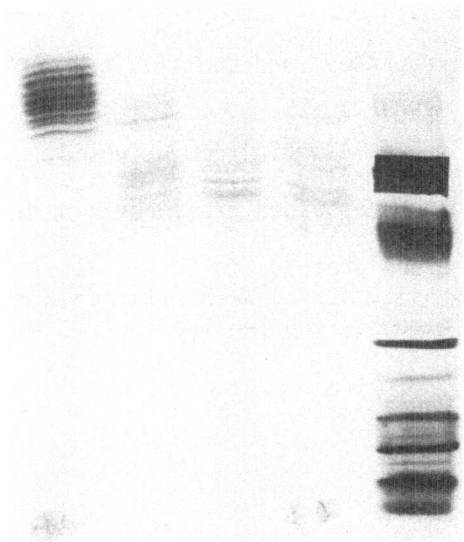

Fig. 3 Isoelectric focussing of porcine urinary kallikrein from
affinity chromatography, of porcine pancreatic and porcine
urinary kallikrein from DEAE-Sephadex chromatography, and
of marker-proteins (from left to right).

Table: Amino Acid Composition of Porcine Kallikreins

Amino Acid	Urinary Kallikrein	Pancreatic Kallikrein
	Moles Amino Acid per Mole Protein	
Asp	29	27
Thr	14	14
Ser	12-14	14
Glu	20-21	23
Pro	16	16
Gly	21	22
Ala	13	13
Val	10	10
Cys 1/2	10	10
Met	4	4
Ile	10-	12
Leu	19	19
Tyr	7	7
Phe	9-10	10
Lys	10	10
His	8	8
Trp		7
Arg	3	3
		229

The enzyme is a glycoprotein and contains hexosamines.

Porcine urinary kallikrein is active in lowering the blood pressure in dogs. The kallikrein from urine is, compared on the basis of equal BAEE-splitting activity, by a factor of 1.7 more active in lowering the dog blood pressure than the pancreatic enzyme.

Acknowledgement: We are grateful to Dr. B. Radola, Technical University Munich-Weihenstephan, for his assistance in conducting the isoelectric focussing.

THE PRIMARY STRUCTURE OF PIG PANCREATIC KALLIKREIN B [+)]

H. Tschesche*, W. Ehret**, G. Godec*, C. Hirschauer**,

C. Kutzbach***, G. Schmidt-Kastner***, and F. Fiedler**

   * Institute of Organic Chemistry, Technical University
     of Munich,
  ** Institute of Clinical Chemistry and Clinical Bio-
     chemistry, University of Munich,
 *** Farbenfabriken Bayer AG, Elberfeld; GFR.

Our studies on the amino acid sequence of pig pancreatic kallikrein B (EC 3.4.21.8) have been performed with a preparation (1) that had been treated with neuraminidase to remove bound sialic acids. After reductive cleavage of the disulfide bridges and carboxymethylation, two peaks of UV-absorbing material could be separated by gel filtration on Sephadex G-75 in 50% acetic acid. According to gel electrophoresis, both were essentially homogeneous. Evidently, pig pancreatic kallikrein is composed of two chains presumably held together by disulfide bridges, as it had already been inferred from the presence of two amino terminal and two C-terminal amino acid residues (2).

ISOLATION OF A- AND B-CHAINS

The larger chain eluted first from the gel column was designated the B-chain (previously β-chain) and the smaller one the A-chain (previously α-chain). When gel filtration of reduced carboxymethylated kallikrein on Sephadex was performed in an

_____

+) This work has been supported by the Deutsche Forschungsgemein-
schaft, Bonn-Bad Godesberg, the Sonderforschungsbereich 51,
München, and the Stiftung Volkswagenwerk, Hannover.

ammonium bicarbonate buffer of pH 7, however, we obtained a surprising result shown in Fig. 1. The smaller A-chain was now eluted
before the B-chain, followed by two minor peaks C and D. These
two minor peaks were eluted in a position where we would have expected the A-chain. Evidently, the A-chain of kallikrein has a
large tendency towards aggregation in usual aqueous solvents.

The carboxymethylated B-chain showed no unusual behavior on
ion exchange chromatography. For the purpose of peptide purification, linear concentration gradients of triethylammonium
acetate (3) at pH 6 on DEAE- or CM-Sephadex columns generally
proved satisfactory. The A-chain, however, resisted all attempts
of rechromatography. It either ran freely through ion
exchange columns or simply could not be eluted even by drastic
means in case it was bound. Only quite recently we found a
system that allowed ion exchange chromatography of the A-chain
as well.

PEPTIDES OF THE A-CHAIN

Fortunately, the A-chain isolated by gel filtration in the
ammonium carbonate system proved pure enough to be used for further
degradation. The A-chain consists of 80 amino acid residues,
including two arginines and three lysines, but does not contain
methionine. Therefore, tryptic hydrolysis was the method of choice.
Four main peaks - II, III, IV-1 and IV-2 - were obtained after gel
filtration of a tryptic digest of the A-chain, as shown in Fig. 2.
Rechromatography of the various peaks on ion exchange columns revealed that the peak designated IV-1 contained two principal
peptides. Thus, 5 tryptic peptides instead of the expected 6
were obtained. One lysyl bond proved resistant to tryptic hydrolysis under the conditions employed.

The alignment of the 5 peptides is shown in the upper part
of Fig. 2. Forty steps of automatic Edman degradation of the A-
chain allowed positioning of the first 3 peptides. Very short
tryptic hydrolysis of the maleylated A-chain (with blocked lysines)
had previously resulted in cleavage of the chain into two peptides,
a large fragment and peptide II containing neither arginine nor
lysine. This result places peptide II at the C-terminus of the A-
chain. The remaining peptide IV-2 has then to be placed immediately
before peptide II, a position confirmed by its C-terminal arginine
residue. Incidentally, as judged from the glucosamine content,
the carbohydrate of the A-chain is located on peptide II. This
is indicated by the circular symbol, Fig. 2. The peptides obtained
proved suitable for sequencer analysis. Only peptide II of the
A-chain containing 27 amino acid residues has not yet been
completely sequenced.

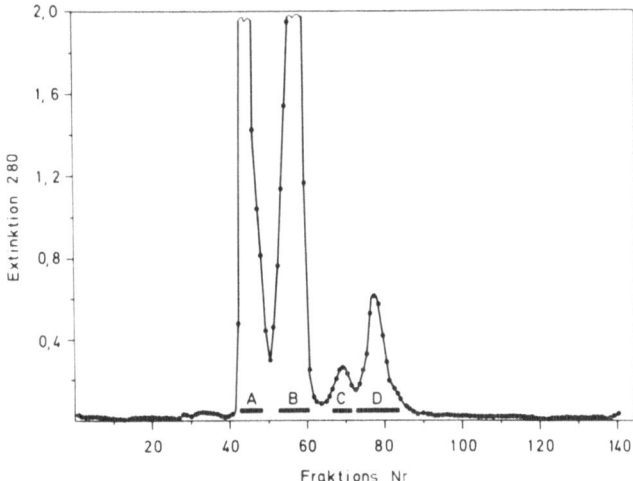

<u>Figure 1.</u>   Gel filtration of reduced and carboxymethylated
             kallikrein B on Sephadex G-75. Column 2 x 200 cm;
             0.1 M ammonium bicarbonate pH 7; 3.8 ml/fraction.

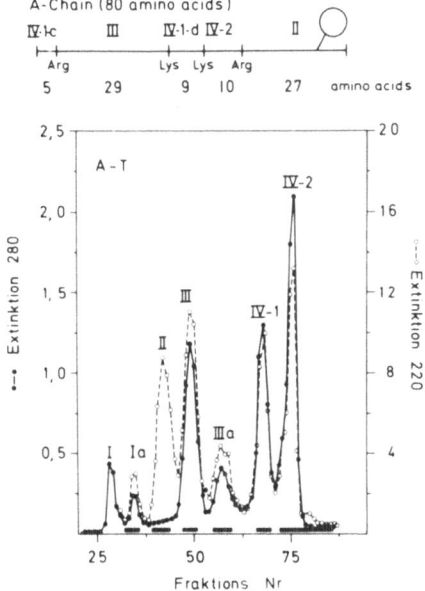

<u>Figure 2.</u>   Fractionation of a tryptic digest of reduced and
             carboxymethylated A-chain of kallikrein on Sephadex
             G-50. Column 0.9 x 140 cm; 0.1 M ammonium bicar-
             bonate pH 8; 1.1 ml/fraction. The alignment of
             the peptides is given in the upper part of the
             figure.

PEPTIDES OF THE B-CHAIN

The larger B-chain, consisting of 149 amino acids, contains the 4 methionine residues of kallikrein. Cleavage with cyanogen bromide yielded the expected 5 peptides. The strong tendency of some of these peptides to form aggregates during gel filtration required 50% acetic acid as solvent, Fig. 3. Peptide II of the B-chain was the only one not containing homoserine and thus derived from the C-terminus. This peptide also contained glucosamine. Peptide I contained the single arginine residue of the B-chain. Tryptic hydrolysis of the maleylated B-chain yielded a large and a small peptide. The latter contained the arginine residue and was thus derived from the N-terminus of the B-chain. Peptide IV-1 from cyanogen bromide cleavage was found to be a constituent of the small arginine-peptide and thus represents the amino terminal part of peptide I.

This result was independently confirmed by sequencing of the intact carboxymethylated B-chain, which gave unequivocal assignment of the first 33 residues. We were fortunate to find additional overlap peptides that allowed the positioning of peptides IV-3 and IV-2. Both peptides were obtained together with peptide IV-1 in peak IV of the gel filtration, Fig. 3. From the 5 peptides forming the B-chain of kallikrein, peptides I and II proved to be too large to be completely sequenced by the Edman procedure in the automatic sequencer. They required further degradation by trypsin. These studies are still in progress.

Of course, this presentation is a rather abridged one. In order to become suitable for sequencer analysis, all the peptides had to be further purified by rechromatography using ion exchange chromatography. Here, especially peptide II generated similar problems as were observed with the entire A-chain. A chromatographic system consisting of 50% acetic acid slightly buffered with 0.05 M sodium hydroxide as solvent and SP-Sephadex C-25 as ion exchanger finally proved suitable for rechromatographies in such difficult cases. Elution was performed with a linear gradient of sodium chloride in the starting solvent. Peptides are usually eluted in the order of increasing number of positive charges. In order to avoid desalting, we sometimes substituted sodium hydroxide and sodium chloride by triethylamine, though the peaks tend to broaden in this system.

GENERAL FEATURES OF THE KALLIKREIN MOLECULE

An overall picture of the kallikrein molecule evolving from our studies is shown in Fig. 4. The main form of kallikrein B consists of two chains held together by disulfide bridges. In analogy to the other members of the family of the serine proteinases

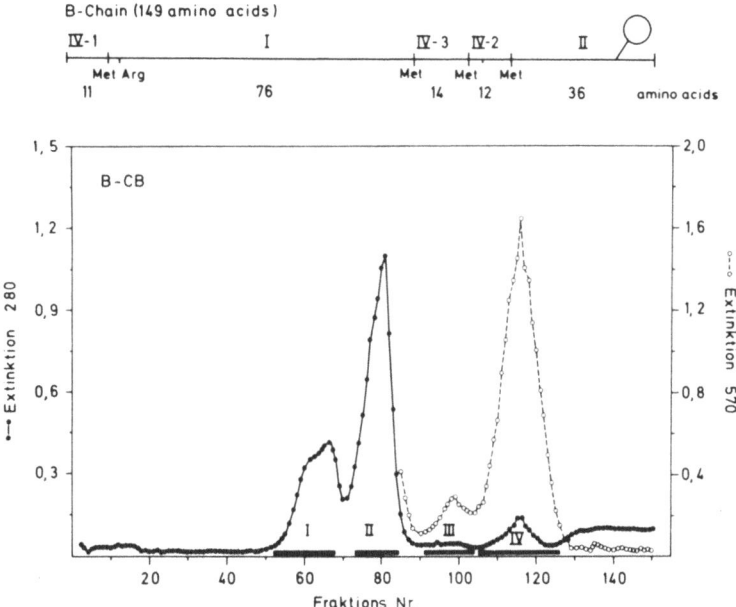

<u>Figure 3.</u>   Fractionation of BrCN-treated reduced and carboxymethy-
           lated B-chain of kallikrein on Sephadex G-75.   Column 2
           x 180 cm; 50% acetic acid; 3.7 ml/fraction.   The align-
           ment of the peptides is given in the upper part of the
           figure.

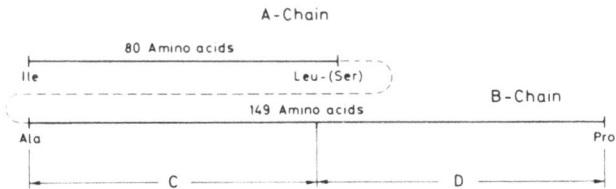

<u>Figure 4.</u>   General features of the molecule of pig pancreatic
           kallikrein B.

it is most probable that native kallikrein - respectively prekallikrein - is synthesized as a single-chain molecule. The N-
terminal isoleucine residue of the A-chain and further 26 amino
acid residues identical with corresponding residues in porcine
trypsin, Fig. 5, require positioning of the A-chain at the amino-
terminus of the presumed single-chain kallikrein molecule. The
split separating the A- and B-chains probably occurred during the
autolytic step in the workup of pancreatic homogenates. Further
degradation has evidently taken place at the site of the split
between the A- and B-chains. About half of the A-chains of our
kallikrein preparation still contained C-terminal serine. The
other half only contained the preceding leucine, since the terminal serine residue had been removed.

Recently the small C and D peaks obtained on gel filtration
in ammonium bicarbonate buffer of reduced and carboxymethylated
kallikrein (Fig. 1) were identified as fragments of the B-chain,
see Fig. 4. Both fragments occur in amounts of 10 - 20% of the
B-chain and indicate additional cleavages in the molecule of
kallikrein. This might possibly explain the observations of
Zuber and Sache (4) who reported the occurrence of at least three
chains in their preparations of kallikreins d_1 and d_2. These
forms of the enzyme, however, only exhibited about half of the
specific activity of our kallikrein preparations.

THE PRIMARY STRUCTURE AND HOMOLOGY TO TRYPSIN

Details of the structure of kallikrein B are presented in
Fig. 5. The sequence is compared to that of porcine trypsin as
determined by Neurath, et al., (5). The numbering system is that
of chymotrypsinogen (6).

The sequence of the A-chain has been almost completed with
the exception of the positioning of 5 residues at the C-terminus.
Homologies are clearly evident. One insertion after position 41
is necessary in order to obtain maximal homology. The identity
of the N-terminal residues, both being isoleucine, has already
been mentioned. Half cystine 22 is part of a disulfide bridge
which was found to be unique for trypsin. Probably the bridge
also exists in kallikrein. This is one of the indications of
a closer relationship between the two enzymes. The other half-
cystines in position 42 and 58 are present as well. Histidine 57
of the active site of all other serine proteinases is also found

---

Figure 5. Partial amino acid sequence of pig pancreatic kallikrein
B as compared to porcine trypsin (5). The numbering
system is that of chymotrypsinogen (6).

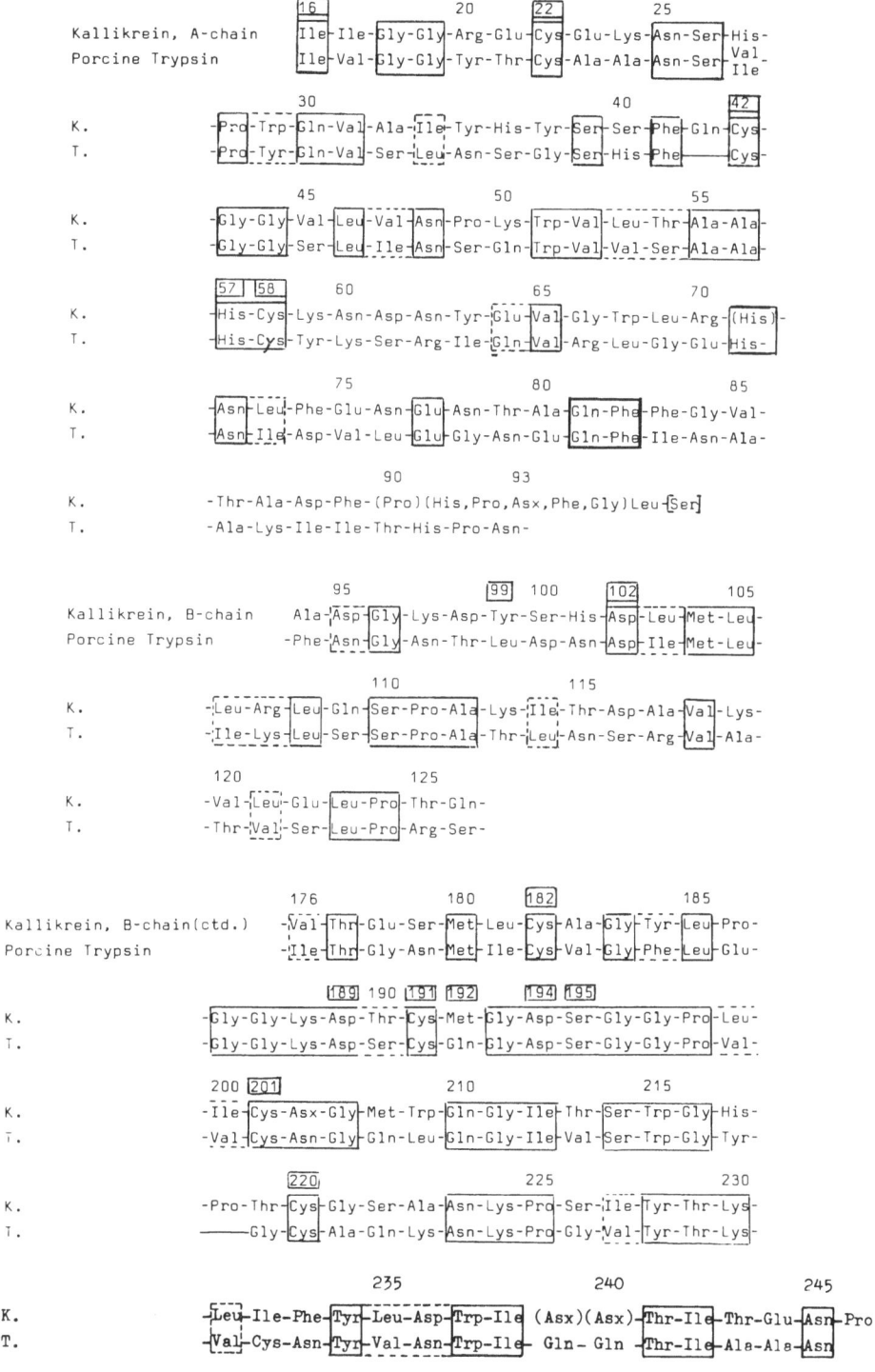

in kallikrein. A region of greater variability in all serine proteinases occurs towards the C-terminus of the A-chain. Here the
alignment might require some adjustment. This part of the kallikrein molecule contains at least 4 more amino acid residues when
compared to trypsin. This includes the C-terminal serine of the
A-chain which was preserved only in about half of the molecules
of our kallikrein preparations as mentioned above.

On the basis of homology one is tempted to conclude that
in the presumed original single-chain kallikrein molecule, the
B-chain closely follows the A-chain. The B-chain contains aspartic
acid 102, one of the residues involved in the charge relay system
(7) of the catalytically active site of the serine proteinases.
Another interesting residue of kallikrein is tyrosine 99 which
substitutes leucine 99 in porcine trypsin. This homologous
residue according to the X-ray work of Blow, et al., (8) makes
numerous contacts with the P_2 residue of soybean trypsin inhibitor.
Substitution of this residue by tyrosine could possibly explain
why kallikrein is highly specific against substrates of the type
-Phe-Arg-X (9), since a favourable tyrosine-phenylalanine interaction seems possible.

In the B-chain of kallikrein, 49 amino acid residues which
follow residue 126 still have to be determined. After this gap,
the sequenced part of the B-chain continues towards the C-terminus.
The four half-cystine residues 182, 191, 201, and 220 are also
homologous to those found in trypsin. Aspartic acid 189 is located in the binding pocket of trypsin (10) and is evidently
responsible for the specificity towards positively charged substrates. The same residue is found in kallikrein and allows to
rationalize the specificity of this enzyme for arginine and - to a
lesser extent - sysine residues (11). Methionine 192 otherwise
is only found in the chymotrypsins, whereas other bovine and porcine
serine proteinases contain a glutamine residue in this position.
Aspartic acid 194 is found in kallikrein as well as in trypsin.
In other serine proteinases it is the residue which forms the
ion pair with the N-terminal isoleucine 16 after activation of
the zymogen (12). Presumably, this residue has the same function
in kallikrein. Finally, in other serine proteinases serine 195
was identified as the active site nucleophile being part of the
aspartic acid 102-histidine 57-serine 195 charge relay system (7).
Evidently this system is also present in kallikrein in a homologous
position. Experimental evidence for the presence of the active
site partial sequence aspartic acid-serine-glycine in pig pancreatic
kallikrein had already been obtained (13).

Kallikrein from porcine pancreas is the first kallikrein for
which structural information is herewith presented. The results
clearly indicate that the enzyme, besides chymotrypsin, trypsin,

and elastase, represents a fourth member of the family of pancreatic serine proteinases. A closer evaluation of the phylo-
genetic relationship within this family of enzymes will have to
be postponed until the sequence is completed. Nevertheless, it is
our general impression that kallikrein - though quite an individual
of its own - more closely resembles trypsin than any other member
of the serine proteinases. Of the 168 amino acid residues posi-
tioned so far, comprising over 70% of the 229 amino acids (2) of
kallikrein, 43% are identical with those of porcine trypsin and
36% with those of porcine elastase. This is about as much as
occurs within the serine proteinase family (14). Comparison
with chymotrypsin A reveals only 29% identity. The alignment of
the amino acid sequence of kallikrein seems to be more favourable
with trypsin than with any other enzyme. This probably includes
the homologous positioning of the five disulfide bridges of
kallikrein with five of the six bridges of trypsin and the homologous position of aspartic acid 189 in the specificity pocket of
trypsin. The relationship between the two enzymes, however, is by
far not as close as that between bovine and porcine trypsins
(82% identical residues (5)) or between bovine chymotrypsin A and
B (78% identical residues (14)).

OUTLOOK

The question still remains to be answered why pancreatic
kallikrein was developed by nature. The enzyme occurs in the gland
in only about 1% of the amount (15) of its most closely related
congener, trypsin, which itself already is a potent kininogenase.
A number of characteristic features distinguish kallikrein from
trypsin:

Prekallikrein is much more readily transformed into active
enzyme than trypsinogen (16). This could lead to speculate on
kallikrein being significant in the early stages of or after
secretion. However, activation of chymotrypsinogen by trypsin
also occurs at a much higher rate than that of trypsinogen (17).
The slow autoactivation of trypsin might thus represent a special
property of this key enzyme in the activation of other zymogens.

The carbohydrate content of kallikrein (2, 18) might render
the enzyme more stable against digestion in the intestine or
facilitate its transport to its site of action.

Finally, the enzyme has a very restricted substrate specificity. The structural basis of this phenomenom still remains to be
elucidated. However, this particular property might be significant
in protecting the enzyme against inactivation, e.g. by serum inhibitors, under conditions where even a hundredfold higher amount of
trypsin becomes inactivated.

ACKNOWLEDGEMENTS

We wish to thank Miss C. Frank for her expert performance of the amino acid analyses after HJ-back hydrolysis of some critical phenylthiohydantoins. The valuable help of Miss G. Puff in the chromatographic procedures and peptide purification is gratefully acknowledged.

REFERENCES

1. C. Kutzbach and G. Schmidt-Kastner, Hoppe-Seyler's Z. Physiol. Chem. 353 (1972) 1099-1106.

2. F. Fiedler, C. Hirschauer, and E. Werle (1975) manuscript in preparation.

3. J. Porath, Nature 175 (1955) 478.

4. M. Zuber and E. Sache, Biochemistry 13 (1974) 3098-3110.

5. M. A. Hermodson, L.M. Ericsson, H. Neurath, and K.A. Walsh, Biochemistry 12 (1973) 3146-3153.

6. B.S. Hartley and D.L. Kauffman, Biochem. J. 101 (1966) 229-231.

7. D.M. Blow, J.J. Birktoft, and B.S. Hartley, Nature 221 (1969) 337-340.

8. R.M. Sweet, H.T. Wright, J. Janin, C.M. Chothia, and D.M. Blow, Biochemistry 13 (1974) 4212-4228.

9. F. Fiedler, International Conference on Chemistry and Biology of the Kallikrein-Kinin-System in Health and Disease, Reston, Virginia, 1974, in press.

10. M. Krieger, L.M. Kay, and R.M. Stroud, J. Mol. Biol. 83 (1974) 209-230.

11. F. Fiedler, G. Leysath, and E. Werle, Eur. J. Biochem. 36 (1973) 152-159.

12. P.B. Sigler, D.M. Blow, B.W. Matthews, and R. Henderson, J. Mol. Biol. 35 (1968) 143-164.

13. F. Fiedler, B. Muller, and E. Werle, Hoppe-Seyler's Z. Physiol. Chem. 352 (1971) 1463-1464.

14. B.S. Hartley, Phil. Trans. Roy. Soc. Lond. B 257 (1970) 77-87.

15. C. Kutzbach and G. Schmidt-Kastner In: Kininogenases-Kallikrein (G.L. Haberland and J.W. Rohen, eds.) F.K. Schattauer Verlag, Stuttgart-New York 1973, pp. 23-35.

16. L.J. Greene, J.J. DiCarlo, A.J. Sussman, and D.C. Bartelt, J. Biol. Chem. 243 (1968) 1804-1815.

17. J.P. Abita, M. Delaage, M. Lazdunski, and J. Savrda, Europ. J. Biochem. 8 (1969) 314-324.

18. H. Fritz, I. Eckert, and E. Werle, Hoppe-Seyler's Z. Physiol. Chem. 348 (1967) 1120-1132.

BOVINE PLASMA HMW AND LMW KININOGENS: ISOLATION AND CHARACTERIZATION

OF THE POLYPEPTIDE FRAGMENTS PRODUCED BY PLASMA AND TISSUE KALLIKREINS

Kato,H., Han,Y.N., Iwanaga,S., Suzuki,T., and Komiya,M.*

Institute for Protein Research, Osaka University

Suita, Osaka-565, Japan

There exist at least two types of kininogens with different
molecular weight in mammalian blood plasmas, which are named high
molecular weight (HMW) and low molecular weight (LMW) kininogens
(1). Although their functions in kallikrein-kinin system remain
to be investigated, it has been speculated that HMW kininogen participates in the intrinsic kinin releasing system and lmw kininogen in the extrinsic kinin-releasing system. Quite recently, a
new function of kininogen has been suggested by findings of
Flaujeac (2), Williams (3), and Fitzgerald (4) traits with a
deficiency of kininogen. These plasmas do not release kinin
appreciably upon incubation of plasma kallikrein and also has a
prolonged activated partial thromboplastin time and inability to
form plasmin. These facts suggest the participation of the kininogen in the intrinsic blood coagulation and fibrinolysis, in
addition to the kinin-forming system.

In order to realize biological functions of kininogens, it
seems to be important to study the molecular structure of
kininogens and to compare two kininogens, HMW and LMW kininogens,
which are supposed to have different functions. In the previous
papers, we reported the purifications and characterizations of
bovine HMW and LMW kininogens (5,6). Later, we also reported that
a few of peptide fragments, in addition to kinin, are liberated
from HMW kininogen on the digestion with plasma kallikrein (7).

---

* Present address: Research and Development Division, Dainippon
  Pharmaceutical Co., Ltd., Enoki-33-94, Suita, Osaka-564.

One of the fragments contained an abnormally high level of histidine and its complete amino acid sequence was established (8).

In this paper, we describe further studies on the chemical compositions of polypeptide fragments produced from HMW kininogen by the action of plasma kallikrein and on the comparison with respect to the gross molecular structures of LMW and HMW kininogens.

MATERIALS AND METHODS

Highly purified HMW kininogen was prepared from fresh bovine plasma by the previous method (5). LMW kininogen was purified according to the revised method using zinc acetate precipitation (9). Bovine plasma kallikrein was prepared from highly purified prekallikrein, by activating it with purified bovine prekallikrein activator (10,11). The specific activity of the kallikrein was 23.5 TAME units per mg protein. Snake venom kininogenase (10 TAME units per mg protein) was purified from the venom of Agkistrodon halys blomhoffii by the method described previously (12). The purified preparations of hog pancreatic and human urinary kallikreins were a generous gift, respectively, from Dr. T. Takami, Central Research Laboratories, Ajinomoto Co., Inc., Kawasaki, and Dr. N. Ogawa, Mochida Pharmaceutical Co., Ltd., Tokyo. Sephadex G-75 and Sephadex G-100 were products of Pharmacia, Uppsala, Sweden. Kinin activity was assayed in terms of its ability to cause smooth muscle contraction of isolated rat uterus (13). For the analysis of amino acid composition, peptides were hydrolyzed in 0.5 ml of constant-boiling HCl in evacuated, sealed tubes at 110°C for 24, 48 and 72 hours, and analyzed with an amino acid analyzer, Model JLC-5AH, Japan Electron Optics, Ltd., by the method of Spackman, et al. (14). The amino-terminal residues of the isolated peptides and whole proteins were determined by Edman's phenylisothiocyanate method (15) and Sanger's DNP method (16). The carboxyl-terminal amino acids were analyzed by hydrazinolysis in the presence of Amberlite CG-50 (17) or by carboxypeptidase A and B. The released amino acids were estimated by amino acid analyzer. For the analysis of carbohydrates, total hexoses were measured by the phenol-sulfuric acid method of Dubois, et al. (18) and hoxosamines by the methods of Gardell (19) and sialic acids by the periodate-thiobarbituric acid method of Warren (20).

SDS-polyacrylamide gel electrophoresis was made according to the method of Weber and Osborn (21) and gels were stained with Coomassie brilliant blue R250. Relative intensity of the bands stained with the dye was estimated, using a Fuji Riken densitometer, Model Fujiox FD-IV.

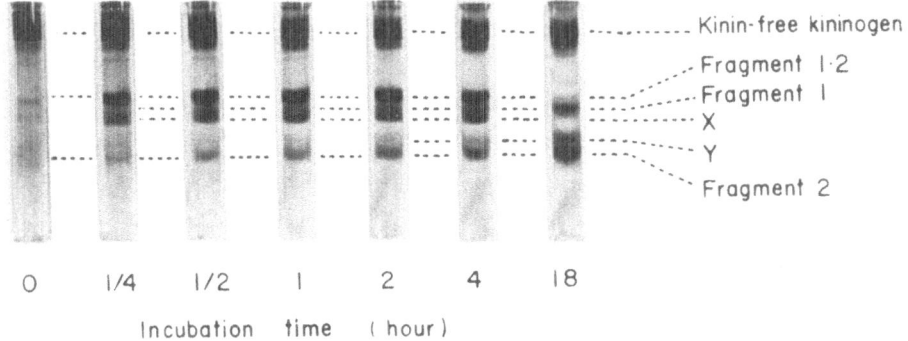

Kinin-free kininogen
Fragment 1·2
Fragment 1
X
Y
Fragment 2

0   1/4   1/2   1   2   4   18

Incubation   time   (hour)

Fig. 1.   SDS-polyacrylamide gel electrophoresis of reaction
products released from HMW kininogen by the action of
plasma kallikrein. HMW kininogen (770 µg) was incubated at 37°C with 0.78 µg of purified kallikrein in
0.35 ml of 0.2 M ammonium bicarbonate buffer, pH 8.0.
At the time indicated, 10 and 16 µl aliquots of the
reaction mixture were taken for kinin assay (Fig. 2)
and for SDS-gel electrophoresis. The electrophoresis
was done at room temperature at a current of 7 mA per
tube for 4 hr., using 10% polyacrylamide gel.

RESULTS

Liberation of Peptide Fragments from HMW kininogen by Plasma Kallikrein

     As reported previously (7), when HMW kininogen was incubated
with plasma kallikrein, two unknown peptide fragments, named
fragment 1 and fragment 2, were produced, in addition to bradykinin. One of the fragments, fragment 2, was a histidine-rich
peptide and its amino acid sequence was recently established (8).
The release of these fragments in the course of digestion of HMW
kininogen with plasma kallikrein was monitored by SDS-polyacrylamide gel electrophoresis. At zero time of incubation, a single
broad kininogen band with a molecular weight of about 76,000 was
detected on SDS-gel (Fig. 1). After incubation for 15 minutes,
the kininogen appeared to have been degraded and two major and one
minor bands newly appeared on the gel. These fragments will be
designated as fragment 1·2, fragment 1 and fragment 2 hereafter.
On digestion for more than 30 minutes, fragment 1·2 seemed to be
degraded gradually, accompanying the increase of intensity of the
bands corresponding to fragment 1 and 2. Moreover, during these
periods of digestion, unidentified fragments, named fragment X and
fragment Y were liberated and the intensity of band of the latter
increased remarkably at later stages. After 18 hrs, the fragment

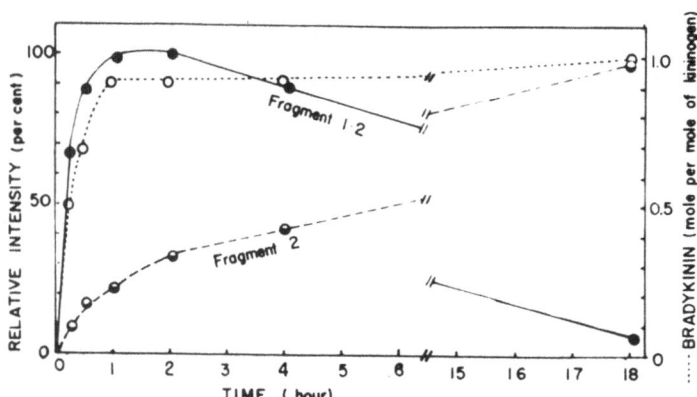

Fig. 2.   Relative rates of liberation of fragment 1·2, fragment
           2 and bradykinin from HMW kininogen by plasma kalli-
           krein. The stained gels in Fig. 1 were scanned by a
           Fuji Riken densitometer, Model Fujiox FD-IV, and the
           relative intensity of the bands was calculated, assuming
           the maximum intensity of each fragment to be 100 per
           cent. The kinin activity was estimated by the contract-
           ion upon isolated rat uterus.

1·2 had almost disappeared, and fragment 1, fragment 2 and fragment Y were accumulated in the digest.

     To estimate the relative rate of release of these fragments
during the digestion, each band stained with Coomassie brilliant
blue on gels was scanned using a densitometer. The results are
shown in Fig. 2. Since fragment 1 and fragment X could not be
clearly resolved on gels, the relative intensities of the bands
corresponding to fragment 1·2 and fragment 2 were compared. The
amount of bradykinin released was also assayed by contraction
upon isolated rat uterus. Fig. 2 clearly indicated that fragment
1·2 is rapidly released in parallel with formation of the kinin,
and that the decrease in amount of fragment 1·2 seemed to be
roughly proportional to the increase in the amount of fragment 2.
The evidence for degradation of fragment 1·2 was also confirmed
by incubating the isolated material with plasma kallikrein. As
shown in Fig. 3, fragment 1·2 was cleaved evidently into fragment
1 and fragment 2 by the action of plasma kallikrein, although the
rate was very slow.

     HMW kininogen was incubated with other kininogenases, such
as, hog pancreatic kallikrein, snake venom, kininogenase from
the venom of Agkistrodon halys blomhoffii and human urinary
kallikrein, and the digests were subjected to SDS-gel electrophoresis. Hog pancreatic kallikrein released a few of peptide

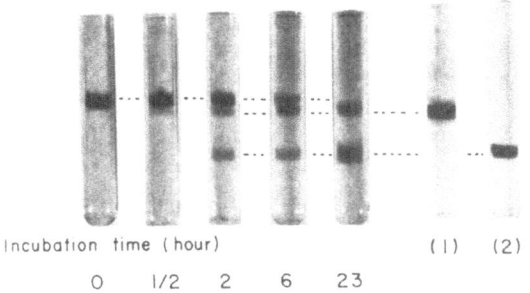

Incubation time (hour)   (I)   (2)

        0   1/2   2   6   23

Fig. 3.   Cleavage of fragment 1·2 into fragment 1 and fragment
           2 by plasma kallikrein. The isolated fragment 1·2
           (40 μg) was hydrolyzed with 2.1 μg of purified kalli-
           krein in 0.4 ml of ammonium bicarbonate buffer, pH 8.0.
           At the time indicated, 100 μl each of the incubation
           mixture was taken and subjected to SDS-gel electro-
           phoresis. Fragment 1 (1) and fragment 2 (2), which
           were isolated previously, were used as reference.

fragments including fragment 1·2, in addition to kinin, with a
weight ratio of enzyme to substrate of 1 to 146. However, the
pattern of the fragmentation differed slightly from that with
plasma kallikrein. On the other hand, snake venom kininogenase
and human urinary kallikrein hardly released peptide fragments
with the weight ratio of enzyme to substrate of 1 to 95 and of
1 to 146, respectively, and two faint bands corresponding to fragment 1·2 and fragment 2 were detected on the SDS-gels after incubation for more than 18 hrs.

Isolation and Chemical Compositions of Peptide Fragments and Kinin-
free Kininogen Produced from HMW Kininogen by the Action of Plasma
Kallikrein

    HMW kininogen (83 mg) was incubated with 78 μg of plasma
kallikrein for 1 hr in 40 ml of 0.2 M ammonium bicarbonate, pH 8.0,
and the digest was applied to a column of Sephadex G-75. The
result is shown in Fig. 4. The kinin-free kininogen, which did
not release kinin upon incubation with plasma kallikrein, was
eluted in a void volume fraction, and one major peak with the absorbance at 280 nm (Fragment 1·2) and bradykinin were separated.
The isolated fragment 1·2 and kinin-free kininogen showed a single
band, respectively, on SDS-gel electrophoresis, as shown in the
same figure. Moreover, the kinin-free kininogen gave two bands in
the presence of 2-mercaptoethanol on SDS-gel electrophoresis,
suggesting that it consists of two polypeptide chains held together

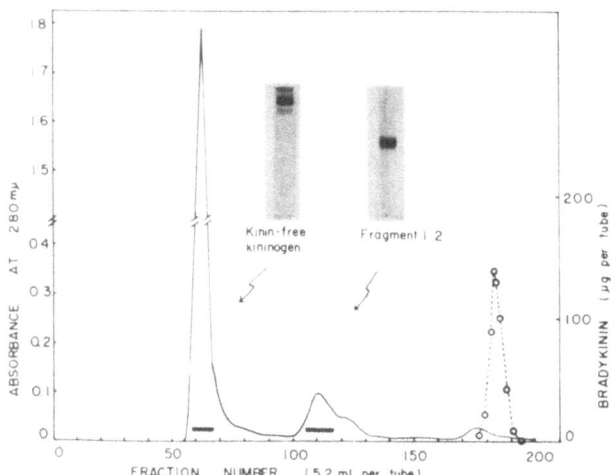

Fig. 4.   Gel-filtration of the reaction products of HMW kininogen
          with plasma kallikrein on a column of Sephadex G-75.
          HMW kininogen (83 mg) was incubated at 37°C with 78 µg
          of purified kallikrein in 40 ml of 0.2 M ammonium bi-
          carbonate buffer, pH 8.0. After 1 hr, DFP was added to
          give a final concentration of 5 x 10^{-3} M and the mixture
          was stood at 37°C for 1 hr and then lyophilized. The
          dried material was dissolved in 5 ml of 0.2 M ammonium
          bicarbonate buffer, pH 8.0, and applied to a column
          (3 x 142 cm) of Sephadex G-75, which had been equilibra-
          ted with the same buffer. Elution was made with the same
          buffer at a flow rate of 35 ml per hr, and the fractions
          indicated by solid bars were combined and lyophilized.
          Aliquots of the pooled fractions were subjected to SDS-
          gel electrophoresis and their electropherograms were
          shown in the same figure.

by disulfide bond. To isolate these polypeptide chains, kinin-
free kininogen was reduced to 2-mercaptoethanol and carboxymethylated by monoiodoacetic acid and the resulting S-alkyl-derivative
was applied to a column of Sephadex G-100. As shown in Fig. 5,
two protein peaks, called heavy chain and light chain, were
separated, and they gave single bands on SDS-gel electrophoresis
as shown in the same figure.

    Table I, II, and III show amino acid compositions and carbo-
hydrate content of all the fragments isolated from HMW kininogen.
Fragment 1·2, fragment 1 and fragment 2 contained extremely high
levels of histidine and glycine and their N-terminal and C-terminal amino acids were serine and arginine, respectively. Moreover, the fragment 1 and fragment 1·2 were found to be glycopep-

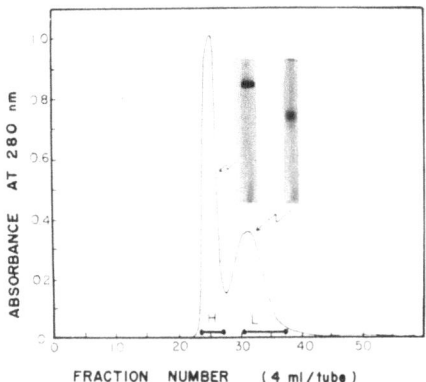

Fig. 5.   Separation of the heavy (H) and light (L) chains con-
          stituting kinin-free HMW kininogen on a Sephadex G-100
          column. The S-alkylated sample (30 mg) dissolved in
          1 ml of 0.2 M ammonium bicarbonate buffer, pH 8.0, was
          applied to the column (2 x 94 cm) and eluted with the
          same buffer at a flow rate of 20 ml per hr. SDS-gel
          (8%) electrophoresis was done at room temperature at
          a current of 8 mA per tube for 4 hr.

tides (Table II). The sum of the total amino acid residues of
fragment 1 and fragment 2 essentially coincided with that of
fragment 1·2, confirming that fragment 1·2 is a precursor peptide
of fragment 1 and fragment 2. Furthermore, the sum of the total
amino acid residues of H- and L- chains derived from kinin-free
HMW kininogen was in good agreement with the total amino acid residues of kinin-free kininogen. The L-chain showed a characteristic composition, in which a sum of five amino acid residues, Asp,
Thr,. Ser, Glu and Pro, comprises 57% of the total residues.
Another characteristic of two chains is the presence of falactosa-
mine in L-chain but not in H-chain. No clear N-terminal residue
reactive to phenylisothiocyanate and 2·4 dinitrofluorobenzene was
detected in H-chain as well as whole HMW kininogen, whereas the
N-terminal threonine was identified evidently on L-chain. The
C-terminal residue of L-chain was determined to be leucine, which
was the same residue as that of whole HMW kininogen.

Hydrolysis of LMW kininogen with Purified Venom Kininogenase from
Snake Venom of Agkistrodon halys blomhoffii

    With the weight ratio of enzyme to substrate of 1 to 115, LMW
kininogen was incubated at 37°C with snake venom kininogenase and
aliquots were taken at the time intervals and subjected to SDS-gel
electrophoresis. As shown in Fig. 6, mobility of the protein band

Table I

Amino Acid Composition (a) of Heavy and Light Chains
of Kinin-Free HMW Kininogen

--- Residues per mole ---

	HMW-Kininogen	Kinin-Free HMW Kininogen	H-chain	L-chain	H + L	Kinin-Free Kininogen + Fragment 1·2 + BK
Asp	63	60	45	15	60	67
Thr	41	40	26	14	40	44
Ser	49	44	32	13	45	51
Glu	64	57	44	14	58	67
Pro	39	35	21	13	34	41
Gly	39	20	17	3	20	40
Ala	31	31	23	7	30	33
1/2Cys	20	18	17	1	18	18
Val	38	35	28	6	34	39
Met	8	6	4	2	6	8
Ile	22	22	17	5	22	23
Leu	36	33	24	9	33	38
Tyr	19	17	14	3	17	18
Phe	20	20	15	5	20	22
Trp(d)	8	6	4	2	6	8
His	28	12	9	2	11	31
Lys	43	35	28	5	33	46
Arg	13	11	9	1	10	15
Total	581	502	377	120	497	609

Table I (cont'd)

N-Terminal	(Ser)	Thr	----	Thr
C-Terminal	Leu(Arg)	Thr		Leu
Molecular weight	76,000(b)	66,000(b)(c)	48,500(c)	16,000(c)

(a) The amino acid compositions were calculated from extrapolated or average values estimated on samples of 24, 48 and 72 hrs hydrolyzates.
(b) Determined by sedimentation equilibrium method.
(c) Calculated from amino acid composition and carbohydrate content.
(d) Determined spectrophotometrically (25).

Table II

Carbohydrate Content of Kinin-Free Kininogen and Fragments
Released from HMW-Kininogen by the Action of Plasma Kallikrein

	HMW-Kininogen	Kinin-Free Kininogen	H-chain	L-chain	Fragment 1
Hexose (%)	4.57	4.97	4.61	6.03	3.73
Galactosamine (%)	1.53	1.43	0	5.15	1.55
Glucosamine (%)	2.12	2.97	4.18	0	0
Sialic acid (%)	4.35	5.45	3.82	10.09	2.09
Total (%)	12.57	14.82	12.61	21.27	7.37

Table III

Amino Acid Composition of Fragments Released from
HMW Kininogen by the Action of Plasma Kallikrein

	Fragment 1·2	Fragment 1	Fragment 2	Fragment 1 + Fragment 2
--- Residues per mole ---				
Asp	7	4	4	8
Thr	4	4	-	4
Ser	6	6	1	7
Glu	10	9	2	11
Pro	3	3	-	3
Gly	20	11	11	22
Ala	1	1	-	1
1/2Cys	-	-	-	-
Val	4-5	4	-	4
Met	2	2	-	2
Ile	1	1	-	1
Leu	5-6	4	2	6
Tyr	1	-	1	1
Phe	-	-	-	-
Trp (b)	2	1	1	2
His	19	10	11	21
Lys	12	6	7	13
Arg	2-3	2	1	3
Total	100-102	68	41	109
N-Terminal	Ser	Ser	Ser	
C-Terminal	Arg	Arg	Arg	
Molecular weight		8,000(a)	4,600	

Amino acid compositions of each fragment were calculated from the
values estimated on samples of 24 hr hydrolyzates, except for that
of fragment 2, which was calculated from the complete amino acid
sequence determined previously (8).

(a) Calculated from amino acid composition and carbohydrate content.
(b) Determined spectrophotometrically (25).

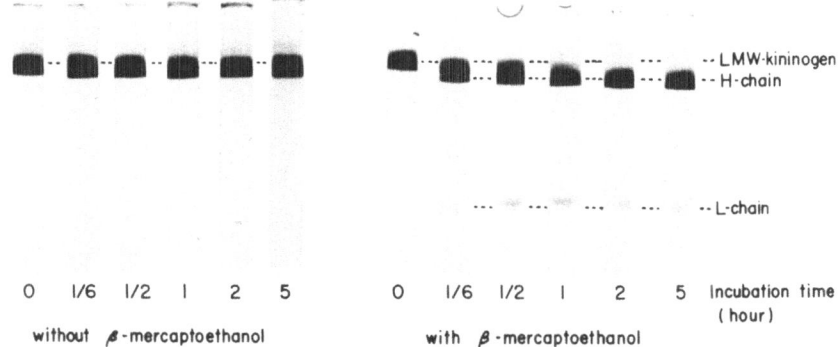

0

| 0 | 1/6 | 1/2 | 1 | 2 | 5 | | 0 | 1/6 | 1/2 | 1 | 2 | 5 | Incubation time (hour) |

without β-mercaptoethanol   with β-mercaptoethanol

Fig. 6.   SDS-polyacrylamide gel electrophoresis of reaction
products of LMW kininogen with snake venom kininogenase.
LMW kininogen (9.2 mg) was incubated at 37°C with 80 µg
of purified venom kininogenase in 4 ml of 0.2 M ammonium
bicarbonate buffer, pH 8.0. At the time indicated,
20 µl aliquots of the reaction mixture were taken and
subjected to SDS-gel (8%) electrophoresis in the presence and absence of β-mercaptoethanol.

corresponding to LMW kininogen did not change during the incubation, and no fragments were detected on the gels before reduction.
However, in the presence of 2-mercaptoethanol, the protein band
of LMW kininogen disappeared and a band with slightly faster
mobility and another faint band were detected on gels. The release of bradykinin reached to maximum within 1 hr, when the kinin
activity was estimated in terms of the contraction of isolated rat
uterus. These results indicated that snake venom kininogenase releases bradykinin, but no other peptide fragments from LMW kininogen, producing kinin-free LMW kininogen, which seems to consist
of heavy and light chains held together by disulfide bond.

The 1 hr digest of LMW kininogen with snake venom kininogenase, treated under the same conditions as mentioned in Fig. 6
was applied on a column of Sephadex G-75 and kinin-free LMW
kininogen was separated from bradykinin. No other peaks with the
absorbance at 280 nm could be detected. The kinin-free LMW
kininogen, which was eluted in a void volume fraction, was reduced
and carboxymethylated and the resulting material was subjected to
gel filtration on a column of Sephadex G-75. As shown in Fig. 7,
two protein peaks were separated, one in a void volume fraction
and another small peak in the retarded fraction. Each protein
peak appeared to be homogeneous on SDS-gel electrophoresis and
their mobilities corresponded to heavy and light chains, respectively.

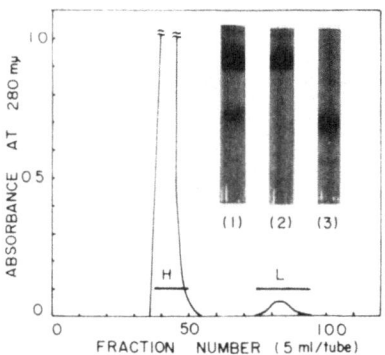

Fig. 7.   Separation of the heavy (H) and light (L) chains of
           kinin-free LMW kininogen on a column of Sephadex G-75.
           Reduced and carboxymethylated kinin-free LMW kininogen
           (140 mg) was applied to the column (3 x 90 cm), equili-
           brated with 0.2 M ammonium bicarbonate buffer, pH 8.0.
           Elution was made with the same buffer at a flow rate of
           30 ml per hr, and the fractions indicated by solid bars
           were combined and lyophilized. The SDS-gel electropho-
           retic patterns of S-alkylated kinin-free LMW kininogen
           (1), H-chain (2) and L-chain (3) were shown in the same
           figure.

     The amino acid analysis on the isolated H-chain and L-chain
showed that the former consists of 344 amino acid residues and the
latter, 50 amino acid residues (Table IV). The partial N-terminal
sequence of L-chain was determined to be Ser-Val-Glx-Val-Met by
dansyl-Edman method, and this sequence was the same as the C-
terminal sequence of kinin-yielding peptide, which was previously
isolated from LMW kininogen by cyanogen bromide treatment (22).

     Although quantitative analyses on carbohydrate content of H-
chain and L-chain are not made yet, hexosamine was not detected
on L-chain by amino acid analysis. The amino acid composition of
H-chain derived from kinin-free LMW kininogen was quite similar
to that of H-chain derived from kinin-free HMW kininogen. Moreover, the two H-chains had the same mobility on SDS-gel electrophoresis.

DISCUSSION
     Bovine HMW kininogen having a molecular weight of 76,000
consists of a single polypeptide chain with a masked N-terminal
residue and C-terminal leucine, and it carries the vasoactive
peptide, bradykinin, in the interior of the chain bridged by a
disulfide bond (6). The SDS-gel electrophoretic analysis of fragmentation of HMW kininogen with plasma kallikrein indicates that

Table IV

Amino Acid Composition of Heavy and Light Chains
of Kinin-Free LMW Kininogen

	LMW-Kininogen	H-chain	L-chain	H + L + BK
	--- Residues per mole ---			
Asp	37	38	-	38
Thr	24	21	4	25
Ser	28	25	5	31
Glu	46	40	10	50
Pro	26	21	5	29
Gly	20	17	4	22
Ala	26	23	5	28
1/2Cys	16	15	1	16
Val	30	28	4	32
Met	5	4	1	5
Ile	15	15	-	15
Leu	23	23	2	25
Tyr	13	13	1	14
Phe	14	14	-	16
Lys	26	25	4	29
His	9	9	2	11
Arg	11	9	2	11
Trp(a)	4	4	-	4
Total	373	344	50	401

Amino acid compositions were calculated from extrapolated or
average values estimated on samples of 24, 48 and 72 hrs
hydrolyzates, except for that of L-chain, which was calculated
from the values of 24 hr hydrolyzate.
(a) Determined spectrophotometrically (25).

HMW kininogen liberates initially a large peptide fragment,
fragment 1·2, together with bradykinin, and then, the fragment
1·2 is cleaved into fragment 1 and fragment 2. Fragment 2 is a
histidine-rich peptide and contains a total of 41 amino acid
residues with the N-terminal serine and C-terminal arginine (8).

Fragment 1 is a glycopeptide containing also high level of
histidine, and the partial N-terminal sequence of Ser-Val-Gln-Val-
Met-Lys-Thr-Glu-Gly is the same as the C-terminal sequence of
CNBr-fragment containing kallidin (6). The N-terminal sequence of
fragment 1·2 is also the same as that of fragment 1 (unpublished).

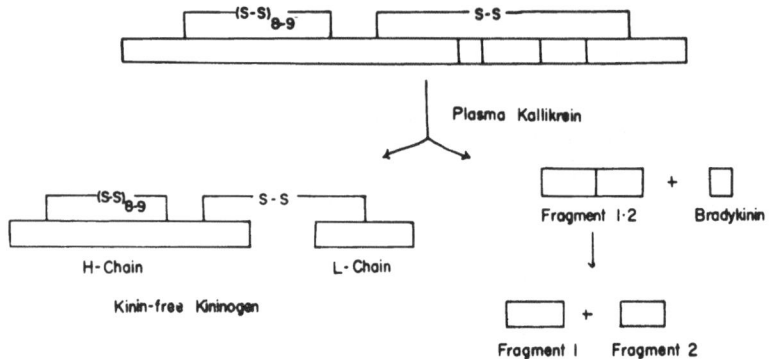

Fig. 8.   Fragmentation of HMW kininogen with plasma kallikrein.

Thus, fragment 1 or fragment 1·2 must be connected with the C-terminus of the kinin along the polypeptide chain of kininogen.

The residual protein, named kinin-free HMW kininogen, which consists of two polypeptide chains of H- and L-chains, has to constitute the N- and C-terminal portions of whole HMW kininogen, because their end groups are identical to those of the mother protein molecule. Since L-chain contains only one half-cystine residue, H- and L-chains constituting kinin-free HMW kininogen are thought to be linked by a single disulfide bridge. Moreover, a sum of the total amino acid residues of H- and L-chains coincides with that of the kinin-free kininogen and also the sum of those of kinin-free HMW kininogen, fragment 1·2 and bradykinin, with those of whole HMW kininogen, as shown in Table I. Thus, it indicates that all the fragments of HMW kininogen produced by plasma kallikrein had been isolated.

Based on these results, it seems now possible to build up a linear peptide sequence of HMW kininogen molecule and its gross structural feature, as shown in Fig. 8. Thus, there should be at least four peptide bond cleavages associated with the kallikreinic digestion of HMW kininogen, yielding the kinin-free HMW kininogen, fragment 1, fragment 2 and bradykinin. There will be minor cleavages of other peptide bonds, because unidentified minor fragments are detected on the SDS-gels. It should be emphasized that peptide fragments are released, besides bradykinin, from HMW kininogen by plasma kallikrein. Although the biological activities of fragment 1·2, fragment 1 and fragment 2, are scarcely known, a preliminary experiment indicates that these retard the generation of plasma kallikrein activity induced by a glass contact activation of Hageman factor (Factor XII) (23).

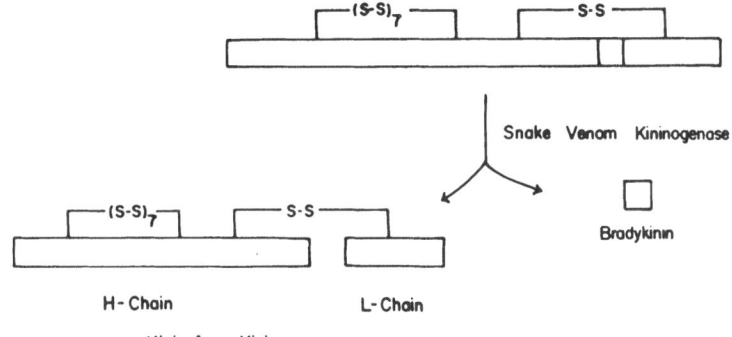

Fig. 9.   Fragmentation of LMW kininogen with snake venom kininogenase.

LMW kininogen as well as HMW kininogen is a glycoprotein with
a molecular weight of 50,000 (24). The N-terminal amino acid of
this kininogen was previously reported to be serine, however,
recent studies show that it may be a masked form, just like HMW
kininogen (unpublished). This suggests that the previously isolated LMW kininogen had suffered from limited proteolysis. Snake
venom kininogenase from the venom of <u>Agkistrodon</u> <u>halys</u> <u>blomhoffii</u>
releases bradykinin, producing kinin-free LMW kininogen which
consists of H- and L-chains held together by disulfide bond. The
L-chain contains one half-cystine residue, therefore, the H-chain
and L-chain are bridged by a single disulfide bond, which is the
same as that of HMW kininogen (Fig. 9).

The amino acid composition and molecular weight of H-chain
derived from LMW kininogen is quite similar to those of H-chain
derived from HMW kininogen, suggesting that they have essentially
the same amino acid sequence. Previously, we have compared peptide maps of HMW kininogen and LMW kininogen and have shown that
almost all of the spots derived from LMW kininogen are included
in the peptide map of HMW kininogen (6). These similarities of
LMW kininogen and HMW kininogen may be due to their heavy chains
having essentially the same amino acid sequences.

<u>ACKNOWLEDGEMENTS</u>

The assistance of Miss Masayo Kitaguchi in amino acid analysis
is appreciated. This work was supported in part by grants from
the Scientific Research Fund of the Ministry of Education of
Japan.

REFERENCES

1. Habermann, E. (1970) in: Handbook of Experimental Pharmacology (Erdos, E.G., ed.) pp. 250-288, Springer-Verlag, Berlin-Heidelberg-New York.
2. Wuepper, K.D., Miller, D.R. and Lacomb, M.J. (1975) Federation Proc. 34, 859.
3. Colman, R.W., Badasarian, A., Talamo, R.C., Seavey, M., Scott, C.F. and Kaplan, A.P. (1975) Federation Proc. 34, 859.
4. Saito, H., Ratnoff, O.D., Waldmann, R. and Abraham, J.P. (1975) J. Clin. Invest. 55, 1082-1089.
5. Komiya, M., Kato, H. and Suzuki, T. (1974) J. Biochem. 76, 811-822.
6. Komiya, M., Kato, H., and Suzuki, T. (1974) J. Biochem. 76, 833-845.
7. Komiya, M., Suzuki, T. and Han, Y.N. (1973) Seikagaku (in Japanese) 45, 682.
8. Han, Y.N., Komiya, N., Iwanaga, S. and Suzuki, T. (1975) J. Biochem. 77, 55-68.
9. Yano, M., Kato, H., Nagasawa, S. and Suzuki, T. (1967) J. Biochem. 62, 386-388.
10. Takahashi, H., Nagasawa S. and Suzuki, T. (1972) J. Biochem. 71, 471-483.
11. Komiya, M., Nagasawa, S. and Suzuki, T. (1972) J. Biochem. 72, 1205-1218.
12. Iwanaga, S., Sata, T., Mizushima, Y. and Suzuki, T. (1965) J. Biochem. 58, 123-129.
13. Yano, M., Nagasawa, S. and Suzuki, T. (1971) J. Biochem. 69, 471-481.
14. Spackman, D.H., Stein, W.H. and Moore, S. (1958) Anal. Biochem. 30, 1190-1206.
15. Edman, P. (1970) in: Protein Sequence Determination (Needleman, S.B., ed.) pp. 211-255, Springer-Verlag, Berlin.
16. Bailey, J.L. (1967) in: Techniques in Protein Chemistry, 2nd ed., pp. 163-182, Elsevier, New York.
17. Braun, V. and Schroeder, W.A. (1967) Arch. Biochem. Biophys. 118, 241-252.
18. Dubois, M., Gilles, K.A., Hamilton, J.K., Rebers, P.A. and Smity, F. (1956) Anal. Chem. 28, 350-356.
19. Gardell, S. (1953) Acta Chem. Scand. 7, 207-215.
20. Warren, L. (1959) J. Biol. Chem. 234, 1971-1975.
21. Weber, K. and Osborn, M. (1969) J. Biol. Chem. 244, 4406-4412.
22. Kato, H., Nagasawa, S. and Suzuki, T. (1967) Biochem. Biophys. Res. Communs. 27, 163-168.
23. Iwanaga, S., Han, Y.N., Komiya, M., Suzuki, T. Katori, N., Ohishi, S. (1975) Life Science 16, 792-793.
24. Nagasawa, S., Mizushima, Y., Sata, T., Iwanaga,S. and Suzuki, T. (1966) J. Biochem. 60, 643-652.
25. Goodwin,T.W. and Morton,R.A. (1946) Biochem.J. 40, 628-632.

PURIFICATION OF KALLIKREIN FROM CAT SUBMAXILLARY GLAND

Chiaki Moriwaki*, Yoshio Hojima* and M. Schachter**

Faculty of Pharmaceutical Sciences, Science University
of Tokyo, Tokyo, Japan*; Department of Physiology,
University of Alberta, Edmonton, Canada**

Cat submaxillary gland has been used in many investigations
on kallikrein-kinin system. Though it has not yet been established,
the physiological functions of kallikreins in various glands, such
as the functional vasodilatation, have been studied mainly in cat
submaxillary gland (1, 2, 3). Furthermore, the secretory cells or
subcellular distribution has been studied in this gland (4).
Meanwhile the isolation of submaxillary kallikrein has not yet
been achieved. In a series of investigation on the proteases in
the rat submaxillary gland, Ekfors, et al. obtained a kallikrein-
like peptidase (5), but the identity of the enzyme with kallikrein
was not clear because of the lack of study on the biological
activity of the preparation. Fiedler, et al. described that hog
submaxillary kallikrein was separated into a number of active
components with isoelectric points in the range pH 3.3 - 4.4 (6),
but the specific activity of their preparation was less than a
half of that of purified hog pancreatic kallikrein. We attempted
the isolation of kallikrein from the cat submaxillary gland and
obtained a highly purified preparation which was homogeneous in
disc electrophoresis.

·Isolation and Purification A typical result of purification
of CSK, cat submaxillary kallikrein, is summarized in Table 1. The
fresh glands were freeze dried and the water soluble fraction was
again lyophilized. Starting from 2.6 g of this fraction which
corresponded to 30 glands, 33.5 g wet weight, acetone fractionation,
DEAE-Sephadex A-50 chromatography, Sephadex G-75 gel filtration and
finally isoelectric fractionation is an Ampholine pH gradient (3.5-
5.0) were carried out. The specific activities of the final
preparation are 1260 KU/mg in the vasodilator assay (7), and 24.5

units/mg in BAEE esterolytic activity assay (8). Its vasodilator
activity is almost equal to that of the most pure hog pancreatic
kallikrein.

On acetone fractionation more than 70% of the activity was
recovered in the precipitate of 50-75% acetone concentration. The
active fraction was suspended, dialysed against 0.05 M Tris-HCl-
0.1 M NaCl buffer and then applied on DEAE-Sephadex A-50 column.
The vasodilator and esterolytic activities were eluted out together
at 0.25 M NaCl concentration (Fig. 1).

Table I. Purification of Cat Submaxillary Kallikrein

Procedure	Total A_{280}	Total Activity		Specific Activity	
		KU	BAEE*	KU/A_{280}	BAEE*/A_{280}
Water extraction	1976 (2600 mg)	33390	605	17.0	0.31
Acetone fractionation 50 - 75 %	195	25160	490	130	2.52
DEAE-Sephadex A-50	46.6	22550	450	484	9.64
Sephadex G-75	20.1	21820	410	1090	20.4
Isoelectric focusing, Sephadex G-50 and lyophilization	12.0 mg	15170	295	1260(/mg)	24.5(/mg)

* BAEE unit : μmoles degraded in 1 min

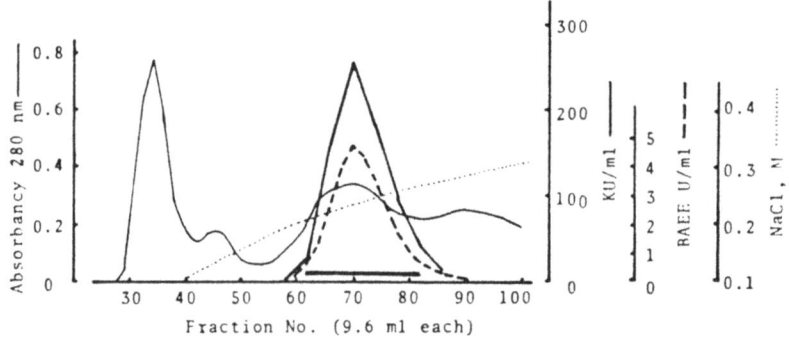

Fig. 1. DEAE-Sephadex A-50 Chromatography of CSK
         (Active fraction from acetone fractionation)
         Elution : 0.05 M Tris-HCl buffer containing
         0.1 M NaCl, pH 7.8, NaCl gradient 0.1 - 0.4 M

The active fractions (No. 62-82) were combined and concentrated by ultra-filtration, and then gel filtered through Sephadex G-75 column (Fig.2). Most of the contaminants could be eliminated by this procedure, and the specific activity elevated to 1100 KU, 2.2 times that of the preceding step.

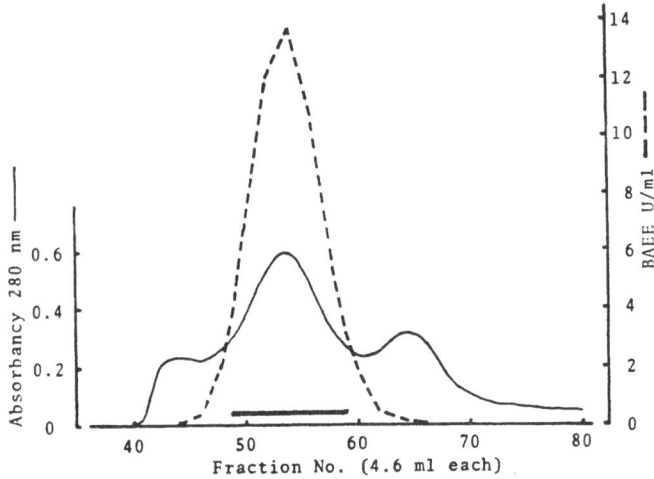

Fig. 2. Sephadex G-75 Gel Filtration of CSK
(Active fraction from DEAE-Sephadex A-50 chromatography)
Elution : 0.02 M ammonium formate, pH 6.0

While the active fraction in Sephadex gel filtration seemed to be free from the contaminants in disc electrophoresis, it was separated into 6 different active components by Ampholine iso-electric focusing like some other glandular kallikreins. All of these fractions with pI values in the range 4.27 - 4.94 gave both vasodilator and BAEE splitting activities (Fig. 3). They (fractions No. 53-82) were combined as the purified CSK because the amount of each fraction was not enough for further experiments. As mentioned above, Fiedler, et al. reported that hog submaxillary kallikrein is separated into 8 active components (pI 3.29 - 4.37), and the present observation is in fairly good agreement with their finding beyond the species difference.

Disc Electrophoresis Disc electrophoresis with 7% polyacryl-amide gel of the active fractions from both Sephadex gel filtration and isoelectric fractionation gave a single protein band, but a broad one, which did not migrate so rapidly as other glandular kallikreins. In order to find out whether the broad protein band was really kallikrein or not, 70 µg of purified CSK was performed electrophoresis in two gel tubes. One gel was stained with

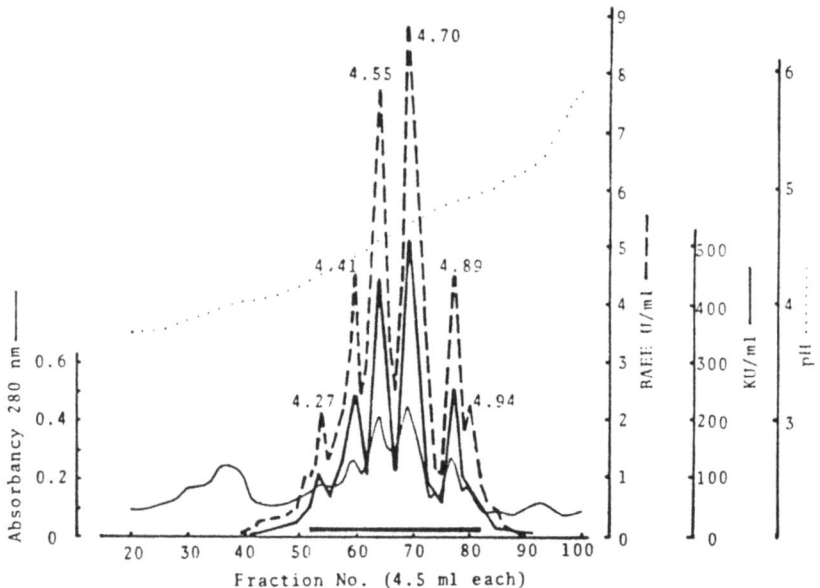

Fig. 3.   Isoelectric Focusing of CSK with Ampholine (pH 3.5-5.0)
          (Active fraction from Sephadex G-75 gel filtration)

coomassie brilliant blue and the other was sliced into 20 fragments
of 3 mm thick. Each slice was homogenized and extracted with 2 ml
of 0.05 M Tris-HCl buffer, pH 8.0, and then its BAEE activity was
determined. The fragments which corresponded to the broad protein
band only possessed the activity.

Properties   Esterolytic activities on BAEE, TAME and BTEE of
purified CSK were 24.5, 11.6 and 0.06 units/mg, respectively. The
activity ratio (BAEE/TAME) is far less than that of pancreatic
kallikrein (9), and is close to that of kallikrein-like peptidase
from rat submaxillary gland (5). The latter enzyme was capable of
hydrolysing N-α-benzoyl-DL-arginine-p-nitroanilide, but the
activity was not detectable in purified CSK.

Trasylol caused weak inhibitory effect on CSK. Only 20% of
decrease in the vasodilator and BAEE esterolytic activities were
found by a treatment of 10 KU of purified CSK with 50 KIU of
Trasylol for 30 min.

The molecular weight of this kallikrein was roughly estimated
to be 50,000 by Sephadex gel filtration. This value is higher than
those of other glandular kallikreins.

Thus the final preparation of cat submaxillary kallikrein is found to be free from contamination of other proteins, but it consists of several multiple forms of kallikrein. Taking account of the broad band in disc electrophoretic pattern and higher molecular weight, it might be supposed that CSK seems to be rich in carbohydrate content. Further data on analysis of CSK will be presented in near future.

In the present investigation, we did not pursue the property of each multiple form. We found previously that there was only one kallikrein component in human mixed saliva (10). The relation between the kallikreins in the salivary glands and in the saliva will be an interesting problem, same as the distribution of it in the gland.

Summary

Cat submaxillary kallikrein was purified from the water extract of the gland by 50-75% acetone fractionation, DEAE-Sephadex A-50 chromatography, Sephadex G-75 gel filtration and Ampholine isoelectric focusing. The final preparation gave the activities of 1260 KU/mg in vasodilator assay, 24.5 and 11.6 units/mg on BAEE and TAME esterolytic assay, respectively. Trasylol gave only weak inhibitory effect on this kallikrein. The isoelectric points of the kallikrein were in the range pH 4.2-5.0, and this kallikrein seemed to consist of several multiple forms with different pI values, like some other glandular kallikreins. It gave a single protein band in disc electrophoresis, while it migrated in retard and formed a broad one. This may be ascribable to the rich carbohydrate content in the kallikrein.

References

1. S.M. Hilton and G.P. Lewis, J. Physiol., 128, 235 (1955); 129, 253 (1955); 134, 471 (1956).

2. K.D. Bhoola, J. Morley, M. Schachter and L.H. Smaje, J. Physiol., 179, 172 (1965); S. Beilenson, M. Schachter and L.H. Smaje, J. Physiol., 199, 303 (1968).

3. K. Gautovik, S.M. Hilton and S.M. Torres, J. Physiol., 197, 22p (1968); K. Gautovic, Acta Physiol. Scand., 76, 191 (1969).

4. K.D. Bhoola, J. Physiol., 196, 431 (1968); K.D. Bhoola and G. Dorey, J. Physiol., 203, 59p (1969); K.D. Bhoola, Biochem. Pharmacol., 18, 1252 (1969).

5. T.D. Ekfors, P.J. Riekkinen, T. Malmiharju and V.K. Hopsu-Havu, Z. Physiol. Chem., 348, 111 (1967).

6. F. Fiedler, B. Muller and E. Werle, Z. Physiol. Chem., <u>351</u>,
    1002 (1970).

7. C. Moriwaki, Y. Hojima and H. Moriya, Chem. Pharm. Bull., <u>22</u>,
    975 (1974).

8. G.W. Schwert and Y. Takenaka, Biochem. Biophys. Acta, <u>16</u>,
    570 (1955).

9. Y. Hojima, C. Moriwaki and H. Moriya, Chem. Pharm. Bull.,
    <u>23</u>, 1120, 1128 (1975).

10. Y. Fujimoto, H. Moriya and C. Moriwaki, J. Biochem., <u>74</u>, 239,
    247 (1973).

MECHANISM OF CLOSTRIPAIN-INDUCED KININ RELEASE FROM HUMAN, RAT AND CANINE PLASMA

B.B. Vargaftig and E.L. Giroux

Centre de Recherche Merrell International

16, rue d'Ankara, 67000 Strasbourg, France

Clostripain (clostridiopeptidase B, E.C. 3.4.4.20) is a thiol proteinase found in extracts from cultures of Clostridium histoly-ticum (Ogle and Tytell, 1953; Labouesse and Gros, 1960), and displays a marked specificity for the carboxyl linkage of arginine (Gros and Labouesse, 1960; Mitchell and Harrington, 1968). Clostripain has been reported to release kinin-like polypeptides directly from bovine or horse kininogen-containing preparations (Prado, et al., 1956; Prado and Prado, 1962). In the course of investigations concerning the haemorrhagic and pro-inflammatory activity of bacterial collagenase (Giroux, Lefort and Vargaftig, 1976) we found that clostripain, a contaminant of one collagenase preparation, displayed indirect kinin-releasing activities which had not been described before. This communication reports our investigation of the mechanism of such release.

METHODS AND MATERIALS

Human, rat and canine plasmas, not contacted with glass, were obtained by centrifugation of venous blood collected with 1/10th of the final volume of a 4% (w.v^{-1}) solution of sodium citrate; they were stored at room temperature. Aliquots of plasma containing 10 mM CaEDTA as kinanase inhibitor (Erdos and Sloane, 1962) were incubated for various intervals with crude clostripain dissolved in Tris buffer (0.1 M, pH 7.6). Incubates were bioassayed on superfused cat ileum strips (Ferreira and Vane, 1967) and occasionally on a rat duodenum or a rat urinary bladder strip (Erspamer, Negri and Piccinelli, 1973). The superfusing Krebs solution contained inhibitors to eliminate the interference of histamine, serotonin, catecholamines or acetylcholine (Vane, 1964 and 1971).

Bradykinin, used as a standard spasmogenic agent, and plasma samples were injected directly onto the cascade of isolated tissues via a lateral T tubing. Inhibitors under investigation were added to plasma before crude clostripain to inhibit the endogenous kinin-releasing system activated by exogenous enzyme. Alternatively, they were incubated with crude clostripain to inhibit its activity. This allowed distinction between inhibition at the kinin cascade level or directly at the exogenous enzyme level. Figure 1 summarizes the procedure and anticipates some results.

Enzymatic activity of clostripain was measured by following the hydrolysis of benzoyl-D, L-arginine-p-nitroanilide : various amounts of enzyme in 1.1 ml of buffer (40 mM morpholino propane sulfonic acid, 10 mM $CaCl_2$, 0.02% NaN_3, adjusted to pH 7.5 with NaOH) containing 5 mM D,L-penicillamine were activated for a few minutes. Two ml of substrate, 1.55 mM benzoyl-D,L-arginine-p-nitroanilide in the same buffer, was added to each enzyme sample. Absorbance at 405 nm was measured at time zero and after 20 min. incubation at $37^\circ C$. Rates of hydrolysis were determined from plots of ΔA 405 vs μg of protein assayed. p-Nitroanilide was used to prepare a standard curve.

Kininase activity was shown by incubation of fixed amounts of the clostripain preparation with increasing amounts of bradykinin and bioassay on cat ileum strips, until a standard contraction, as induced by a bradykinin reference without clostripain, was obtained.

The following materials were used: collagenase CLS-EF, which will be called crude clostripain, and carboxypeptidase B (CBX-B) from Worthington; collagenase ref. 15642, which will be called purified collagenase, and benzoyl-D,L-arginine-p-nitroanilide hydrochloride (BAPNA) from Boehringer Mannheim; pancreatic or parotid gland protein protease inhibitors: Trasylol[R] (0.15 µg/KIE, kindly provided by Dr. N. Bhargava, Organon, Oss, The Netherlands), Zymofren[R] from Specia, and Iniprol[R] from Choay; soybean (SBTI), ovomucoid (OMTI) and lima bean (LBTI) trypsin inhibitors, dithiothreitol (DTT), trypsin grade III, morpholino propane sulfonic acid (MOPS) and polyarginine (approx. mol. wt. 58,000) from Sigma; dexamethasone phosphate (Soludecadron[R] and indomethacin from Merck, Sharp & Dohme; aspirin as a lysine salt (Aspegic[R] from Laboratoires Egic; phenylbutazone from Midy; hexadimethrine bromide from Abbott and from Aldrich; NaEDTA and CaEDTA from Koch-Light; carrageenin (Viscarin brand) from Marine Colloids; bradykinin from Sandoz; pancreatic kallikrein (Kalleone[R] retard) from Bayer; tosyllysinechloromethylketone (TLCK) from Serva, D,L-penicillamine, from Aldrich.

Figure 1

Interference of Various Drugs with Release of Kinin-Like Activity
from Rat Plasma by Crude Clostripain

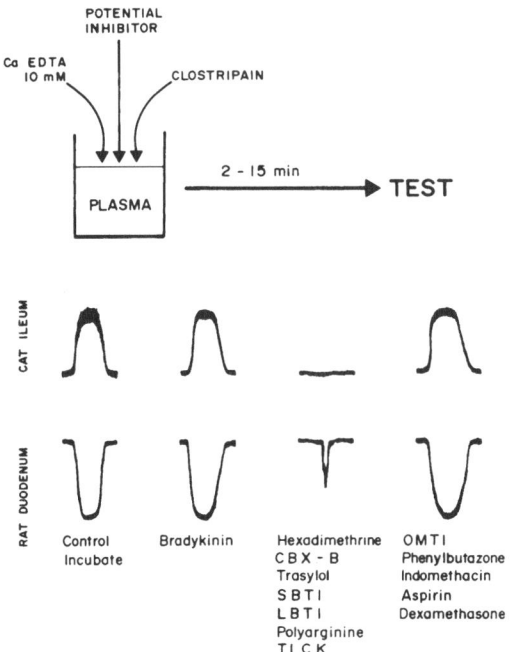

Diagrammatic representation of the procedure used to demonstrate
release of kinin-like activity from plasma and of results obtained
by bioassay on a cat ileum strip (upper tracings) and on a rat
duodenum (lower tracings), as compared to the effects of synthetic
bradykinin. Inhibitors effective on rat and on human plasma are
listed, as well as substances that failed to inhibit kinin release.
These materials, except for polyarginine and TLCK, were added to
plasma prior to addition of crude clostripain.

RESULTS

1. Crude Clostripain Triggers Release of Kinin-Like Activity
    from Native Plasma.

Addition of 1-2.5 mg of crude clostripain per ml of dog, human
or rat plasma was followed by the appearance within 2-15 minutes of
kinin-like activity as detected by a contracting effect on cat ileum
and rat urinary bladder strips, and by a relaxing effect on rat

duodenum. Characteristics of this activity were similar to those
of synthetic bradykinin:

A. Crude clostripain-plasma incubates contracted the rat
stomach strip after a short relaxation (in similar conditions prostaglandins induce only contractions), contracted the gerbil colon,
and displayed no activity on the rabbit aorta strip which is sensitive to prostaglandin endoperoxide precursors ("rabbit aorta
contracting activity", Piper and Vane, 1969; Vargaftig and Dao,
1971).

B. The kinin-like activity was completely absent in presence
of the kinin-destroying enzyme carboxypeptidase B (Erdos, McMennamin
and Wohler, 1962); this is illustrated in figure 2.

C. Incubates of native plasma (human, dog or rat) with crude
clostripain lost the kinin-like activity within 30 to 60 minutes
despite presence of 10 mM CaEDTA, which inhibited plasma kininases.
This was due to kininase activity present in crude clostripain
(figure 3). Kininase activity prevented quantitative evaluation of
kinin activity released in terms of bradykinin equivalents.

D. The yield of kinin-like activity was the same whether
obtained from native or from platelet rich plasma, thus ruling out
any influence of prostaglandins. Involvement of prostaglandins in
the kinin-releasing activity was further ruled out by the lack of
effect of prostaglandin synthetase inhibitors on the release
process.

2. Release of Kinin-Like Activity by Crude Clostripain from
    Human and Rat Plasma Is Due to Activation of Endogenous
    Kinin-Releasing Mechanisms, whereas Release from Dog
    Plasma Is Direct.

Release of kinins by clostripain has been suggested to be due
to plasminogen activation (Lewis, 1960), but Prado and Prado (1962)
demonstrated that clostripain released kinin activity both from
heated and from native horse plasma. Soybean trypsin inhibitor
failed to prevent this release from either substrate. It was
concluded that clostripain releases kinins by splitting kininogen
directly. Our results with human or rat plasma do not support this
conclusion, whereas results with dog plasma are in full agreement
with it:

A. Human, rat or dog plasmas were heated for 3 hours at 56°C
or for 20 minutes at 61° C, to destroy prekallikrein or both
prekallikrein and Hageman Factor, respectively (for a discussion
of these procedures, see Eisen and Vogt, 1970). Heated rat or human
plasma did not release kinin-like activity upon addition of crude

Figure 2

Inhibition by Carboxypeptidase B of the Kinin-Like Activity
Released by Crude Clostripain from Human Plasma

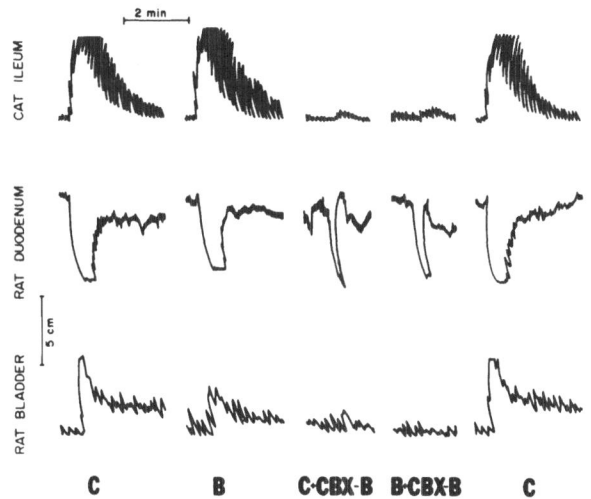

Recordings are illustrated of contractions or relaxations of assay
tissues upon superfusion with: incubates of human citrated plasma
and 2.5 mg.ml^{-1} of crude clostripain (C); 40 ng.ml^{-1} of synthetic
bradykinin (B); of C and of B with 0.3 µg.ml^{-1} of carboxypeptidase
B. Kinin-like activity was released in C, contracting the cat ilium
(upper trace) and the rat bladder (lower trace) strips, while relaxing the rat duodenum. This activity was suppressed in presence of
the kinin-destroying enzyme carboxypeptidase B added to crude clostripain-plasma incubates (C & CBX-B) or to bradykinin solution
(B + CBX-B). A small short-lasting relaxation remaining on the rat
duodenum was also obtained with unactivated plasma, and resulted
from the assay conditions. Vertical scale: contraction of the
assay tissue with a 10-fold recorder amplification. Horizontal
scale: time.

clostripain, whereas release from dog plasma was in fact increased
by heat treatment. As illustrated in figure 4, heated rat plasma
did not release kinins upon incubation with low concentrations of
trypsin or upon agitation with a magnetic bar. Both these procedures are known to release kinins indirectly, through activation
of endogenous mechanisms (for a discusstion, see Vogt, 1966, and
Eisen and Vogt, 1970).

Figure 3

Kinin-Like Activity Induced in Rat Plasma by Crude Clostripain
Containing Kininase as a Contaminant

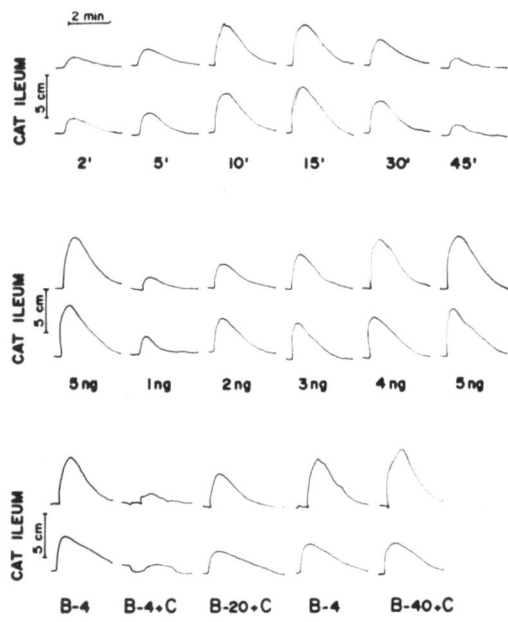

Incubates were bioassayed on two strips of cat ileum. Sensitivity
of the recorder was adjusted to obtain a full scale contraction
in response to 5 ng of synthetic bradykinin; 0.15 ml of incubates
of plasma plus crude clostripain were assayed. Upper Panel:
Mixtures of rat plasma with 1.25 mg.ml^{-1} of crude clostripain were
incubated at room temperature for various time intervals, as indicated. The maximum of activity occurred at 15 min., was decaying
at 30 min. and was almost nil at 45 min. Center Panel: A dose-
response scale for synthetic bradykinin. Lower Panel: A mixture
of 4 ng of bradykinin, 10 mM CaEDTA and crude clostripain, 500
µg.ml^{-1}, was bioassayed after five minutes incubation. Kininase
activity having been demonstrated (B-4+C), 20 and 40 ng of bradykinin were incubated with the same amount of crude clostripain
(B-20+C and B-40+C, respectively). In the presence of crude clostripain, 40 ng of bradykinin was required in order to obtain contractions of cat ileum matching those obtained by bioassay of
4 ng of bradykinin in the absence of crude clostripain (B-4).

Figure 4

Reduction of Release of Kinin-Like Activity by Heating
Plasma and by Pre-Treatment of Rat with Carrageenin

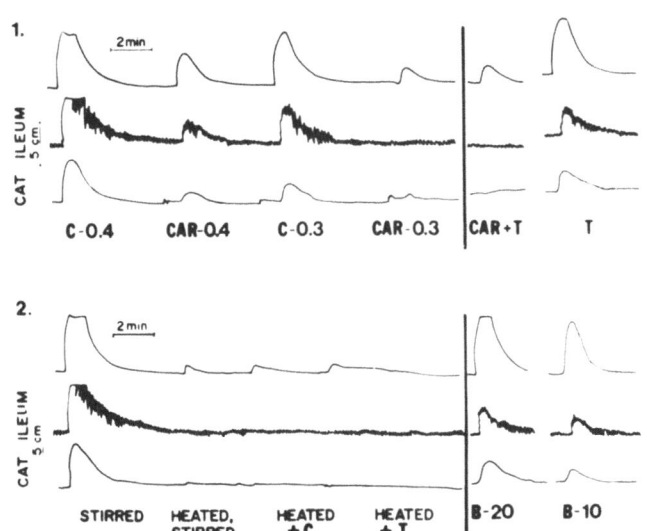

Recordings of contractions of superfused cat ileum strips are
illustrated as follows: Panel 1: Rat plasma was incubated with
1.25 mg.ml^{-1} of crude clostripain. Volumes of 0.3 ml and 0.4 ml
were bioassayed (C-0.3 and C-0.4, respectively). Plasma obtained
from carrageenin-treated rats was incubated with crude clostripain
and assayed under similar conditions, as indicated by CAR-0.3 and
CAR-0.4. Less kinin-like activity was obtained from plasma collected from carrageenin-treated rats. Release of kinin activity by
2.5 µg.ml^{-1} of trypsin was reduced in plasma collected from a
carrageenin-treated rat (CAR+T) as compared to normal plasma (T).
Panel 2: Plasma stirred with a metallic bar (2 min., 1100 rpm)
generated kinin-like activity (STIRRED) whereas no such activity
was obtained from heated (3 h, 56°C) plasma (HEATED, STIRRED).
Similar treatment abolished the ability of the rat plasma to generate
kinin-like activity when incubated with crude clostripain
(2.5 mg.ml^{-1}) or with trypsin (2.5 µg.ml^{-1}), as indicated by HEATED
+ C and HEATED + T, respectively. Contractions caused by 10 and
20 ng of synthetic bradykinin (B-10 and B-20, respectively) are
illustrated for reference. Scales as in figure 2.

B.   Release of kinin-like activity from rat or human plasma was prevented by the addition, one minute before the crude clostripain, of any of the three mammalian protein protease inhibitors and SBTI and of LBTI, whereas OMTI was ineffective (figure 5; concentrations in table I). This pattern of inhibitory effect is in agreement with the presumed inhibition of plasma kallikrein, except for the effect of LBTI (Back and Steger, 1968). None of these inhibitors prevented release of kinin-like activity from dog plasma (figure 6).

C. Implication of endogenous kinin-releasing mechanisms led us to test hexadimethrine, a specific blocker of the activation of Hageman Factor (Eisen, 1964). As shown in figure 7, addition of 100-250 µg.ml^{-1} of hexadimethrine to rat plasma resulted in complete suppression of generation of kinin-like activity. Results with human plasma were less predictable, as inhibition varied between 50 and 100%, depending upon the individual plasma. In contrast, inhibition by hexadimethrine of crude clostripain-induced kinin release was not observed in dog plasma.

Figure 5

Inhibition by the Mammalian Protein Protease Inhibitor Iniprol[R] of Release of Kinin-Like Activity from Rat Plasma by Crude Clostripain

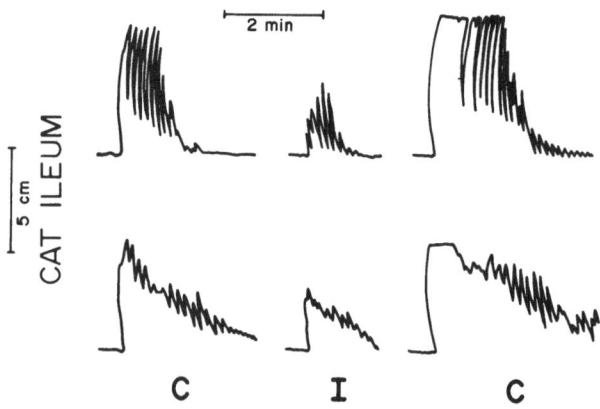

Incubates of rat plasma containing 10 mM CaEDTA with 1.25 mg.ml^{-1} of crude clostripain were bioassayed in the absence (C) and in the presence (I) of 5000 U.ml^{-1} of Iniprol [R]. Inhibition of generation of kinin-like activity was observed. Complete inhibition could be obtained with higher concentrations of the inhibitor (not shown). Scales as in figure 2.

Table I

Interference of Potential Inhibitors of Release of Kinin-Like
Activity from Plasma by Crude Clostripain

POTENTIAL INHIBITOR	INHIBITORY CONCENTRATION[1]	
	human/rat plasma	dog plasma
SOYBEAN TRYPSIN INHIBITOR	0.1	(1.25)
LIMA BEAN TRYPSIN INHIBITOR	2.5	(2.5)
INIPROL [R]	5,000 U	(10,000 U)
TRASYLOL [R]	0.25	not performed
ZYMOFREN [R]	1,250 U	(2,500 U)
HEXADIMETHRINE	human: 1 rat: 0.5	(2)
OVOMUCOID TRYPSIN INHIBITOR	1.25	(1.25)
POLYARGININE	(0.025)[2]	(0.025)[2]
CARBOXYPEPTIDASE B	0.035	0.035
INDOMETHACIN	(1)	(1)
ASPIRIN	(1)	(1)
DEXAMETHASONE	(1)	(1)
PHENYLBUTAZONE	(1)	(1)

(1) Amount per ml (in mg or otherwise indicated) of potential inhibitor required to prevent generation of kinin-like activity by 1.25-25 $mg.ml^{-1}$ of crude clostripain. Sensitivity of the recorder was adjusted to obtain a full scale deflection equivalent to contraction of the isolated cat ileum by 20-30 $ng.ml^{-1}$ of synthetic bradykinin. Experimental samples were 0.4 ml of plasma. When inhibition was not observed, the highest amount of potential inhibitor tested is indicated in parentheses.

(2) Polyarginine was added to plasma 20 minutes before crude clostripain and failed to inhibit formation of kinins.

Figure 6

Failure of Protein Protease Inhibitors to Affect the Release of Kinin-Like Activity from Dog Plasma by Crude Clostripain

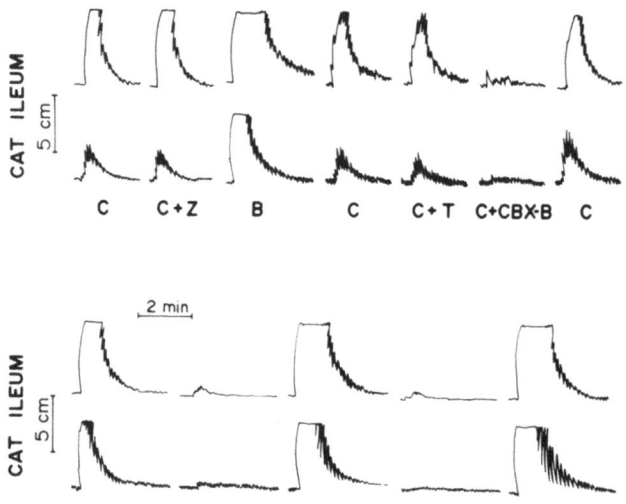

Incubates of dog plasma containing 10 mM CaEDTA with 2.5 mg.ml^{-1} of crude clostripain were bioassayed in the absence (C) and in the presence of Zymofren[R] (Z, 2,500 U.ml^{-1}), of Trasylol[R] (T, 1.24 mg.ml^{-1}) and of carboxypeptidase B (CBX-B, 3.5 µg.ml^{-1}). Contraction induced by bradykinin (B, 40 ng) is included as a reference. Neither Zymofren nor Trasylol[R] inhibited release of kinin-like activity. Similar incubates with 0.005 U.ml^{-1} of pancreatic kallikrein were bioassayed in the absence (K) and in the presence of Zymofren[R] (K+Z, 250 U.ml^{-1}) or of carboxypeptidase B (K+CBX-B, 3.5 µg.ml^{-1}). Zymofren[R] fully inhibited release of kinin.

Figure 7

Inhibition by Hexadimethrine Bromide of Release of Kinin-Like
Activity from Rat Plasma by Crude Clostripain

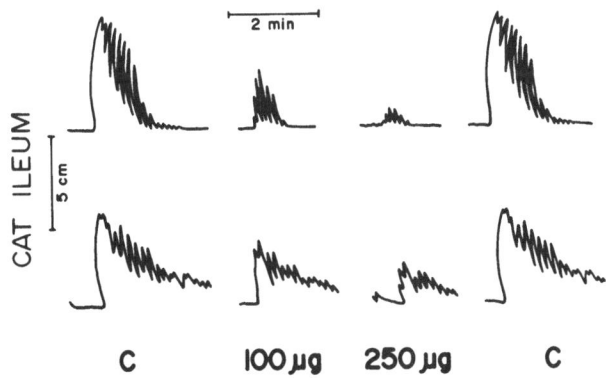

Incubates of rat plasma containing 10 mM CaEDTA and 1.25 mg.ml^{-1} of
crude clostripain were bioassayed in the absence (C) and in the
presence of 100 and 250 µg per ml of hexadimethrine, which inhibited
generation of kinin-like activity. Scales as in figure 2.

D. Treatment of rats by the i.p. route with carrageenin removes
from the animals a factor necessary for the full development of
inflammatory (aspirin-sensitive)oedema (Vargaftig et al., 1970);
kininogen is depleted by such treatment (Rothschild, 1967). Plasma
collected from carrageenin-treated rats did not sustain kinin
release upon agitation, or addition of small amounts of trypsin or
of crude clostripain (figure 4). It thus appeared that prior
depletion of kinin-producing components from blood prevented release
of kinin activity by crude clostripain, although this procedure did
not establish which factor was suppressed among those required for
successful triggering of kinin release. Prior depletion of kininogen
would diminish crude clostripain-induced generation of kinin-like
activity either by a direct or by an indirect mechanism.

E. Three non-steroidal acidic anti-inflammatory agents (phenylbutazone, indomethacin and aspirin) which are recognized prostaglandin synthetase inhibitors (Vane, 1971) and thus are effective as
inhibitors of generation of prostaglandins, of their immediate endoperoxide precursors and of other pharmacologically active substances

formed from arachidonic acid (Vargaftig and Dao, 1971; Vargaftig
and Zirinis, 1973; Hamberg, et al., 1974; Hamberg and Samuelsson,
1974; Vargaftig, Tranier and Chignard, 1974; Willis, 1974; Hamberg,
1975; Vargaftig and Chignard, 1975), failed to inhibit formation
of kinin-like activity from rat or human plasma when added up to
2.5 mg.ml^{-1}. Dexamethasone phosphate, in similar conditions, was
also ineffective.

   3. Clostripain Is the Enzyme in Collagenase CLS-EF Responsible
       for Initiating Kinin Generation in Human, Rat and Dog
       Plasma.

   Clostripain is not a major component of the ammonium sulfate-
precipitated fraction of culture filtrates which is used as crude
C. histolyticum collagenase, since 10-15 fold increases in specific
activity have been reported (Labouesse and Gros, 1960; Mitchell and
Harrington, 1968) upon purification of clostripain from this
material. However, kinin release, as well as the amidase activity
of the crude collagenase proparation were markedly enhanced by
thiols (dithiothreitol and penicillamine), consistent with our
implication of clostripain as the factor responsible for induction
of kinin-like activity in plasma. Other evidence that clostripain
is responsible for kinin release in our system is as follows:

   A. Treatment of crude clostripain with the chloromethyl ketone
derivative derived from α-N-tosyl-L-lysine (TLCK), as described by
Porter, Cunningham and Mitchell (1971), resulted in blockade of the
kinin-releasing activity, as measured on dog (figure 8) or on rat
plasma, i.e. for direct and for indirect release, respectively.
This is expected if inhibition occurs at the clostripain level and
not within the kinin cascade. TLCK is reported to specifically
inactivate clostripain in crude preparations of C. histolyticum
collagenase (Porter, Cunningham and Mitchell, 1971).

   B. Treatment of crude clostripain with an equal amount, by
weight, of polyarginine for two minutes resulted in disappearance
of the ability to trigger kinin release and to split the synthetic
substrate. Blockade was already apparent when polyarginine was
added to crude clostripain at 1/20th of its weight, provided incubation lasted 10 minutes (figure 9). Polyarginine is known to be
a potent inhibitor of clostripain (Mitchell and Harrington, 1968).

   C. Kinin-releasing activity of crude clostripain was thermo-
labile, as was the amidase activity. Half-lives upon heating tended
to be shorter for amidase activity (table II).

   D. Amidase activity of crude clostripain was found to be
1.0 μmol of nitroanilide product.min^{-1}.mg^{-1}. A sample of purified
collagenase from Boehringer Mannheim had little clostripain activity (less than 10^{-2} μmols product formed.min^{-1}.mg^{-1}) and did not

Figure 8

Suppression by TLCK of the Ability of Crude Clostripain to
Release Kinin-Like Activity from Dog Plasma

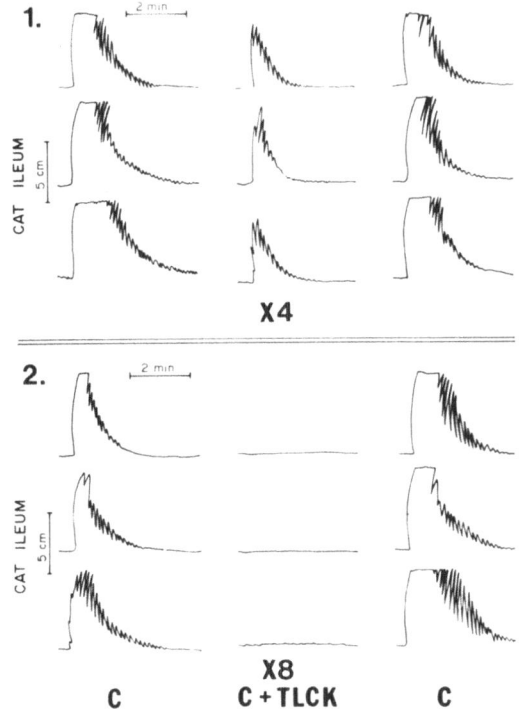

Plasma was incubated with crude clostripain in which 75% (panel 1,
indicated as X4) or 95% (panel 2, indicated as X8) of the amidase
activity was eliminated by TLCK. In both panels the two outside
tracings indicate the kinin activity of control crude clostripain-
plasma incubates. Scales as in figure 2.

Figure 9

Suppression of the Ability of Crude Clostripain to Release
Kinin-Like Activity upon Incubation with Polyarginine

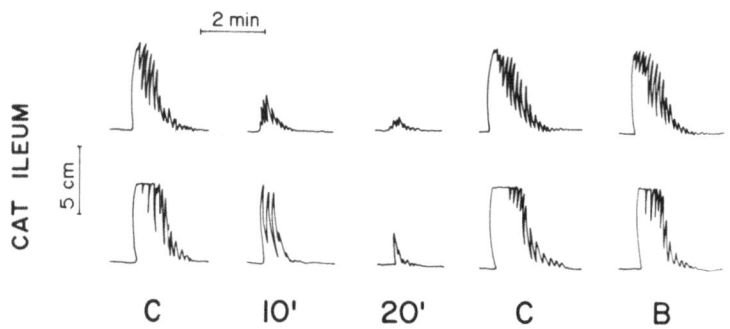

Incubates of rat plasma containing 10 mM CaEDTA and 1.25 mg.ml^{-1}
of crude clostripain, indicated as C, were bioassayed and the contractions observed were compared to those evoked by crude clostripain incubated in similar fashion with plasma, but pre-incubated
for ten or twenty minutes with polyarginine (25 µg for 500 µg of
crude clostripain), indicated as 10' and 20', respectively. Incubation for 20 minutes completely prevented the release of kinin
activity. Tissue response to 20 ng of bradykinin is indicated (B).

release kinin-like activity. In contrast to their effects upon
release of kinin activity from rat or human plasma, the mammalian
protein protease inhibitors, SBTI and LBTI failed to prevent the
amidase activity of crude clostripain (table III). TLCK inhibited
amidase activity of the crude clostripain preparation (table IV).

E. In preliminary experiments all characteristics of kinin
release by crude clostripain, as reported here, were reproduced
with a pure clostripain, recently available from Worthington:
indirect kinin release from human and rat plasmas, direct release
from dog plasma, and the appropriate inhibition pattern. The only
difference was that pure clostripain did not destroy bradykinin,
as did the crude preparation. However, bradykininase activity is
not attributable to clostripain (Prado and Prado, 1962; Mitchell,
1968).

Table II

Half-Lives of the Amidase Activity and of the Kinin-Releasing
Activity of Crude Clostripain after Thermal Treatment

ACTIVITY	TEMPERATURE	TIME REQUIRED FOR SUPPRESSION OF HALF THE ACTIVITY
AMIDASE	42°C	stable
	56°C	15 min.
	70°C	4 min.
KININ RELEASE	42°C	stable
	56°C	21-36 min.
	70°C	9-14 min.

Half-lives were determined from semi-logarithmic plots of activity
vs duration of heat treatment. Kinin release was obtained in rat
plasma, and the values are the range of results of three experiments.

DISCUSSION

Clostripain appears to release kinins from plasma of different
species either by a direct mechanism (dog and horse) or by an indirect mechanism (rat and human). An indirect release mechanism is
suggested by failure of heated plasma to sustain release of kinins,
and by effectiveness of various protein protease inhibitors which
do not inhibit amidase activity. Release of kinins proceeds by
various pathways and may involve four critical starting points:
activation of Hageman Factor, activation of prekallikrein (prekininogenase), activation of plasminogen, or direct splitting of
kininogen. The latter mechanism was ruled out as a principal explanation of our observations on rat and human plasmas. Effectiveness
of hexadimethrine in human, and particularly in rat plasma, suggested that clostripain might activate Hageman Factor, thus triggering
the kinin-releasing cascade. This would provide a general explanation for the effectiveness of protein protease inhibitors and of
SBTI which inhibit generation of kinins in plasma at the levels of

Table III

Inhibition of Amidase Activities of Trypsin and of
Crude Clostripain

POTENTIAL INHIBITOR	AMOUNT (in µg) REQUIRED FOR INHIBITION	
	TRYPSIN	CRUDE CLOSTRIPAIN
SOYBEAN TRYPSIN INHIBITOR	2.1	(10)
LIMA BEAN TRYPSIN INHIBITOR	1.1	(5)
INIPROL (R)	170 Units	(20,000 Units)
HEXADIMETHRINE	(1000)	(1000)
OVOMUCOID TRYPSIN INHIBITOR	3.5	(20)
POLYARGININE	(20)	1.6

Trypsin (2 µg) and crude clostripain (8 µg), were assayed for amidase activity after pre-incubation with various amounts of inhibitors.
Plots of activity vs amount of inhibitor added were extrapolated to
calculate the amount of inhibitor necessary to completely suppress
amidase activity. When inhibition was not observed, the highest
amount of potential inhibitor tested is indicated in parentheses.

Table IV

Inhibition of Amidase Activity of Crude Clostripain by TLCK

TLCK ADDED (µg per mg crude clostripain)	RELATIVE AMIDASE ACTIVITY
---	100
0.7	24
0.8	11
1.0	4

Crude clostripain was activated in 10 mM DTT and treated with
aqueous TLCK.

activation and/or action of Hageman Factor and/or kallikrein (Eisen and Vogt, 1970; Trautschold and Werle, 1961; Kassell, 1970). These inhibitors failed to inhibit the direct kinin release from dog plasma. Activation of Hageman Factor is furthermore suggested by the effectiveness of LBTI in suppressing kinin generation in rat or human plasma, since LBTI does not block prekallikrein or kallikrein, but prevents activation of Hageman Factor (Schoenmakers et al., 1965; Cochrane and Wuepper, 1971). Lima bean trypsin inhibitor also blocks plasmin (Back and Steger, 1968), thus our suggestion of a dominant importance for Hageman Factor must remain a hypothesis.

Vogt (1966) proposed that functionally different kinin genera-ting systems exist in human, rat and dog plasmas, such that dog plasma has only the so-called kininogenase I, which is not activated by glass or other stimuli of Hageman Factor, and that kininogenase II, present in rat or human plasma, is absent from the dog. More-over, since dog plasma forms kinins when incubated with pancreatic kallikrein, whereas rat plasma fails to do so, it appears that dog contains kininogen I, whereas in rats only system II is complete. Human plasma falls in between, since it contains both systems I and II. One might hypothesize that clostripain releases kinin activity from native rat plasma by activating the Hageman Factor-activated kininogenase II system which is fully inhibited by hexadimethrine. Release from human plasma should follow a similar pathway, compli-cated by the presence of the Hageman Factor-independent kininogenase I system which accounts for some variation in the potency of hexadi-methrine in blocking release of kinin activity. Failure to activate indirectly the release of kinin from dog plasma is explained by absence of the Hageman Factor-dependent pathway, whereas kininogen I is present and is a substrate for clostripain acting directly as a kininogenase. Presumably horse plasma resembles dog plasma in this respect, thus explaining the before-mentioned observation of Prado and Prado (1962). Our observations are essentially consistent with Vogt's (1966) construct; however, they do not eliminate other interpretations. Recently functionally defined kininogenase II was demonstrated in dog plasma (Nakahara, 1974), contradictory to the earlier hypothesis (Vogt, 1966). Others (Jahrreiss and Habermann, 1971) have not found it necessary to postulate the existence of multiple kinin-forming systems in plasmas. At least two kininogens may be purified from human plasma (Habal et al., 1974; Guimaraes et al., 1974).

Several exogenous proteases may induce kinin activity in plasma (for review, see Prado, 1970); trypsin appears to demonstrate direct and indirect kinin release (data summarized by Vogt, 1966) similar to clostripain. Many inhibitors of trypsin activity are also inhibitors of endogenous proteases in the kinin cascade, while clos-tripain is not inhibited by typical trypsin inhibitors. In addition, clostripain has a much greater enzymatic specificity than has

trypsin (Ogle and Tytell, 1953). These factors and the pharmacological activity attributable to its enzymatic activity indicate clostripain may be a valuable tool for further investigating the role
of Hageman Factor in coagulation, kinin release, complement activation and possible interaction with platelets leading to building-
up of pro-inflammatory mediators.

ACKNOWLEDGEMENTS

The excellent technical assistance provided by Mrs. M.L. Part is
gratefully acknowledged. We also thank the useful comments on this
text made by Dr. J. Koch-Weser (Centre de Recherche Merrell International, Strasbourg, France).

REFERENCES

Back, N. and Steger, R. (1968), Fed. Proc., 27 96-99
Cochrane, C.G., and Wuepper, K.D. (1971), in Immunopathology of
     Inflammation (B.K. Forscher and J.C. Houck, eds.), Exerpta
     Medica, Amsterdam, p. 137-145
Eisen, V. (1964), Br. J. Pharmacol., 22 87-103
Eisen, V., and Vogt, W. (1970), in Handbook Exp. Pharmacol. 25
     (E.G. Erdos, ed.), Springer, Berlin, p. 82-130
Erdos, E.G., McMennamin, M.A., and Wohler, J.R. (1962), Life
     Sci., 1 765-769
Erdos, E.G., and Sloane, E.M. (1962), Biochem. Pharmacol.,
     11 585-592
Erspamer, G.F., Negri, L., and Piccinelli, D. (1973), Arch.
     Pharmacol., 279 61-74
Ferreira, S.H., and Vane, J.R. (1967), Br. J. Pharmacol.,
     29 367-377
Giroux, E.L., Lefort, J., and Vargaftig, B.B. (1976), submitted
     for publication
Gros, P., and Labouesse, B. (1960), Bull. Soc. Chim. Biol.,
     42 559-568
Guimaraes, J.A., Lu, R.C., Webster, M.E., and Pierce, J.V.
     (1974), Fed. Proc., abstract 2431
Habal, F.M., Movat, H.Z., and Burrowes, C.E. (1974), Biochem.
     Pharmacol., 23 2291-2303
Hamberg, M., (1975), Proc. Nat. Acad. Sci., in press
Hamberg, M., and Samuelsson, B. (1974), Proc. Nat. Acad. Sci.,
     71 3400-3404
Hamberg, M., Svensson, J., Wakabayashi, T., and Samuelsson, B.
     (1974), Proc. Nat. Acad. Sci., 71 345-349
Jahrreiss, R., and Habermann, E. (1971), Arch. Pharmacol.,
     269 85-100

Kassell, B. (1970), in Methods in Enzymology 19 (G.E. Perlmann
     and L. Lorand, eds.), Acad. Press, New York, p. 844-852
Labouesse, B., and Gros, P. (1960), Bull. Soc. Chim. Biol.,
     42 543-558
Lewis, G.P. (1960), Physiol. Rev. 40 647-676
Mitchell, W.M. (1968), Science, 162 374-375
Mitchell, W.M., and Harrington, W.F. (1968), J. Biol. Chem.,
     243 4683-4692
Nakahara, M. (1974), Biochem. Pharmacol., 23 3009-3015
Ogle, J.D., and Tytell, A.A. (1953), Arch. Biochem. Biophys.,
     42 327-336
Piper, P.J., and Vane, J.R. (1969), Nature, 223 20-35
Porter, W.H., Cunningham, L.W., and Mitchell, W.M. (1971),
     J. Biol. Chem., 246 7675-7682
Prado, J.L. (1970), in Handbook Exp. Pharmacol. 25 (E.G. Erdos,
     ed.), Springer, Berlin, p. 156-192
Prado, J.L., Monier, R., Prado, E.S., and Fromageot, C. (1956),
     Biochim. Biophys. Acta, 22 87-95
Prado, J.L., and Prado, E.S. (1962), An. Acad. Bras. Cien.,
     34 51-55
Rothschild, A.M. (1967), in Int. Symp. Vaso-Active Polypep-
     tides: Bradykinin and Related Kinins (M. Rocha e Silva and
     H.A. Rothschild, eds.), Edart, Sao Paulo, p. 197-203
Schoenmakers, J.G.G., Matze, R., Haanen, C., and Zilliken, F.
     (1965), Biochim. Biophys. Acta, 101 166-176
Trautschold, I. and Werle, E. (1961), Z. Physiol. Chem.
     325 48-59
Vane, J.R. (1964), Br. J. Pharmacol., 23 360-373
Vane, J.R. (1971), Nature New Biol., 231 232-235
Vargaftig, B.B., Bhargava, N., de Vos, C.J., and Bonta, I.L.
     (1970), Advan. Exp. Med. Biol., 8 477-485
Vargaftig, B.B., and Chignard, M. (1975), Agents and Actions,
     5 137-144
Vargaftig, B.B., and Dao, N. (1971), Pharmacology, 6 99-108
Vargaftig, B.B., Tranier, Y., and Chignard, M. (1974),
     Prostaglandins, 8 133-156
Vargaftig, B.B., and Zirinis, P. (1973), Nature New Biol.,
     244 114-116
Vogt, W. (1966), in Hypotensive Peptides (E.G. Erdos, N. Back
     and F. Sicuteri, eds.), Springer, Berlin, p. 185-192
Willis, A.L. (1974), Prostaglandins, 5 1-25

ALGOGENIC ACTIVITY OF HUMAN PLASMA FOLLOWING MUSCULAR WORK

Vecchiet, L., Dolce, V., Galleti, R.

Institute of Sports Medicine

Chieti University, Italy

In a series of research conducted to interpret the physiopathologic mechanisms associated with the onset of pain in muscles that had been subjected to a determined type and intensity of work, it had been noticed that the intradermic injection of "pre-active" plasma after stress, unlike plasma from the same subject at rest, determines recurrent pain, secondary hyperalgesia, and itch (1). The 12 minute "activate plasma*" drawn after a period of stress trial determines recurrent pain of higher intensity and longer duration, a wider secondary hyperalgesia, and itch.

---

* Note: Regarding the "activation" concept, plasma, serum, inflammatory fluids (as blister fluid), if kept in siliconized glass, does not show any algogenic activity if applied on a blister base induced by contharidin or injected intradermally. Instead, it provokes appreciable pain after glass contact (3-5). Such pain appears after a 2 minute glass contact period, reaches its highest effect after a 12 minute glass contact, and then diminishes to zero if the contact period reaches or exceeds 17 minutes (6). An explanation of this phenomenon, as provided by Armstrong, Margolis, and others (7-12), suggests that the glass surface adsorbs the Hageman factor and activates it to its enzymic form which proceeds to activate pre-kallikrein to kallikrein forming plasma kinins from kininogen substrate. The kinins, thus, are responsible for the initiation of pain and the decline of the algogenic activity is due to the destruction of kinin by serum kininases.

On the basis of the knowledge that kinin release may be responsible for recurrent pain and hyperalgesia, the plasma from patients before and after stress was studied for smooth muscle stimulating activity (SMSA) using the isolated guinea pig ileum (2). It was shown that plasma drawn after the stress stimulus had increasing SMSA compared to plasma from non-stressed subjects and even non-activated plasma after stress had, in some instances, some SMSA. By using specific inhibitors as anticholinergics, antihistamines, and anti-serotonen agents, the SMSA was shown to be a slow reacting kinin-like substance.

The present study was carried out to determine plasma kininogen levels before and after stress so as to estimate the role played by the vasopeptide kinin system in this phenomenon.

MATERIALS AND METHODS

The research was conducted in 10 healthy, untrained males between the ages of 10-20 years. Each subject underwent a series of stress trials using the Dargatz cyclo-ergometer (13-14). The trials were rectangular tests of increasing intensity starting with 100 watts and increasing the power by 10 watts each session. Pre-stress conditions for the subjects included no food 4 hours before the test, light clothing dress, no cigarette smoking one hour before, no previous heavy work, a tranquil environment at temperature 15-20°C and humidity less than 70%. So as to obtain normal support of the feet on the pedals, the subject was required to keep the correct position on the cyclo-ergometer with control of the saddle height (6). Each trial lasted 30 minutes without the onset of pain. The above high intensity tests were carried out at 48 hour intervals till the critical stress state was achieved; i.e., when muscular pain in the limbs began to be felt in 10-20 minutes. The last test then was repeated during the following days at least twice to check the reproducibility of the phenomenon.

Both arterial and venous blood samples were drawn immediately before and after a critical stress period. Before the test, two polyethylene cannulae were fixed respectively in the radial artery and superficial vein of the forearm or of the elbow turn. With a plastic syringe containing 20 units/ml heparin, 10 ml of blood was withdrawn and placed into a pre-cooled polyethylene test tube. Hematocrit determinations were carried out on all blood samples. The blood samples were centrifuged for 20 minutes at 3000 rpm, the plasma collected in polyethylene tubes, and frozen immediately at lower than -20°C. At the time of kininogen assay, the plasmas were thawed by bringing to ambient temperature.

The assay was carried out in the following fashion:

The pH of 2.8 mls of the plasma (0.2 ml had been removed for bacteriologic studies) was adjusted to 7.3 - 7.8 by the addition of 0.06 ml / NaOH (if necessary, 1-2 drops of 1N HCl were added). The solution then was buffered at pH 7.8 with 0.5 ml Tris buffer, 0.2M. The resulting suspension was incubated with 0.2 mg crystalline trypsin (Worthington Labs., Freehold, N.J.) for 30 minutes at room temperature. Enzyme action was stopped by the addition of 5 ml boiling absolute ethanol. The tubes then were plunged in bain-marie at 70°C, and evaporated to dryness in Petri dishes at an oven temperature of 40° - 50°C.

Table 1

Plasma kininogen levels in patients before and after stress

Subject No.	Power (Watts)	Latent Period Of Pain Onset	PLASMA KININOGEN γ/ml			
			Arterial Blood		Venous Blood	
			N.V.	F.V.	N.V.	F.V.
1	104	12'26"	2.0	4.75	2.25	4.75
2	136	16'35"	2.50	3.75	2.50	5.00
3	115	18'05"	2.50	3.75	2.75	5.00
4	104	11'43"	2.50	3.50	2.50	4.50
5	115	14'38"	1.75	3.00	2.00	3.25
6	125	15'19"	2.00	3.50	2.25	4.05
7	104	12'30"	3.00	4.75	3.00	6.00
8	136	17'54"	2.25	4.00	2.50	4.25
9	115	19'00"	1.50	3.25	1.75	3.50
10	115	18'48"	2.75	4.50	2.75	5.00
M			2.275	3.875	2.425	4.575
DS			0.462	0.623	0.374	0.790
t			*	8.12 / o	1.271	8.63 / 2.802
P			*	< 0.001 / o	>0.10	< 0.001 / < 0.0125

* N.V. = Normal value (before stress)
   F.V. = Final value (after stress)

The material, suspended in 5 ml Ringer solution, was bioassayed for SMSA on the isolated perfused guinea pig ileum in accordance with established techniques. A 2 cm piece of ileum was used suspended in 5 ml of oxygenated Tyrode solution maintained at a 36°C temperature. The bath also contained 1 ml of diphenhydramine HCl (Benadryl, Park Davis, Chicago, Ill.) at a concentration of 10^{-8}g/ml, and 1 ml methyl sergide bimaleate (Sandoz, Hanover, N.J.) at a concentration of 10^{-9}g/ml per liter Tyrodes. Contractions were registered on a smoked kymograph after the addition of 0.1 ml of the preparation. Heights of contraction were compared to synthetic bradykinin (Sandoz) as a reference standard. The bath was washed after each test to restore the muscle to its previous state. A double ileum system was used and the results analyzed statistically.

RESULTS·

Table 1 and Figure 1 summarize the results. Listed in Table 1 are the single determinations of arterial and venous plasma kininogen values before (N.V.) and after (F.V.) the critical stress, the mean of the values, standard deviation, and t test. In Figure 1, the mean kininogen values of before and after stress are plotted. It

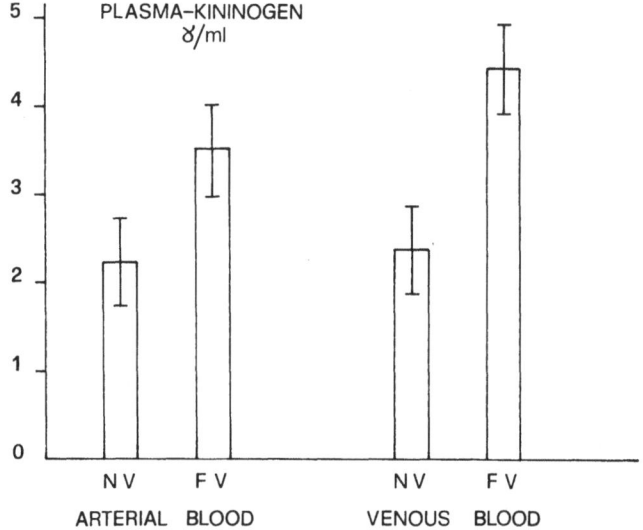

Figure 1. Graphic presentations of venous and arterial plasma kininogen levels in patients before and after stress.
N.V. = normal value (before stress)
F.V. = final value (after stress)

can be seen that before stress there was no difference in the plasma kininogen levels. However, after stress, the concentration of kininogen in both the venous and arterial blood increased with generally higher levels in the venous blood.

DISCUSSION AND CONCLUSIONS

The study has demonstrated that there was no significant difference in the plasma kininogen levels between the arterial and venous blood. In the condition in which the subject is required to perform work resulting in muscle pain, there occured a frank significant increase in both arterial and venous plasma kininogen levels. Furthermore, this increase was greater in the venous blood than arterial blood.

It is hoped that this data might provide some interpretation and explanation for the muscle pain due to stress.

REFERENCES

1. Vecchiet,L., Fini,F., Branzi,G.C., Matassi,L.; Med. Sport, 9, 223, 1969.

2. Vecchiet,L., Matassi, L., Buzzelli, G., Fini, F., Branzi, G.C.; Sett. Med., 56, 823, 1968.

3. Argent, D.E., Armstrong, D., Jepson, J.B., Keele, C.A., Phillips, L.A.; J. Physiol., 124, 18, 1954.

4. Armstrong, D., Jepson, J.B., Keele, C.A., Stewart, J.W.; J. Physiol., 129, 80, 1955.

5. Galletti, R., Marra, N., Vecchiet, L.; Rass Neurol. Veg., 15, 200, 1960.

6. Marra, N., Vecchiet, L., Galletti, R.,; Rass. Neurol. Veg., 15, 227, 1960.

7. Armstrong, D., Jepson, J.B., Keele, C.A., Stewart , J.W., 135, 350, 1957.

8. Margolis, J.,; Ann. N.Y. Acad. Sci., 104, 133, 1963.

9. Lewis, G.P.; Metabolism, 13, 1256, 1964.

10. Keele, C.A., Armstrong, D.; "Substances producing pain and itch". Arnold E., London 1964.

11. Zachariae H., Malmquist, J., Cates, J.A.; J. Physiol., <u>190</u>, 81, 1967.

12. Masson, P.L.; La Ricerca, <u>2</u>, 389, 1972.

13. Vecchiet, L., D-lce, V., Fini, F., Branzi, G.C.; Sports Med., <u>13</u>, 3, 1973.

14. Vecchiet, L., Dolce, V., Fini, F., Branzi, G.C.; Medecine du Sport, <u>2</u>, 46, 1972.

PROGRESS ON BIOCHEMICAL URINARY KALLIKREIN TEST

G. Porcelli

Centro Chimica Recettori

Ist. Chimica, Fac. Med. Universita Cattolica, Roma

In the last few years researches on the clinical implications of human urinary kallikrein, were extensively developed by the methods of Beaven,et al (1), Trautschold and Werle (2), and Siegelman, et al. (3).

In all those methods the catalysing power of kallikrein esterase activity to hydrolyse synthetic substrates, such as Benzoyl-Arginine-Methyl-Ester (B.A.M.E.), Benzoyl-Arginine-Ethyl-Ester (B.A.E.E.) and Tosyl-Arginine-Methyl-Ester (T.A.M.E.), was measured from the quantity of liberated methanol or ethanol.

Two moments of the enzymatic hydrolysis are considered in those methods, the initial and the final steps.

According to Schwert and Takenaka (4), spectrophotometric measurement of BAEE hydrolysis at 253 nm consents to determine continuously the esterasic kinetics, and this system is generally adopted for biological liquids.

After some experience in this field (5), we have developed about 3 years ago, a new method to assay esterase activity of human urinary kallikrein, using BAEE as substrate and controlling in all instances the enzymatic kinetic spectrophotometrically.

MATERIALS AND METHODS

We have used BAEE "Cyclo Chemical U.S.A.", 18/32 dialysis membranes Scientific Instrument Centre Ltd. All chemicals were reagent grade.

Apparatus: spectrophotometric measurements were taken with Beckman, "ACTA III-C" with cuvettes set by LAUDA Ultrathermostat at 25°C. Centrifugation were performed with refrigerated centrifuge "Christ".

Buffer solution: enzymatic determinations were made in TRIS-HCl 0.1 M at 8.0 pH.

Preparation of urine samples and spectrophotometric measurement: 100 ml of -10°C acetone were added to 50 ml of a 24 hr. urine sample. The solution thus obtained was poured in equal amounts into 2 - 100 ml centrifuge tubes and left standing 30' in refrigerator: After centrifugation at 5,000 rpm for 15', 5 ml of H_2O were added to the precipitate and then 1 ml of cold acetone.

This turbid solution, poured in a 7 ml centrifuge tube after centrifugation at 5,000 rpm for 15' yielded a clear solution which was then dialyzed against running water for 20 hours.

The opalescence which resulted from the dialysis was removed by centrifugation at 8,000 rpm for 30' and after measuring the exact volume, esterase activity was determined on 1 ml of the solution.

The following solutions were prepared for spectrophotometric measurements of kallikrein esterase: a mixture made up of 2 ml of buffer, 0,5 ml of a solution $3X\ 10^{-3}$ M of BAEE dissolved in the same buffer and 1 ml of H_2O was poured in the reference cuvette. A similar mixture was poured in the sample cuvette, replacing 1 ml of H_2O with 1 ml of the final extract of the urine sample.

Kallikrein esterase often exhibits a latency period before kinetics becomes constant. Hence spectrophotometric measurement of enzymatic activity is performed both graphically and on digital with control at first.

Once the enzymatic activity has become stable, the digital control of D.O. increment at 253 mμ for 5' is enough.

Esterase Units of the urine sample: the following formula is used to determine kallikrein amount in esterase units contained in the urine sample:

$$\frac{\Delta\ O.D._s. \times V._{f.e.} \times V_{tot.}}{\Delta\ O.D._{st.} \times T \times V_s.} =$$

where $\Delta O.D._s$.   is O.D. increment at 253 nm of the sample;

$V_{f.e}$ is the volume of the final urine extract;

V_{tot} is the volume of 24 hr. urine;

$\Delta O.D._{st}$.   is the O.D. increment at 253 nm of a highly purified sample of urinary kallikrein isolated from 100 lt of human urine (6) and of another sample of the same enzyme prepared according to the technique described in (5) from 5 lt of human urine. Such value is = 0.014 and is equivalent to a O.D. increment at 253 nm which results from hydrolysis of 0.05 µMoles of BAEE/min;

T   is the time in minutes for spectrophotometric measurement of constant kinetics;

V_s is the volume of urine sample taken for the analysis (50 ml).

RESULTS AND DISCUSSION

The handicap to determine spectrophotometrically the esterase activity of urinary kallikrein by BAEE, was always the high absorbance of urinary sample at 253 nm.

Our successful direct urinary esterase assay on BAEE depends largely on performance of the spectrophotometer used which consents to determine, for an optical density up to 1.500 at 253 nm, 0.001 increments per minute for about one hour and with considerable accuracy.

With this method the amount of kallikrein in a sample of 24 hours urine of healthy male subject, aged 35, ranged between 24 and 27 E.U./24 hr.

Urinary kallikrein in normal woman, 27 yrs. old, assayed every 5-6 days, presents significant variations related to the menstrual cycle: i.e. marked increases in enzyme excretion during the ovulatory and premenstrual periods.

Figure 1 shows Kallikrein E.U./lt. of first sample of morning urine in the same normal subject (age 21 years) during the menstruation cycle.

A sample of 24-hour urine tested ten times was reproducible with an average deviation of less than o.1%.

Table 1

Kinetics on Digital System for Essential Hypertensive Patients

Patient number	Δ O.D. 0'-5'	Δ O.D. 5'-10'	Δ O.D. 10'-15'	E.U. 0'-5'	E.U. 5'-10'	E.U. 10'-15'
1	0,000	0,000	0,000	0	0	0
2	-0,028	0,000	0,002	Neg.	0	3
3	0,004	0,008	0,008	5	10	10
4	0,004	0,007	0,005	9	15	11
5	-0,009	0,000	0,004	Neg.	0	14
6	-0,100	-0,021	-0,001	Neg.	Neg.	Neg.
7	0,000	0,000	0,003	0	0	6
8	0,000	0,003	0,001	0	3	1
9	0,007	0,006	0,004	13	10	7
10	0,014	0,018	0,016	48	61	55
11	0,002	0,003	0,004	3	5	6
12	-0,032	-0,004	0,000	Neg.	Neg.	0
13	-0,044	-0,001	0,002	Neg.	Neg.	2
14	0,006	0,010	0,010	5	9	9
15	0,011	0,009	0,010	33	27	30

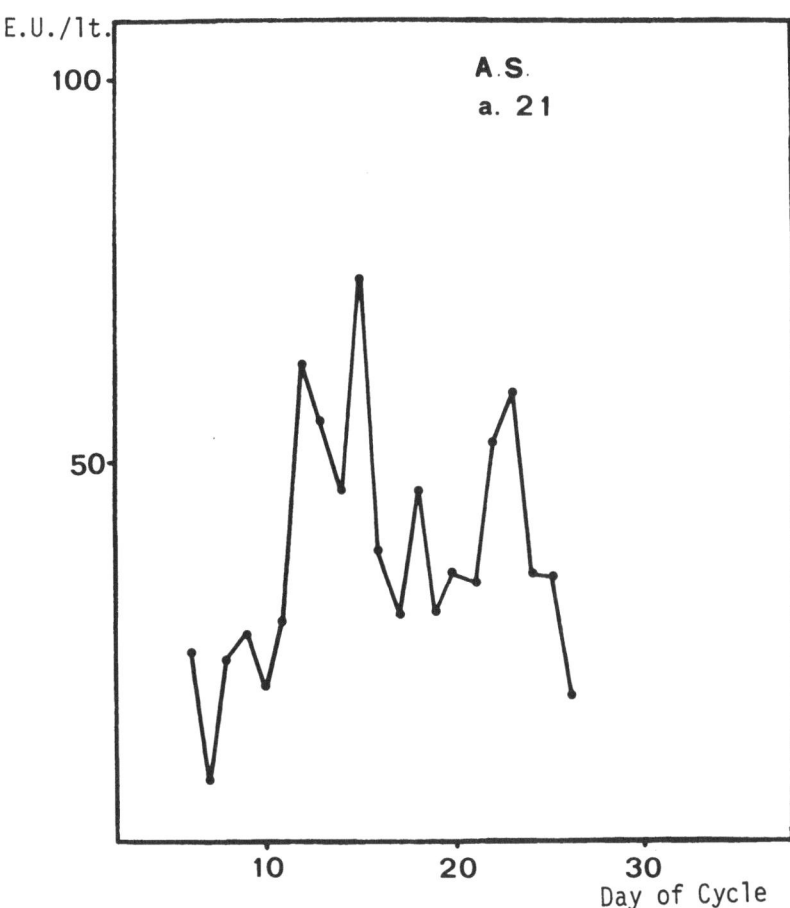

Figure 1. First sample of morning urine in the same normal subject, aged 21 years, during the menstruation cycle. Amount of kallikrein in E.U./lt.

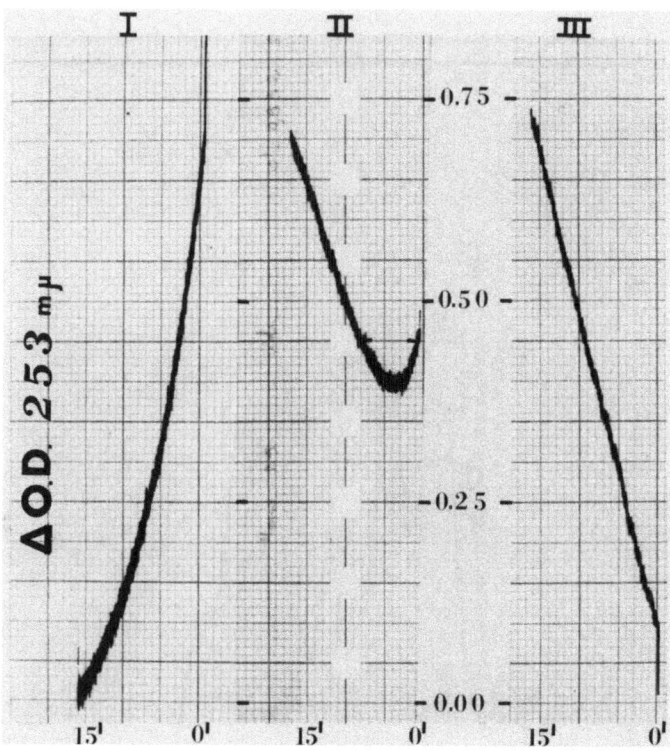

Figure 2. Kinetics hydrolysis of BAEE by the respective urinary extracts of three different subjects. (I) Corresponding to an essential hypertension patient: instead of going up, the kinetics decreases. (II) Corresponding to a patient who was diagnosed essential hypertension, but whose blood pressure was normal when the sample of urine was taken for the assay. (III) Corresponding to a normal person.

Urinary kallikrein, measured with this method, decreased in subjects with essential hypertension (7).

A significant lower kallikrein activity in the urine spontaneously hypertensive rats as compared to the normotensive ones was evidenced also (8).

For urine sample of essential hypertensive subjects the spectrophotometric measurement of urinary kallikrein kinetics is particularly advantageous.

At this subject Figure 2 shows the kinetic curves at 253 nm of BAEE hydrolysis with final urinary extracts of three different subjects.

In Table 1 are reported kinetic measurements on digital system of BAEE hydrolysis at 253 nm with final urinary extract of several hypertensive patients.

ΔO.D. at 253 nm for patient number 2,5,6,7,12 and 13 in the first five minutes is negative and then variable.

For other samples the O.D. increments are very low, except for n°10 and n°15 whose diagnosis of essential hypertension was in contrast with results. Successive renographyes in those patients have evidence renal diseases.

The new method described in this paper was developed in our laboratory about three years ago, and never raised any problem as far as urine samples of normal and pathologic subjects were concerned. It is easy to execute and provides accurate results, which makes it competitive with the other methods.

When a highly purified sample of kallikrein, prepared from 100 lt of human urine (6) or when a semi-purified sample of the same enzyme prepared according to the same technique (5) from 5 lt of urine, hydrolyses 1.5 Moles of BAEE an O.D. increment of 0.420 at 253 nm was obtained. This value related to the hydrolysis of 0.05 moles of substrate is equivalent to O.D. increment of 0,014 which is arbitrarily defined as Esterase Unit of human urinary kallikrein. The Esterase Unit (E.U.) is equivalent to about 7.4 Frey Units.

During spectrophotometric measurement of urinary kallikrein it is essential to check that kinetics be constant. Latency times, before the enzymatic hydrolysis becomes constant vary from one individual to another; at times it takes less than 1 minute from the start of measurement, occasionally it may take 5'.

Thus, paper recording combined with digital reading is suggested to confirm the linear character of the kinetics.

REFERENCES

1. Beaven V.H., Pierce J.V., Pisano J.J., Clin. Chim. Acta, <u>32</u>, 67 (1971)
2. Trautschold I., Werle E., Hoppe-Seyler Z. Physiol. Chem. <u>325</u> 48 (1961)
3. Siegelman A.M., Carlson A.S., Robertson T., Arch. Biochem. and Biophys. <u>97</u>, 159 (1962)
4. Schwert G.W., Takenaka Y., Biochim. Biophys. Acta, <u>16</u>, 570 (1955)
5. Porcelli G., Corxatto R.H., Porcelli F., Adv. Exper. Med. and Biol., <u>21</u>, 135 (1972)
6. Porcelli G., Marini-Bettolo G.B., Croxatto R.H., Di Iorio M., Ital. J. Biochem. <u>23</u>, 44 (1974)
7. Greco A.V., Porcelli G., Croxatto R.H., Ghirlanda G., Min. Med. <u>65</u>, 3058 (1974)
8. Porcelli G., Bianchi G., Croxatto R.H., Proc. Soc. Exptl. Biol. Med. <u>149</u>, 983 (1975)

BIOCHEMICAL ACTIONS OF FIBROBLAST KININ-FORMING PROTEASE (1)*

Hsin C. Li, William F. McLimans*, and Nathan Back

Department of Biochemical Pharmacology, School of
Pharmacy, State University of New York and Department
of Cell Physiology*, Roswell Park Memorial Institute,
Buffalo, New York

Both a neutral (1) and acid (2,3) protease capable of forming
kinins from a variety of mammalian substrates have been isolated
and purified from the transplanted rodent Murphy-Sturm lymphosarcoma (MSLS). The MSLS tissue was comprised of a neterogeneous
population of tumor cells and fibroblasts. Initial studies with
a pure cell line of mouse fibroblasts grown in stationary cell
culture identified the presence of a kinin-forming protease active
optimally at pH 4.0.

In a continuing investigation into chemical mediators (with
specific reference to protease kinin-forming systems) in neoplastic
tissue, the kinin-forming acid protease from the rodent fibroblast
L-929 was isolated in large quantity, purified, and various biochemical parameters studied.

METHODS AND RESULTS

Cell Culture

One hundred mls (6×10^5 cells/ml) of mouse fibroblast cells
L-929 were cultured continously in Spinner flasks in Minimum
Essential Medium containing 10% fetal calf serum and 0.4% lactal-
bumin. The pH was controlled automatically between pH 7.2 - 7.48
and cell population maintained between 2000,000 - 1×10^6 cell/ml

(1)*
Supported in part by USPHS grant #HE-11492

medium. Cell viability, determined by trypan blue exclusion test
(5), was estimated between 85-98%.

Initial Isolation

For the initial isolation studies, 300-500 mg of L929 cells
were centrifuged at 3000 rpm, sonicated 5 times for 1½ minutes
each time, centrifuged for 15 minutes at 10,000 rpm, and the supernatant dialyzed for 48 hours against a 0.01 M phosphate buffer,
pH 6.8, 0.1 M NaCl, 1mM EDTA. Eighteen mls was obtained with a
protein concentration of 5.9 mg/ml. Initial protease activity was
measured on a denatured hemoglobin substrate by incubating 2 ml of
the supernatant with 4 ml of the substrate for 60 minutes. After
addition of 4 mls 10% trichloracetic acid and filtration through
a Whatman #1 filter, absorption readings were made on a Gilford
spectrophotometer at 28 mµ. Appropriate control tubes were run
and gave an extinction reading of 0.914 while the sonicated dialysate tubes read at an E of 1.097. An active protease thus was
confirmed. Incubation of the dialysate with rat plasma resulted
in a carboxy-peptidase-sensitive smooth muscle stimulating activity
as measured on the isolated perfused rat uterus.

Purification on a G-200 Sephadex Column (2.5x90cm). 10^9 cells
were homogenized for 8 minutes, the homogenate dialyzed 18 hours
against a 0.01 M phosphate buffer, pH 6.8 in 0.1 M NaCl, 1mM EDTA,
and centrifuged 45 minutes at 12,000 rpm. The protein concentration was 6.38 mg/ml. The dialysate was placed onto the G-200
Sephadex column and the eluent fractions assayed for kinin-forming
activity as described previously (4). The specific activity,
calculated in terms of ng bradykinin per mg protein preparation
using synthetic bradykinin as the reference standard, was 520.7 ng/
mg from the pooled fractions 25-41 with a 99% yield. The specific
activity of the initial L929 dialysate was 220.5 ng/mg; thus, a
2.4 fold purification was achieved.

Purification on Hydroxylapatite Column (2x30 cm). 17 ml of
the above preparation, 3.8 mg/ml, was applied onto a hydroxylapatite
column equilibrated with an 0.01 M phosphate buffer, pH 6.8,
0.1 M NaCl, 1mM EDTA linear gradient was used after the first peak
was eluted and eluents assayed for kinin-forming activity found in
fractions 49-64. The pooled fractions, concentrated to 20 ml, had
a specific activity of 649.0 ng/mg, a 25% yield with a 2.9 fold
purification.

Cysteine Activation. The hydroxylapatite-purified protease
(0.65 mg protein/ml) was dialyzed for 18 hours at 4° against 500 ml
of 0.01 M phosphate buffer, 0.1 M KCl containing 5 mM cysteine.
This increased the specific activity from 649.0 to 1064.8 ng kinin
per mg protein.

Purification on DEAE-A50 Ion Exchange Column (1x20 cm). The
cysteine-activated protease solution (11 ml, 0.73 mg/ml) was applied
onto a DEAE-A50 column equilibrated with 0.01 M phosphate buffer,
0.1 M KCl and 2.5 mM mercaptoethanol. The initial eluating buffer
was 50 ml of the 0.01 M phosphate buffer followed by 150 ml of the
equilibrating buffer and then a linear gradient of 0.01 M phosphate
buffer, 1.0 M KCl, 2.5 mM mercaptoethanol. The specific activity
of the enzyme eluated (0.73 mg/ml) from the column first without
applying a salt gradient was 2062.5 ng/mg, a 9.4 fold purification
with a final yield of 14%.

Purification of rat plasma kininogen. For further pH profile
and enzyme kinetic studies, rat plasma kininogen was isolated and
purified from rat plasma applied onto a DEAE-A50 column (25x30 cm)
and onto a G-100 Sephadex column (2.5x90 cm). A major peak was
found in fractions 55-63 from the DEAE-A50 column with a specific
activity of 77.4 ng bradykinin/mg protein. The fractions 15-17
from the Sephadex column following application of both protein
peaks from the previous column yielded a specific activity of 112.2
ng bradykinin/mg protein.

Molecular Weight Determinations of Protease and Kininogen.
Both the purified acid protease and kininogen were subjected to
Sephadex G-200 gel filtration for molecular weight determination.
The columns (1x57 cm) were calibrated with the following known
molecular weight markers: aldolase, ovalbumin, chymotrypsinogen,
ribonuclease. The void volume (Vo) was determined with dextran
blue. The total column volume (V_t) was calculated on the basis
of the column height and elution volume (Ve) values determined
by applying the standards and test preparations onto the columns
and pooling the eluent from the first tube to the maximum peak
consecutively. Peak maxima for the test preparations were determined by appropriate bioassay technique. The partition coefficient
(Kav) thus was able to be calculated. The molecular weight for
the acid protease was estimated at 39,000 while the molecular
weight for the peak II kininogen was estimated at 110,000.

pH Profile for Acid Protease. The pH profile for the kinin-
forming activity of the DEAE-A50 purified acid protease on the
purified rat kininogen substrate was determined in a pH solution
ranging from 1.0 - 12.0. The incubation mixture, consisting of
0.2 ml of the kininogen (1.76 mg/ml) 0.2 ml of the acid protease
(0.60 mg/ml) and 0.3 ml of the respective buffer, was incubated for
15 hours at 37°, then boiled for 15 minutes, neutralized to pH 7.8
with 0.2 ml 1.0 M Tris buffer, and assayed for kinin. The effective
pH range was quite narrow (3-5) with the optimum at 4.0. At
pH 4.0, 137 ng kinin/mg substrate per mg enzyme was generated.

Kinin Release with Respect to Enzyme Concentration and Time.
The kinin released from 0.075 mg kininogen following incubation at
pH 4.0 with acid protease concentrations ranging from 0.019 mg to
0.120 mg for 0.5, 1, 2, 4, and 8 hours respectively was studied.
With a fixed substrate concentration, kinin formed was directly
proportional to the enzyme concentration. Thus, following 8 hours
of incubation, 0.012 mg of enzyme formed 9.0 ng kinin, 0.038 mg
of enzyme formed 4.0 ng kinin, and 0.019 mg of enzyme formed 1.75
ng kinin.

Subcellular localization of acid protease activity. Ultra-
centrifugal cell fraction was carried out with a dialyzed homogenate
of 10^9 cells. The precipitate 1500 g fraction was collected after
15 minutes centrifugation. The 10,000 g precipitate was obtained
after 20 minutes centrifugation of the supernatant. The resulting
supernatant was identified as the extralysosomal fraction. The
respective fractions were reconstituted in 0.01 M phosphate buffer,
pH 6.8 and protease kinin-forming activity determined by incubating
aliquots together with rat plasma containing 1,10-phenanthroline
and Trasylol. Kinin formed was assayed on the isolated rat uterus.
The major portion of the protease activity (61.5%) was in the 10,000
g cell supernatant fraction (calculated at the end of 48 hours incubation). The 1500 g precipitate fraction contained 38.5% of the
activity.

DISCUSSION

The present study provides additional information regarding the
kinin-forming protease in rodent fibroblasts (4). The protease was
purified 10-fold by gel filtration and ion-exchange column techniques.
Optimum activity was achieved at pH 4.0. Kinin formation was
enzyme concentration-dependent. The apparent molecular weight
of the protease was found to be approximately 39,000, agreeing
closely to 37,000 found for spleen cathepsin D (6) and 36,000 for
muscle cathepsin D (7). Similar to rabbit lysosomal acid protease
(8) and the Murphy-Sturm lymphosarcoma kinin-forming acid protease
(2), the fibroblast protease was activated by 5mM cysteine. The
similarity between this acid protease kinin-forming system and that
found in rabbit polymorphonuclear leukocytes (9) has been discussed
previously (4). The major difference between these two proteases
is the site of cellular localization.

The purified rat plasma kininogen molecular weight was
estimated by G-200 Sephadex column technique to be 110,000. The
literature apparently does not record any previous molecular weight
studies with rat plasma kininogen. As reported initially by
Jacobsen (10), rat plasma does contain two molecular species of

kininogen. Jacobsen and Kriz (11) subsequently estimated the high molecular weight of human kininogen (I) to be 108,000 ± 10,000.

Fibroblast proliferation occurs at the transplant site during the initial growth phase following tumor transplantation (12). Fibroblasts localized between the growing edges and necrotic areas of solid tumor transplants were found by histochemical techniques, to contain a cathepsin-like activity (13). During regression of the rodent Jensen sarcoma, cathepsin levels in the growing region of the tumor were higher than those in non-regressing tumors (14). It has been suggested that the invasiveness of human gynecological tumors may be associated with cathepsin-like enzyme activity (15). Thus, while the functional role of fibroblasts and associated protease activity is obscure, evidence does suggest some involvement in tumor invasiveness, regression, and connective tissue proliferation.

SUMMARY

Purification and further characterization of a kinin-forming acid protease in a mouse fibroblast L929 stationary cell culture line was carried out. Supernatants of dialyzed fibroblast homogenates digested denatured hemoglobin at pH 4.0. The supernatant was fractionated on a G-200 Sephadex column, hydroxylapatite column and finally on a DEAE-A50 Sephadex ion exchange column. A 9.4 fold purification was achieved with a 13.8% yield. The enzyme had a specific activity of 2062 ng kinin per mg protein when measured on a purified rat kininogen using the isolated rat uterus as the bioassay tissue. The protease had a pH optimum of 3.8-4.0. Molecular weights of the enzyme and substrate estimated on a G-200 Sephadex column were 39,000 and 110,000 respectively. Kinin formation was a function of both incubation time and enzyme concentration. Protease activity was localized primarily in the 10,000 g supernatant cell fraction (61.5%) with the 1500 g precipitate cell fraction containing 38.5% of the activity.

REFERENCES

1. N. Back and R. Steger. in Bradykinin and Related Peptides. Adv. Exptl. Med. & Biol. 8, Eds. F. Sicuteri, M Rocha e Silva, & N. Back, pg. 225, 1970.

2. N. Back & R. Steger, in Vasopeptides: Chemistry, Pharmacology, and Pathophysiology. Adv. Exptl. Med. & Biol. 21. Eds. N. Back & F. Sicuteri. pg. 417, 1972.

3. J.H. Ihm, R. Steger, & N. Back. Fed. Proc. 34: 508, 1975.

4. N. Back & R. Steger. Proc. Soc. Exp. Biol. Med. 143: 769, 1973.

5. A.M. Pappenheimer, J. Exp. Med. 25: 633, 1917.

6. V. Turk, I. Kreger, F. Gubensek & P. Lebez, Enzymologia 36: 182, 1969.

7. K. Fukushima, G.H. Gnoh, & S. Shinano. Agri. Biol. Chem. 35: 1495, 1971.

8. S. Wasi, R. Murray, D. MacMorine, & H. Movat. Brit. J. Exp. Pathol. 47: 411, 1966.

9. L. M. Greenbaum, R. Freer, J. Chang, G. Semento, and K. Yamafuji. Brit. J. Pharmacol. 36: 623, 1960.

10. S. Jacobsen, Brit. J. Pharmacol. 28: 64, 1966.

11. S. Jacobsen and M. Kriz. Brit. J. Pharmacol. 29: 25, 1967.

12. H. Grossfeld, M.L. Crossley, & J.B. Allison, Cancer Res. 23: 770, 1963.

13. R. Hess, Cancer Res. 20: 940, 1960.

14. R.F. Kampschmidt and D. Wells. Cancer Res. 28: 1938, 1968.

15. C.E. Blackwood, I. Mandl, and M. E. Long, Am. J. Obst. & Gynec. 91: 419, 1965.

ADRENERGIC AND CHOLINERGIC CONTROL OF THE ACTIVATION OF THE KALLI-KREIN-KININ SYSTEM IN THE RAT BLOOD

A.M. Rothschild, J.C. Gomes and A. Castania

Department of Pharmacology, School of Medicine of

Ribeirao Preto, USP, Brazil

Sympathomimetic amines activate the kallikrein system of rat blood, causing up to 50% lowering of kininogen, transient kinin release and transient benzoyl arginine ethyl ester (BAEE) hydrolase activity. The action of catecholamines mimics and could be a model for the study of kallikrein activation and kinin release observed following nerve stimulation (Hilton & Lewis [1], Gautvik, Kriz, Lund-Learsen and Waaler [2], Inoki, Toyoda & Yamamoto [3], Turker & Turker [4], Inoki, Hayashi, Kudo, Matsumoto & Yamamoto [5]). Catecholamine activation of the kininogen-consuming process has the following characteristics:

a) reproducible in vitro in rat whole oxaleted blood (6);
b) not obtained in cell-free plasma nor in plasma containing either platelets, eosinophils, lymphocytes or erythrocytes (7);
c) effectiveness: epinephrine > nor-epinephrine; isoprenaline ineffective, does not block the action of epinephrine (6);
d) inhibited by either alpha or beta-adrenergic antagonists, the former being more potent (6);
e) inhibited by acetylsalicylic acid (Aspirin), bovine kallikrein inhibitor (Trasylol) or soy bean trypsin inhibitor (SBTI) (6,7).
f) reproducible in rat plasma treated with rat peritoneal fluid cell (PFC) suspensions exposed to epinephrine for 2 min.; not obtained with untreated PFC; after activation by epinephrine, PFC can be centrifuged and washed without loss of their acquired activity (8);
g) not obtained when PFC free of mast cells are added to plasma in the presence of epinephrine (8);
h) inhibited by dibutyril cyclic-AMP, 5×10^{-5}M (9);

i) possibly associated with mast cell vacuolization and intracellular granule retraction, a phenomenon observed in epinephrine
or nor-epinephrine-treated rat mesentery mast cells (10) which
is inhibited by Aspirin (8), at the same concentrations which
block kininogen depletion;

j) epinephrine activation of kallikrein in the presence of
PFC is not accompanied by the release of histamine from such cells.
Increased amounts of histamine are however observed in the tissues
of epinephrine-treated rats (11, 12); they are to be attributed
to enhanced, short-term synthesis of histamine induced by epinephrine, (Rosengren & Svensson) (13);

k) kininogen depletion and mast cell vacuolization apparently
identical to those produced by catecholamines, are shown in rats
treated with carbamylcholine, a cholinergic agonist. The effect
on kininogen can also be shown in vitro, in oxalated blood incubated for 5 min. with carbamylcholine. This excludes reflexly
released catecholamines as mediators of kallikrein activation in
carbamylcholine treated rats.

In conclusion: a kininogen-consuming, kallikrein-activating
and, in those instances in which it has been looked for (8, 14),
Kinin-generating system, is activated in rat blood by either adrenergic or cholinergic agonists. The system bears a resemblance
to the immunogenic SRS-A and histamine releasing system of human
lung (15), which is also activated by alpha-adrenergic or cholinergic agonists and exhibits a negative sensitivity to cyclic-AMP.
It is to be noted however, that kallikrein-activation by epinephrine in the intact rat occurs without concomitant release of histamine.

The nature of the cellular activating process which precedes
the formation of kallikrein probably via pre-kallikrein activation,
remains unknown. Preliminary experiments indicate sensitivity
to Trasylol but not to SBTI, even though plasma kininogen
depletion induced by epinephrine in whole blood is inhibited by
the soy bean blocker which probably acts on kallikrein proper.
Other data, obtained with peritoneal fluid cells treated with
epinephrine have failed to reveal increased activity of such cells
on acetyltyrosine ethyl ester (ATEE) and no acquired ability to
hydrolyse BAEE or ALME (acetylysin ethyl ester) or AGLME (acetyl-
glycil-lysil methyl ester), respectively plasmin and plasminogen
activator substrates.

REFERENCES

1. Hilton, S.M., Lewis, G.P.: The relationships between glandular
    activity, bradykinin formation, and functional vasodilation
    in the submandibular salivary gland. J. Physiol. (Lon.)
    134: 471-478 (1956).

2. Gautvik, K., Kriz, M., Lund-Larsen, K., Waaler, B.A.: Sympa-
    thetic vasodilation, kallikrein release and adrenergic
    receptors in the cat submandibular salivary gland. Acta
    physiol. scand. 90, 438-444 (1974).

3. Inoki, R., Toyoda, T., & Yamamoto, I.: Elaboration of a Brady-
    kinin-like Substance in dog's canine pulp during electrical
    stimulation. Naunyn-Schmiedegerg's Arch. Pharm. 279, 387-398
    (1973).

4. Turker, M.N. and Turker, R.K.: A study on the peripheral
    mediators of dental pain. Experientia 30, 932-933 (1974).

5. Inoki, R., Hayashi, T., Kudo, K., Matsumoto, K., & Yamamoto,
    I.: Effect of analgesics on the release of bradykinin-like
    substance and kinin forming enzyme in rat's paw. Comm. VI
    Intern. Congr. Pharmacol., Helsinki, 1975.

6. Castania, A., Rothschild, A.M.: Lowering of kininogen in rat
    blood by adrenaline. Inhibition by sympatholytic agents,
    heparin and aspirin. Brit. J. Pharmacol. 50, 375-383 (1974).

7. Rothschild, A.M., Cordeiro, R.S.B., Castania, A.: Lowering
    of kininogen in rat blood by catecholamines. Involvement
    of non-eosinophil granulocytes and selective inhibition by
    Trasylol. Naunyn-Schmiedeberg's Arch. Pharmacol. 282,
    323-327 (1974).

8. Rothschild, A.M., Castania, A., Cordeiro, R.S.B.: Consumption
    of kininogen, formation of kinin and activation of arginine
    ester hydrolase in rat plasma by rat peritoneal fluid cells
    in the presence of l-adrenaline. Naunyn-Schmiedeberg's Arch.
    Pharmacol. 285, 243-256 (1974).

9. Rothschild, A.M.: Mechanism of action of Aspirin. Comm. VI
    Intern. Congr. Pharmacol. Helsinki, 1975.

10. Oliveira Antonio, M.P., Rothschild, A.M.: Effects of cate-
    cholamines on rat mesentery mast cells. Nature (Lond), 218,
    382-384 (1968).

11. Oliveira Antonio, M.P., Fernandes, F., Rothschild, A.M.:
    Increased lung histamine content and mast cell degranulation
    evoked by epinephrine in the rat. V. Intern. Congress
    Pharmacol. Abstracts Volunt. Papers, p. 8, San Francisco,
    1972.

12. Gomes, J.C. and Rothschild, A.M., unpublished.

13. Rosengren, E. and Svensson, S.E.: Histamine formation in rat gastric mucosa and lung after injecting reserpine or adrenaline. Br. J. Pharmac. 37, 659-665 (1969).

14. Cordeiro, R.S.B., Doctoral Dissertation, Ribeirao preto, 1975.

15. Kaliner, M., Orange, R.P. and Austen, K.F.: Immunological release of histamine and slow reacting substance of anaphylaxis from human lung. J. exp. Med. 136, 556-567 (1972).

Aided by Fundacao de Amparo a Pesquisa do Estado de Sao Paulo (FAPESP), Grant 73/685.

PREKALLIKREIN AND KALLIKREIN INHIBITOR IN LIVER CIRRHOSIS AND

HEPATITIS

Fanciullacci M., Galli P., Monetti M.G., Pela I., and
Del Bianco, P.L.

Department of Clinical Pharmacology
University of Florence, Italy

Direct animal evidence has demonstrated that plasma kininogen
and prekallikrein (kallikreinogen) are synthesized in the liver (1,
2). In the human too, some components of the kallikrein-kinin
system are probably synthesized in the liver. In hepatic cirrhosis,
plasma kininogen was lowered, while it was found at a normal level
in viral hepatitis (3). Besides this, a reduced plasma algogenic
and kinin activity was also reported in cirrhosis (4,5).

Probably, prekallikrein is also produced in the liver. Severe
parenchimal liver diseases, such as cirrhosis, hepatic lymphoma,
and acute hepatitis, were associated with low levels of plasma
kallikrein (6,7).

In aiming to obtain further information on the kallikreinogen-
kallikrein enzyme system in an occurence of serious hepatic damage,
the plasma prekallikrein and kallikrein inhibitor have been evaluated
in patients with hepatic cirrhosis and acute icteric viral hepatitis.

MATERIAL AND METHODS

Plasma prekallikrein and kallikrein inhibitor have been evaluated with the kaolin-contact method (8,9,10). The kaolin activated arginine esterase activity found with this technique has
been shown to be related to plasma kallikrein activity. 20 patients
hospitalized for cirrhosis of the liver, ranging from 43 to 78 years
of age, were studied. Altogether, 30 determinations have been
evaluated in cirrhosis before therapy. The measurements have been
assayed in all patients as soon as hospitalized, and in 10 patients,
the determination was repeated two days later. After a month of

conventional therapy, the assays were repeated once again in these 10 patients. In addition, 12 patients hospitalized following acute icteric viral hepatitis were also observed. Plasma prekallikrein and kallikrein inhibitor were measured in these patients immediately upon hospitalization, and in 10 patients, the dosages were repeated two days later, but before therapy. Altogether 22 determinations were carried out. During the first month of the disease, in 3 cases of hepatitis treated with levulose infusions, serum bilirubin and transaminases, as well as plasma prekallikrein and kallikrein inhibitor were assayed every 5 to 7 days. As controls, 9 healthy volunteers, from 25 to 48 years of age were studied.

RESULTS

1.) In the normal group, plasma levels of prekallikrein and kallikrein inhibitor resulted similar to those previously reported (8,9, 11,12).

2.) The spontaneous plasma arginine esterase activity was not statistically different from normals in both cirrhosis and hepatitis patients.

3.) In cirrhosis, the average of all samples collected before therapy indicated that, when compared with normals, the plasma prekallikrein level is statistically lower (Table 1, Fig. 1). Also arginine esterase activity obtained 5 minutes after kaolin contact resulted statistically lowered. However, the decrease was proportional to that of the prekallikrein; and the inhibitor, when considered in unit value, is not statistically different from the normals (Table 2). After a month of conventional therapy, the prekallikrein and kallikrein inhibitor increased about 15%; however, the difference of the levels before and after therapy was not statistically significant.

4.) In the viral hepatitis group, a statistically low level of prekallikrein was also observed (Table 1., Fig. 2). The kallikrein inhibitor was not statistically different from normals (Table 2). The patients studied for a month showed a progressive increase of prekallikrein by about 100%. The increase of prekallikrein constantly corresponded to a decrease of serum bilirubin and transaminases (Fig. 3).

5.) Prekallikrein in hepatitis was a little higher than in cirrhosis but the difference was not statistically significant.

6.) In both cirrhosis and hepatitis, the first determination of plasma prekallikrein and kallikrein inhibitor yielded the same results as those obtained two days later.

TABLE 1

Plasma Prekallikrein

Groups	n⁰ Patients	n⁰ Det.	* Prekallikrein (moles/ml/hr)	P value
Normal	9	9	98 ± 4	--
Hepatic cirrhosis	20	30	35 ± 6	< 0.001
Hepatitis	12	22	46 ± 6	< 0.001

* - Mean ± S.E.

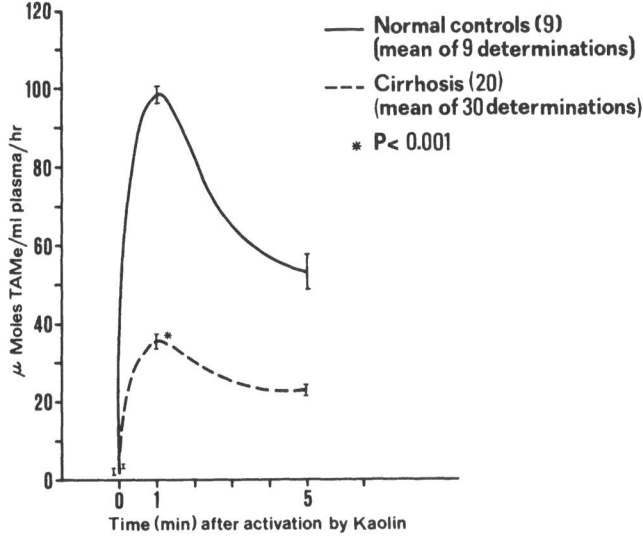

Figure 1. The plasma of the cirrhosis patients exhibits a statistically reduced ability to activate esterase at 1 minute from the kaolin contact, in comparison with normal subjects. The esterase activity at 5 minutes from plasma kaolin contact also appears statistically lowered. However, this decrease seems to be a consequence of the lowering of the 1 minute activated esterase; in fact, the plasma kallikrein inhibitor of the cirrhosis group, when considered in unit value, is not statistically different from the normal value.

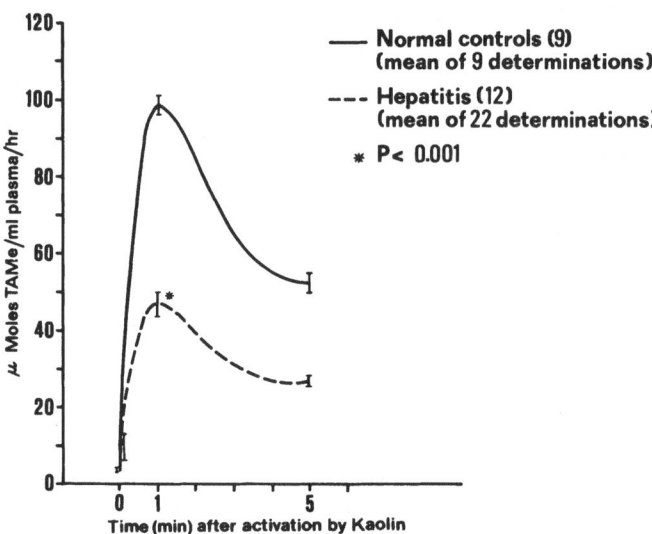

Figure 2. The plasma of the hepatitis group shows alterations
of the kallikrein activation by kaolin contact,
similar to those observed in cirrhosis.

TABLE 2

Plasma Kallikrein Inhibitor

Groups	N⁰ Patients	n⁰ Det.	Kallikrein inhibitor * (moles/ml/hr)	P	Kallikrein inhibitor (unit)	P
Normal	9	9	52 ± 6	--	0.91	--
Hepatic cirrhosis	20	30	22 ± 1	< 0.005	0.67	n.s.
Hepatitis	12	22	26 ± 2	n.s.	0.68	n.s.

* - Mean ± S.E.

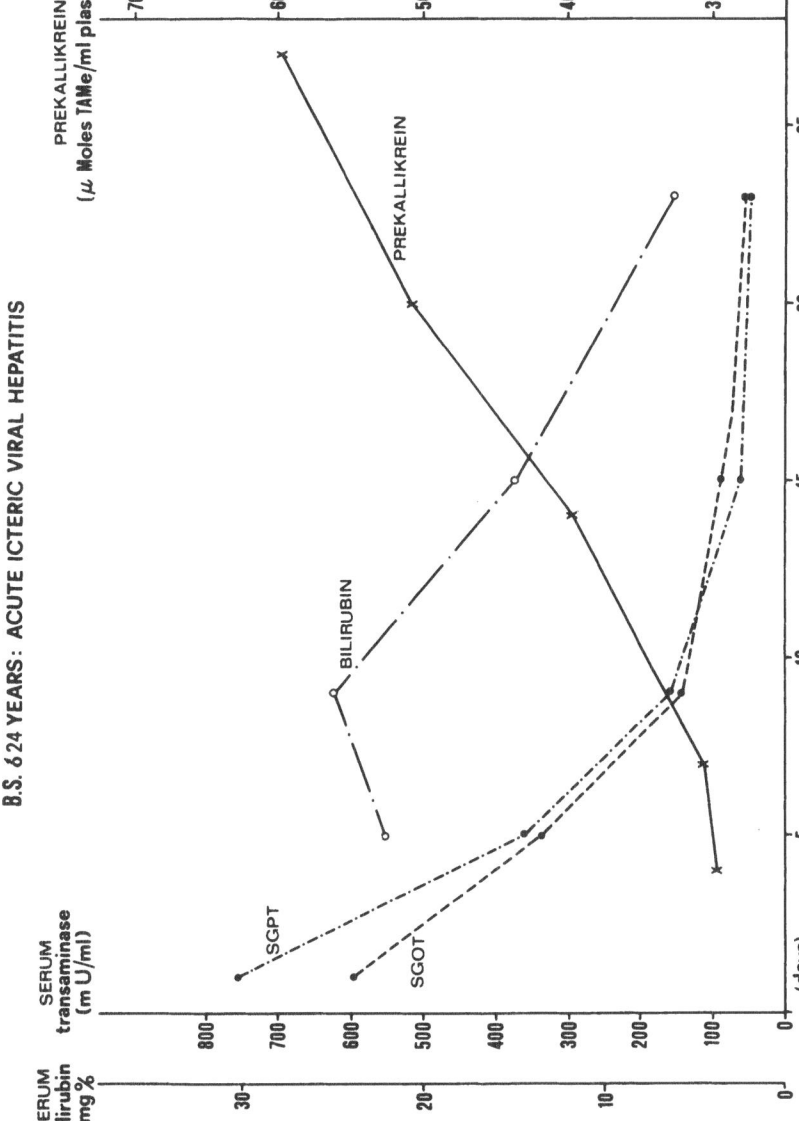

Figure 3.   A typical example of the plasma prekallikrein changes during the clinical improvement of a case of viral hepatitis. During the period of observation, plasma kallikrein increased about 100%. In every determination, the increase of the prekallikrein constantly corresponded to a decrease of bilirubin and transaminases.

COMMENT

The present results seem to demonstrate, even though indirectly, the generation of kallikrein precursor from the liver, and confirm the implication of the kallikreinogen-kallikrein system in cirrhosis and viral hepatitis.

Assays of the Hageman factor, carried out by Colman and co-workers (6), in human hepatic cirrhosis, were normal, thereby including the deficiency of this factor as the mechanism for the reduced one minute esterase activation by Kaolin contact. The most acceptable interpretation of these findings is that the abnormally low plasma prekallikrein is a consequence of reduced production; prekallikrein is probably synthesized in the liver, and cirrhosis compromises the cell function devolved on the generation of the prekallikrein enzyme.

Therapy does not produce an important increase of plasma prekallikrein, while it can increase low kininogen (3). Low prekallikrein could also be due to an increased kallikrein function, and thus augment the release of kinin; on the other hand, previous observations showed that the plasma kinin level in patients with hepatic cirrhosis is normal (3).

The results obtained in hepatitis may be due to a reduced synthesis of prekallikrein in the liver. An in vivo activation of plasma prekallikrein to kallikrein does not seem acceptable; however, this possibility is not excluded. Perhaps the viral disease damages the hepatic cells devolved on the synthesis of plasma prekallikrein. Since the plasma kininogen in viral hepatitis was normal, these data support the hypothesis that the production of plasma kininogen and of prekallikrein in the liver represents two different enzyme syntheses; however, only one is involved in hepatitis, and both are involved in cirrhosis. In addition, the lowering of the kaolin activatable esterase may be due to other mechanisms aside from the prekallikrein consumption or generation: for instance, it may be due to a partial loss of the Hageman factor.

The low level of plasma prekallikrein in icteric hepatitis cannot be attributed to the abnormal serum bilirubin; in fact, other authors reported normal prekallikrein levels in patients with obstructive jaundice (6).

So, the reduction of the prekallikrein seems closely correlated to the disfunction of the hepatic cell. In fact, a constant increase of the prekallikrein during the improvement of hepatitis was observed. The increase of the prekallikrein is correlated with the decrease of serum bilirubin and transaminases. During the first month of the disease, prekallikrein is increased by about 100%, however, without reaching a normal level, such as for bilirubin and transaminases. The period necessary to reach complete recovery of plasma prekallikrein has still to be defined.

From this point of view, the evaluation of plasma prekallikrein could acquire some significance, along with the conventional enzymatic examination, in the diagnosis and evolution of acute icteric viral hepatitis.

SUMMARY

Plasma prekallikrein (kallikreinogen) and kallikrein inhibitor, assayed with the kaolin activable esterase method, have been evaluated in 20 patients with hepatic cirrhosis, in 12 cases with jaundice from acute viral hepatitis, and in 9 normal. A significant reduction of the plasma prekallikrein in cirrhosis has been found. A lowering of plasma prekallikrein has also been observed in viral hepatitis; in this condition, however, the modifications were less important than those obtained in cirrhosis.

In three cases of hepatitis, the behaviour of the plasma prekallikrein and kallikrein inhibitor have been controlled during the period of the disease and compared with the behaviour of some conventional parameters, such as serum transaminases and bilirubin. An important increase of the prekallikrein level has been observed during the improvement of hepatitis. These data confirm the implication of the prekallikrein-kallikrein system in severe liver diseases, and indirectly points out the role of the liver in maintaining the physiological balance of the kallikrein system.

REFERENCES

1. Bryan R.F., Rayan J.W., and Niemeyer R.S.: Bradykininogen synthesis by liver., Adv. Exp. Med. Biol., 21, 43, 1972.

2. Werle F.T., Vogel R., and Kaliampetson G.: Uber das Kallikrein der Darmawand und seine Beziehung zum Blutkallikreingehalt bei Störungen der Darmunfunktion, in Second World Congress of Gastroenterology, Munich, 1962, Eds. Schmidt E., Tomenius J., and Watkinson G.; Karger, Basel, 1963, p. 788.

3. Del Bianco P.L., Fanciullacci M., and Frarchi G.: Plasmatic kininogen in acute hepatitis and in liver cirrhosis., Adv. Exp. Med. Biol., 21, 453, 1972.

4. Galletti R., Marra N., Matassi L., and Vecchiet L.: Decrease of skin algogenic reactivity and plasma algogenic activity in patients with hepatic cirrhosis., Lo Sperimentale., 117, 371, 1967.

5. Galletti R., Matassi L., Chiarini P., Vecchiet L., Buzzelli G.,
    and Marra N.: Plasma kinin activity in cirrhotic subjects.,
    Lo Sperimentale., 118, 253, 1968.

6. Colman R.W., Mason J.W., and Sherry S.: The kallikreinogen-
    kallikrein enzyme system of human plasma. Ann. Int. Med., 71,
    763, 1969.

7. Forrell M.M.: Unterschungen über das Kallikreinogen im Serum
    des gesunden und kranken Menschen und seine Beeinflussung
    durch die Nebennierenrinde. Schweiz. Med. Wochenschr., 87,
    822, 1957.

8. Sherry S., and Colman R.W.: Observation on the plasma kallikrein-
    ogen (prekallikrein)-kallikrein enzyme., Trans. Ass. Am.
    Physicians 81, 40, 1968.

9. Colman R.W., Mattler L., and Sherry S.: Studies on the pre-
    kallikrein (kallikreinogen)-kallikrein enzyme system of human
    plasma. I. Isolation and purification of plasma kallikreins.,
    J. Clin. Invest., 48, 11, 1969.

10. Colman R.W., Mattler L., Sherry S.: Studies on the prekallikrein
    (kallikreinogen) kallikrein enzyme system of human plasma. II.
    Evidence relating the kaolin activated arginine esterase to
    plasma kallikrein., J. Clin. Invest., 48, 23, 1969.

11. Sicuteri F., Antonini F.M., Del Bianco P.L., Franchi G., and
    Curradi C.: Prekallikrein and kallikrein inhibitor in plasma
    of patients affected by recent myocardial infarction. Adv.
    Exp. Med. Biol., 21, 445, 1972.

12. Fanciullacci M., Franchi G., Curradi C., and Sicuteri F.:
    Kallikreinogen and kallikrein inhibitor in cerebral stroke.
    Protides of the biological fluids - 20th Colloquium. Ed. H.
    Peters., Pergamon Press, Oxford and New York, 1973, p. 345.

This work was supported by a grant from the National Research
Council of Rome.

ISOLATION OF PORCINE SUBMAXILLARY KALLIKREIN

M. Lemon, B. Forg-Brey and H. Fritz

Institut für Klinische Chemie und Klinische Biochemie

8 Munchen 2, Nussbaumstrasse, 20, Germany

The relatively early interest in pancreatic kallikrein has led to the ready availability of this enzyme in a pure form. As a result, much more is known of the chemistry of pancreatic kallikrein (for example, see Kutzbach & Schmidt-Kastner, 1973) than of submaxillary or urinary kallikrein.

We describe here the preparation of kallikrein from the porcine submaxillary gland, and present some preliminary results concerning the properties of the enzyme. Kallikrein was assayed either by directly following the hydrolysis of N^{α}-benzoyl-1-arginine-ethyl ester (BAEE) at 253 nm (Trautschold & Werle, 1961) or using the combined test with BAEE and alcohol dehydrogenase (Bhoola & Dorey, 1971). One unit is defined as the activity hydrolyzing 1 μmole of BAEE per minute.

Preliminary Isolation Procedure

The initial steps of the isolation are shown in Fig. 1. 40,000 units of kallikrein were isolated from 8 kg of tissue, the yield being 61% compared to the activity in the neutralized tissue supernatant.

Application of Affinity Chromatography

Kallikrein was further purified by chromatography over trasylol-linked sepharose resin. Trasylol was coupled to CNBr-activated sepharose 4B for 2½ hours in a 200 mM sodium citrate buffer at pH 5.5, containing 700 mM NaCl. At this pH, the coupling efficiency of the resin is relatively low. 14 IU (about

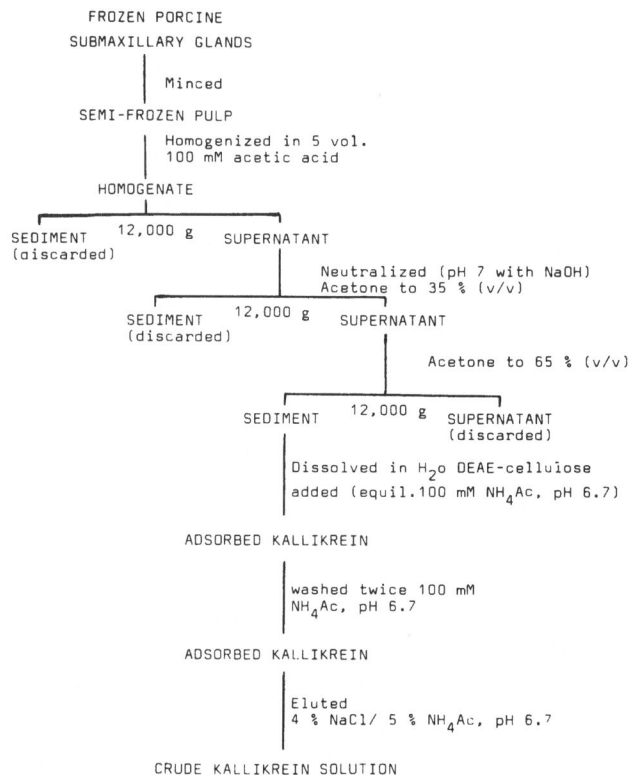

FROZEN PORCINE
SUBMAXILLARY GLANDS
|
| Minced
|
SEMI-FROZEN PULP
| Homogenized in 5 vol.
| 100 mM acetic acid
|
HOMOGENATE

SEDIMENT   12,000 g   SUPERNATANT
(discarded)
                    | Neutralized (pH 7 with NaOH)
                    | Acetone to 35 % (v/v)
                    |
        SEDIMENT   12,000 g   SUPERNATANT
        (discarded)
                            | Acetone to 65 % (v/v)
                            |
            SEDIMENT   12,000 g   SUPERNATANT
                                    (discarded)
            | Dissolved in H₂O DEAE-cellulose
            | added (equil.100 mM NH₄Ac, pH 6.7)
            |
    ADSORBED KALLIKREIN
            | washed twice 100 mM
            | NH₄Ac, pH 6.7
            |
    ADSORBED KALLIKREIN
            | Eluted
            | 4 % NaCl/ 5 % NH₄Ac, pH 6.7
            |
    CRUDE KALLIKREIN SOLUTION

Fig. 1. Initial steps in the isolation of porcine submaxillary
         kallikrein.

0.5 μmole) of trasylol were bound per gram of sepharose resin.
However, although the binding of trasylol can be considerably
enhanced by increasing the pH of the coupling buffer, the kalli-
krein-binding capacity of the resin is not correspondingly im-
proved, presumably because of steric hindrance between adjacent
trasylol molecules. We are at present testing high-capacity
resins made by coupling guanidinated trasylol to sepharose and
cellulose resins via a 6 or 12 carbon bridge.

Crude kallikrein is loaded onto the affinity column in a
buffer of high ionic strength (100 mM triethanolamine at pH 7.8,
containing 1 M NaCl) to minimize non-specific binding. After
extensive washing with this buffer to remove non-specifically
bound material, the kallikrein is eluted with 500 mM benzamidine
in 100 mM triethanolimine buffer, pH 6.45, containing 400 mM NaCl.
The eluate can be freed from benzamidine by ultrafiltration,

followed by gel filtration.

In a typical experiment, using a 10.5 cm x 2 cm column, operated at a flow-rate of 12 ml. hr $^{-1}$, 1470 units of kallikrein were bound from an applied 1700 units (spec. act., 8.2 units. ml^{-1}. E$^{1cm-1}_{280}$). 94% of the bound kallikrein, with a specific activity of 68 units. ml^{-1}. E $^{1cm}_{280}$ $^{-1}$, was recovered after elution and removal of benzamidine.

Chromatography on DEAE-sephadex

The kallikrein after affinity chromatography was freed of remaining contaminants, mainly nucleic acids, by elution from a DEAE-sephadex column using a convex ammonium acetate gradient. The elution pattern is shown in Fig. 2.

The marked peak at 253 nm occuring in fractions 27-35 is presumably due to nuclic acids not removed by the affinity chromatography step. Protein was eluted in a single peak in which absorption at 280 nm corresponded well with kallikrein activity.

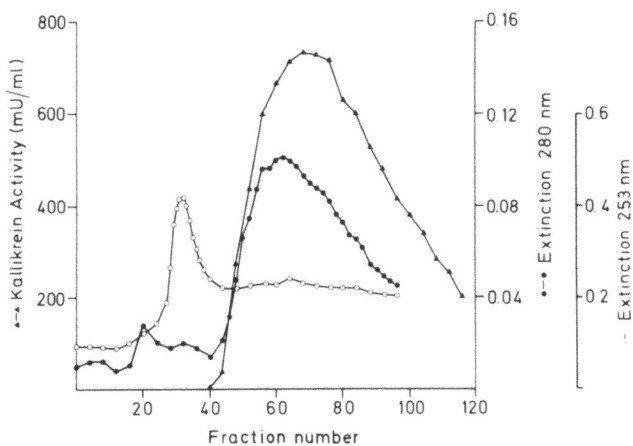

Fig. 2. DEAE-sephadex chromatography of porcine submaxillary kallikrein. The kallikrein was dissolved in 100 mM ammonium acetate (pH 6.7) and loaded onto a 55 x 1.8 cm column of DEAE-sephadex A-50 equilibrated with the same buffer. The kallikrein was eluted on a convex ammonium acetate gradient made by passing 800 mM ammonium acetate (pH 6.7) into a closed vessel containing 150 ml of 100 mM ammonium acetate (pH 6.7) (Fiedler, Hirschauer & Werle, 1970). 8 ml fractions were collected. Flow-rate was 9 ml per hr.

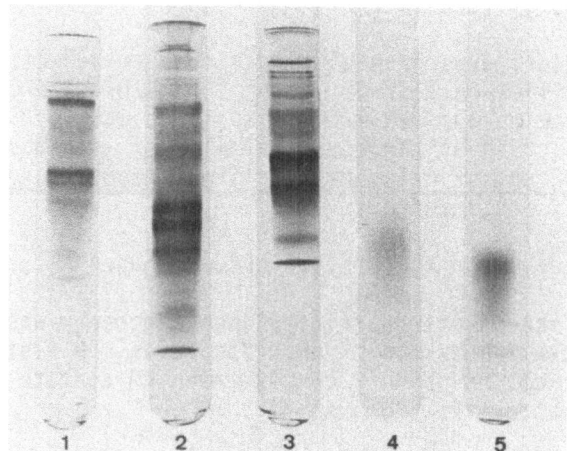

<u>Fig. 3.</u> Disc gel electrophoresis of the kallikrein preparations.
Gels (6 x 60 mm, 10% polyacrylamide discs) were run at
pH 8.9, at a current of 5 mA per gel. Samples were applied
at the top (cathode). Samples are: 1, neutralized supernatant of tissue homogenate; 2, 65% acetone precipitate;
3, DEAE-cellulose eluate; 4, after affinity chromatography;
5, after DEAE-sephadex chromatography.

Disc Gel Electrophoresis Studies

To check the homogeneity of the isolated kallikrein, the
enzyme was subjected to electrophoresis on 10% polyacrylamide discs,
both in the presence and in the absence of sodium dodecylsulphate
(SDS). Gel electrophoresis without SDS is rather unsuited to pig
submaxillary kallikrein. The kallikrein moves as a single diffuse
band, presumably because of the presence of a highly variable sugar
content (Fig. 3). The behaviour of the gel electrophoretic pattern throughout the isolation procedure is also shown.

After treatment with 1% SDS and 1% β-mercaptoethanol at 100°C,
however, the electrophoretic behaviour of kallikrein is markedly
altered (Fig. 4). In the affinity chromatography eluate there
are 4 major bands. The most slow-moving of these is usually absent from the kallikrein after chromatography on DEAE-sephadex.
Nevertheless, the component is not a contaminant, since if treatment with 1% SDS and 8 M urea for 12 hours at room temperature is
substituted for treatment with 1% SDS at 100°C, then the slow-
moving component is apparent even in the most highly purified
samples (see Fig. 4). The exact relationship between the slow-
moving component and the other components is not certain. Using

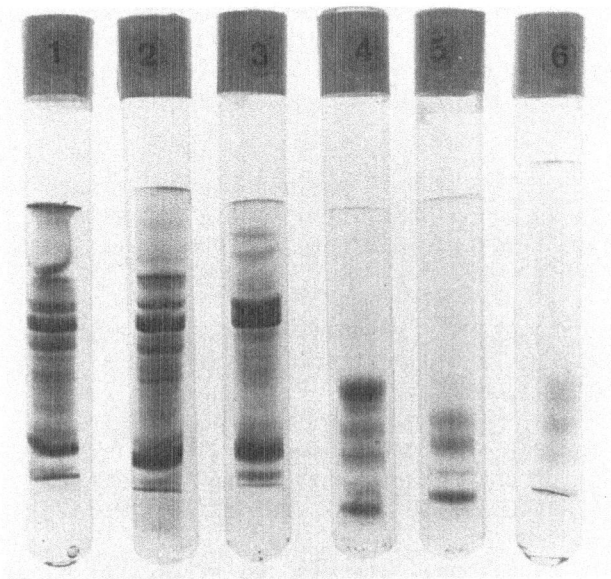

<u>Fig. 4.</u> SDS gel electrophoresis of the kallikrein preparations.
Samples were treated with 1% SDS and 1% β-mercaptoethanol
for 2 min at 100°C, and run at pH 8.9 on 6 x 60 mm 10%
polyacrylamide discs containing 1% SDS. The current was
5 mA per gel. Samples were applied at the top (cathode).
Samples are: 1, neutralized supernatant of tissue homogenate; 2, 65% acetone precipitate; 3, DEAE-cellulose
eluate; 4, after affinity chromatography; 5, after DEAE-
sephadex chromatography; 6, as 5, but treatment with urea
and SDS at 21°C substituted for treatment with SDS at
100°C.

marker proteins of known molecular weight, the molecular weights
of the 4 major bands are estimated to be 32,000 , 28,000 , 25,000
and <15,000. The fastest-running component lies in a poorly-re-
solved region almost on the salt boundary. It is possible to
define an upper limit to its molecular weight, but not an accurate
value.

Properties of the Porcine Submaxillary Kallikrein

The desalted and lyophylized kallikrein from the DEAE-
sephadex chromatography was used as the kallikrein preparation for
the following studies.

Isoelectric point. Isoelectric focussing on 5% polyacrylamide discs, using pH 3-6 Ampholine (LKB Products, Stockholm),
gave an isoelectric point of 3.8. This is in agreement with the
value previously obtained on a sucrose gradient (Fiedler, Muller
& Werle, 1970).

Biological activity. In the dog blood-pressure test, the
same reduction in blood-pressure was obtained with 50 mU, 50 mU
and 30 mU respectively of pancreatic, submaxillary and urinary
kallikrein.

Kinetic parameters. The kallikrein has a specific activity
of 193 units per mg Folin protein (with bovine serum albumin as
a standard) or 97.3 units. ml^{-1}. $E_{280}^{1cm\ -1}$.

The K_m for BAEE was calculated as 114 µM from a Lineweaver-
Burke plot, using BAEE concentrations from 50-500 µM. The corresponding V_{max} was 0.9 x 10^6 units per mg Folin protein.

Trasylol inhibition. Trasylol in sufficient concentration
almost completely inhibited the kallikrein (Fig. 5). Taking the
50% inhibition point, the molecular ratio of trasylol to trasylol
to kallikrein is approximately 1.2 : 1.

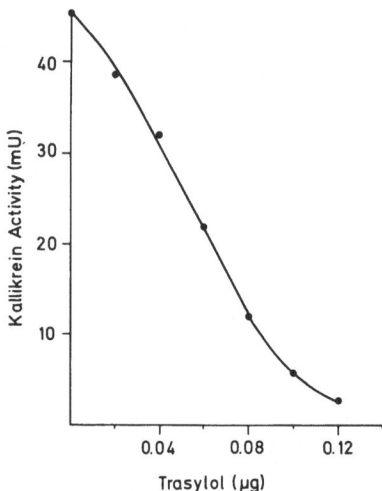

Fig. 5.   Inhibition of porcine submaxillary kallikrein by trasylol.
           The kallikrein (44.4 mU) was incubated with the inhibi-
           tor for 10 min. prior to addition to the BAEE in the
           assay cuvette. Assay was at 25°C in 100 mM Tris-HCl,
           pH 7.8. BAEE hydrolysis was monitored at 253 nm.

Table 1

Amino acid composition of porcine submaxillary kallikrein

	mol/mol*		mol/mol		mol/mol
ASP	27	ALA	13	TYR	7
THR	15	CYS	8	PHE	10
SER	14	VAL	10	LYS	3
GLU	22	MET	3	HIS	7.5
PRO	15	ILE	11	ARG	3
GLY	22	LEU	16.5		

* calculated as described in the text.

Amino Acid Composition

The composition calculated from single hydrolyses performed for 20, 40 and 79 hr. is shown in Table 1. Tryptophan was not determined, and no correction was made for incomplete oxidation of cystine to cysteine. Since the molecular weight of the protein chain of submaxillary kallikrein is not known with certainty, the data obtained for pancreatic kallikrein (Fiedler, Hirschauer & Werle, manuscript in preparation) were used to convert the results of the analysis to residues per kallikrein molecule. In view of the close similarity between the properties of pancreatic and submaxillary kallikrein, this seems to be a justifiable procedure.

Discussion

It is now clear that submaxillary and pancreatic kallikreins resemble each other closely over a broad spectrum of criteria. Doses of pancreas and submaxillary kallikrein which have the same esterase activity have almost identical biological activity. Esterase activities, trasylol inhibition, inactivation by DFP (Fiedler, Muller & Werle, 1970) and the isoelectric focussing patterns (Fiedler, Muller & Werle, 1970; Fiedler, Hirschauer & Werle, 1970) expose only minor differences between the two enzymes. It is therefore hardly surprising that the amino acid compositions of pancreatic (Fiedler, Hirschauer & Werle, manuscript in preparation) and submaxillary kallikrein are almost identical.

　　　M. Lemon has a Scholarship in the Royal Society European
Science Exchange Programme. We are grateful to Bayer AG for
providing facilities for the initial steps in the kallikrein
isolation.

References

Bhoola, K.D. and Dorey, G. (1971). Br. J. Pharmac. _43_, 784-793.
Fiedler, F., Hirschauer, C. & Werle, E. (1970). Hoppe-Seyler's
　　　Z. Physiol. Chem. _351_, 225-238.
Fiedler, F., Muller, B. & Werle, E. (1970). Hoppe-Seyler's Z.
　　　Physiol. Chem. _351_, 1002-1006.
Kutzbach, C. & Schmidt-Kastner, G. (1973). _In_ "Inininogenases",
　　　Haberland, G.L. & Rohen, J.W. (eds), F. K. Schattauer
　　　Verlag (Stuttgart-New York). pg. 23-35.
Trautschold, I. & Werle, E. (1961). Hoppe-Seyler's Z. Physiol.
　　　Chem. _325_, 48-59.

KININASE II (ANGIOTENSIN CONVERTING ENZYME) AND ENDOTHELIAL CELLS IN CULTURE

Una S. Ryan, J.W. Ryan and A. Chiu

Papanicolaou Cancer Research Institute and University

of Miami School of Medicine, Miami, Florida, 33136, USA

It is now well recognized that the lungs process the circulating vasoactive polypeptides, bradykinin and angiotensin I; the former being inactivated while the latter is activated (Ferreira & Vane, 1967; Ng & Vane, 1967; Ryan et al., 1968; 1970b, 1971, 1972). Previously (Ryan et al., 1968, 1969, 1970a & b, 1971; Smith & Ryan, 1972, 1973a), we have postulated that the enzymes responsible for the metabolism of these polypeptides are situated on or close to the luminal surface of the pulmonary endothelial cells. Over the past seven years much evidence from our laboratory (see references above) and those of others (Bakhle, 1968; Sander & Huggins, 1971; Lanzillo & Fanburg, 1974; Soffer et al., 1974) have supported this hypothesis. Recently (Dorer et al., 1972, 1974) have shown that the enzyme that activates angiotensin I (by conversion to angiotensin II) is also responsible in part for the inactivation of bradykinin. As described in the accompanying paper (Ryan, J.W., this volume), we have raised antibodies to this enzyme and are using the antibodies labelled for immunocytochemistry in efforts to provide a definitive test of our hypothesis. This report represents a fine focus on the localization of kininase II using a specific cell type in culture namely, pulmonary endothelial cells.

MATERIALS AND METHODS

Isolation of Cells and Cell Culture

Segments of bovine aorta and pulmonary artery were obtained from a slaughterhouse. Aorta and pulmonary artery of pig and rabbit were obtained by dissection in our laboratory. The vessels were rinsed in sterile phosphate-buffered saline (PBS), pH 7.4, which contained 200 U/ml penicillin, 200 mcg/ml streptomycin, and 325 mcg/ml fungizone. The vessels were stored in PBS at $4^{\circ}C$ from 1-4 h. Cells were obtained by an adaptation of the method of Maruyama (1963), as modified by Jaffe et al. (1973) and Gimbrone, et al. (1974). All openings in the vessel were closed by ligation or by clamping with small hemostats. The vessels were cannulated and perfused with approx. 200 ml Dulbecco's PBS with calcium and magnesium to remove all traces of blood. The lumen was filled with PBS containing 0.2% collagenase (type CLS, Worthington Bio-chem. Corp.). Both ends of the vessel were clamped shut. Sus-pended by its ends, the vessel was placed in PBS and incubated at $37^{\circ}C$ for 15 min in a water bath. After incubation, the effluent was collected into centrifuge tubes and the cells were sedimented at 2500 rpm at $4^{\circ}C$ for 10 min. The pellets were washed once with 3 ml of medium 199 with 20% fetal calf serum, and the cells were resuspended by trituration in 1 ml of fresh culture medium. The yield from this procedure was in the range of $0.5 - 1.5 \times 10^6$ cells. The cell suspension was divided equally among plastic tissue culture flasks, 25 cm^2 (Falcon-T25). Sufficient medium 199, con-taining fetal calf serum (FCS), was added to make a final volume of 5 ml/flask. The medium contained the antibiotics listed above and was supplemented with 2 mM L-glutamine. The flasks were incubated at $37^{\circ}C$ and were fed daily for the first 3 days and every 48 h thereafter. Small clusters of cells coalesced and grew to form confluent monolayers by 7 days. The cells were identified and characterized as endothelium by ultrastructural and biochemical criteria (to be described below). Endothelial cells prepared by this method can be cultured successfully for periods of up to 28 days.

Electron Microscopy and Immunocytochemistry

Electron Microscopy. Endothelial cells were prepared for examination in the electron microscope, either as monolayers (i.e. still attached to the culture flask) or as pellets. In the latter case, cells were removed from the culture flasks by washing with 0.25% trypsin and were collected by centrifugation. The cells were fixed in 2.5% glutaraldehyde in 0.5 M cacodylate buffer at pH 7.4 for 30 min to overnight. After washing in cacodylate buffer, the cells were post-fixed in 1% osmium tetroxide, dehydrated in an ethanol series and embedded in Spurr's low viscosity embedding medium. Sections were cut on an LKB Ultrotome III, mounted on un-supported copper grids and examined in a Philips 301 electron microscope.

Immunocytochemistry. The purification of antibodies and the method of conjugation of antibodies to 8-MP is described in the accompanying article (Ryan, J.W. et al., this volume). Encothelial cells were incubated for the immunocytochemical localization of kininase II, either as monolayers or as pellets (see above). The cells were washed three times with medium 199 without fetal calf serum (fetal calf serum may contain kininase II). In order to obviate the disadvantages of aldehyde fixation for immunocytochemical studies, the cells were treated unfixed, all incubation solutions being made up in medium 199. Alternatively, they were fixed in paraformaldehyde-picric acid (Stefanini et al., 1967). The period of fixation varied from 30 min to several days. Prior to incubation the cells were soaked with 1% sodium borohydride to reduce free aldehyde groups and Schiff bases (Kraehenbuhl et al., 1974).

Experiments were designed to use both direct and indirect methods of localization. In the direct method, the cells were first incubated with normal goat serum to cover non-specific sites, then with 8-MP conjugated to anti-kininase II IgG. In the indirect method, the cells were first incubated with unlabelled anti-kininase II followed by incubation in a second antibody (rabbit anti-goat IgG) labelled with 8-MP. In both instances the micro-peroxidase moiety was reacted with 3,3'-diaminobenzidine and H_2O_2 in the presence of imidazole. In some experiments the cells were fixed in glutaraldehyde after incubation with labelled antibody to stabilize the immunogens. As a control for the direct method, cells were incubated with unlabelled antibody before incubation in labelled specific antibody. As a control for the indirect method, the step involving incubation in specific antibody was replaced by incubation in buffer. In order to test for intrinsic peroxidase activity, controls were run without 8-MP. In addition, some controls omitted DAB or H_2O_2.

Immunofluorescent microscopy. Endothelial cells were examined as monolayers. The procedure was similar to that described above for the electron microscopic immunocytochemical localization of kininase II except that the antibodies, both specific and non-specific, were labelled with the fluorescent markers fluorescein and MDPF (Hoffmann-La Roche), and the material was examined in a Zeiss fluorescence light microscope.

Assay for kininase II using $(^{125}I)Tyr^8$-bradykinin. Details of the assay have been published (Chiu et al., 1975). In brief, kininase II is measured by its ability to catalyze the formation of $(^{125}I)Tyr$-Arg.

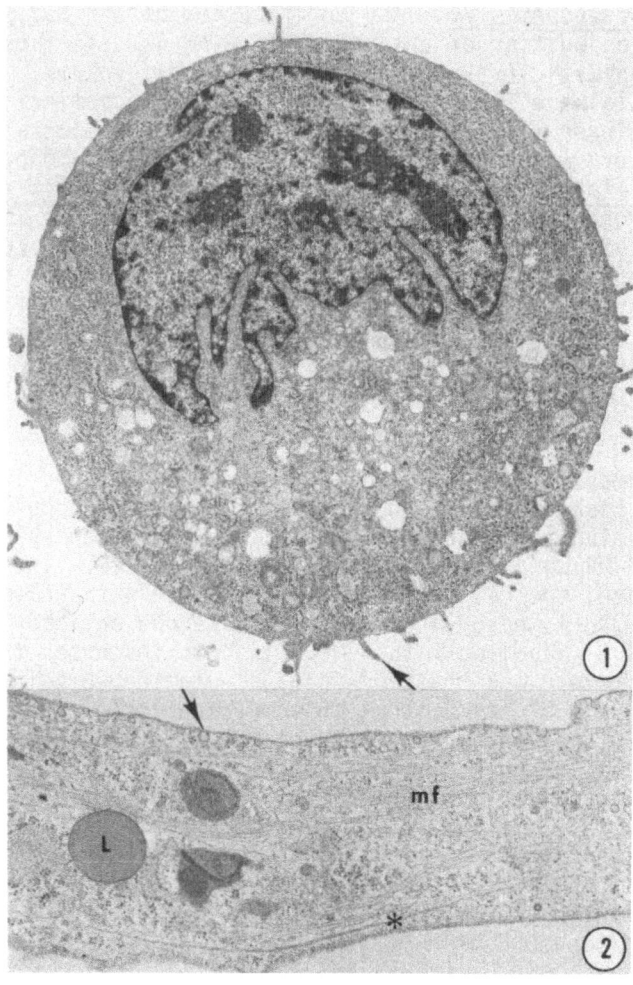

Fig. 1. Rabbit pulmonary vein endothelial cell which had been removed from the culture vessel by shaking with trypsin and collected by centrifugation. The spherical appearance of the cells after this treatment is to be contrasted with the flattened appearance of the cells when growing as a monolayer (Fig. 2). Endothelial projections (arrow) can be seen at the periphery.
X   5,100

Fig.2. Cow pulmonary artery endothelial cell from a culture which Was prepared for electron microscopy as a monolayer. The cells are flattened and grow as a single sheet. Caveolae are abundant on the upper surface of the cell (arrow). Microfilaments (mf), microtubules (asterisk) and lipid droplets (L) are frequently found. These features are shown in greater detail in Figs. 4-8 which all illustrate cells in culture. Pulmonary artery endothelial cells in situ show the same features (Fig. 3).   X 17,000

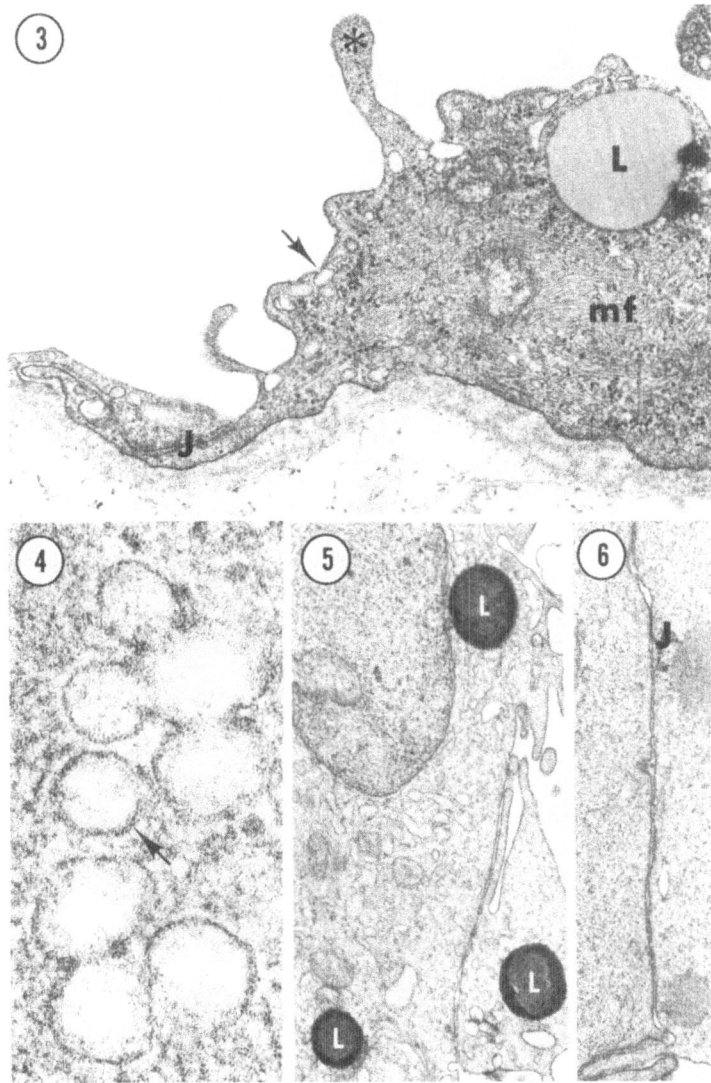

Figs. 3-6. A dog pulmonary artery endothelial cell in situ is
illustrated in Fig. 3. Many of the most striking characteristics
of endothelial cells as they exist in the vessel wall are exempli-
fied by endothelial cells in culture, e.g. endothelial projections
[(asterisk) cf Fig. 1], lipid droplets [(L) cf Figs. 2 and 5],
caveolae [(arrow) cf Figs. 2 and 4], microfilaments [(mf) cf Fig.
2]and tight junctions [(j) cf Fig. 6]. Figs. 4-6 are all taken
from cow pulmonary artery endothelial cells in culture.

Fig. 3 X   28,000   Fig. 5 X   15,000
Fig. 4 X   153,000   Fig. 6 X   16,000

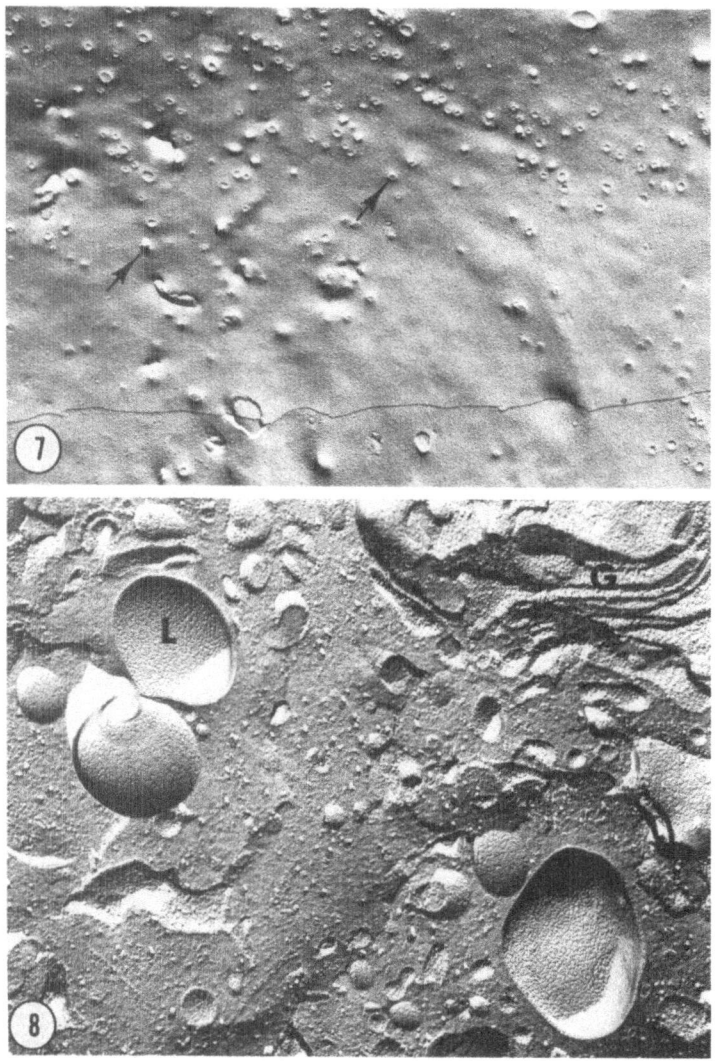

Figs. 7 and 8. Cultures of cow pulmonary artery endothelial cells were fixed with glutaraldehyde, scraped from the culture flasks with a rubber policeman and freeze-fractured in a Balzers 360 M freeze-etch microtome as described previously (Smith, et al., 1973b). Fig. 7 is a replica of the inner aspect of the outer leaflet of an endothelial plasma membrane fractured en face. The wide expanse of membrane exposed by this technique shows large numbers of caveolae (arrows). Fig. 8 represents a fracture through the cytoplasm of the endothelial cell and shows a Golgi apparatus (G) and lipid droplets (L). Fig. 7   X 12,000   Fig. 8   X 41,000

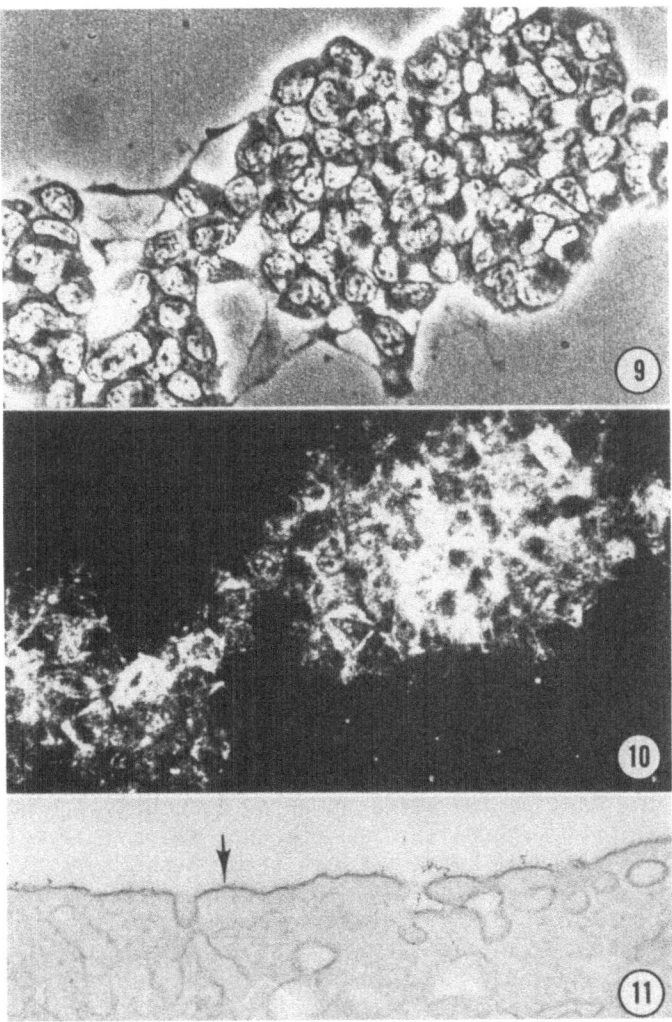

Figs. 9 and 10. A group of pig pulmonary artery endothelial cells was photographed first by phase contrast light microscopy to show general morphology (Fig. 9). The same group of cells was then incubated with anti-kininase II coupled to MDPF as described in the text. The resulting blue-green fluorescence was originally photographed under dark-field illumination in color and is reproduced here in black and white (Fig. 10). The fluorescence outlines the endothelial cells. Figs. 9 and 10 X 2,200

Fig. 11. Portion of a pig aortic endothelial cell from a culture which had been incubated with anti-kininase II-8-MP as described in the text. The reaction product, oxidized 3,3'-diaminobenzidine indicating sites of kininase II, is localized along the plasma membrane and associated caveolae (arrow). Fig. 11 X 58,000

RESULTS AND DISCUSSION

To test further our hypothesis that kininase II is localized on the plasma membrane of pulmonary endothelial cells, we began efforts to maintain pulmonary endothelial cells in culture. However, like many other groups, we have the problem of identifying the cells after they have been removed from the vessels. In the case of human endothelium, blood group antigens can be used as an aid to identification (Jaffe et al., 1973); but in studies of cow, pig, and rabbit endothelium, where well-characterized blood group antibodies are not available, we have been obliged to rely entirely on morphological criteria. We have examined thin sections and freeze-fracture replicas of our cultures and find that the ultra-structural features characteristic of the cells in culture (Figs. 1, 2, 4-8) are the same as those of endothelial cells in situ (Fig. 3.) Caveolae are abundant, particularly when the cells are sectioned as a monolayer (Figs. 2 and 4). The extent of the caveolae is best seen in freeze-fractures in the plane of the plasma membrane (Fig. 7). Lipid droplets are also a prominent feature (Figs. 2 and 3) and can be seen to be released into the culture medium (unpublished observations). Large numbers of micro-filaments can be seen (Fig. 2), frequently in extensions of the cells. Other cytoplasmic components of the cells, such as mito-chondria, Golgi apparatus, rough endoplasmic reticulum and coated pits are illustrated in thin sections (Fig. 1) and in replicas of freeze-fractured cells (Fig. 8). Weibel-Palade bodies occur but are not numerous. None of the characteristics cited above is alone sufficient to identify the cells as being endothelial. However, taking the several organelles into account, the cell types found in the tunica intima of large vessels (fibroblast, smooth muscle and endothelium) have features quite distinct from one another. Abundant micropinocytotic vesicles (caveolae) are found in endo-thelial cells but less frequently in smooth muscle of fibroblast. Lipid is also frequently found in endothelium, but not in fibro-blast or smooth muscle. Myofilaments are common in both smooth muscle and endothelium; however, the "attachment bodies" (dense bodies) found within the myofilaments of smooth muscle are not found in endothelium. The glycogen appearing in some of the cultured cells is not normally a characteristic of endothelium. The presence of glycogen is, however, known to be a characteristic of injured cells and is a frequent phenomenon in tissue culture, even in cells that do not normally contain glycogen (Nigam & Cantero, 1972).

Tight junctions between adjacent cells (Fig. 6), the abundance of caveolae, the prominent Golgi complexes, the frequent presence of lipid droplets, and the perinuclear region rich in mitochondria lead us to believe that these are indeed endothelial cells. These cells may be slightly transformed by the stress of being cultured, as indicated by the presence of glycogen and vacuoles, but nonetheless they retain their basic morphology and characteristics. Some of our cultures resulting from prolonged collagenase treatment showed a different morphology. The cells were larger and grew in multiple layers (endothelial cells grow as a monolayer). They contained abundant filaments and flask-shaped caveolae. We have tentatively identified them as smooth muscle cells.

Before attempting to localize kininase II by immunocytochemistry, it was necessary to show the presence of the enzymic activity in endothelial cell cultures. Previously, we have shown that endothelial cells of the mainstem pulmonary artery of cow and rabbit are capable of converting angiotensin I to angiotensin II (Ryan & Smith, 1973) and of degrading $(^{125}I)Tyr^8$-bradykinin to yield $(^{125}I)Tyr$-Arg (Chiu et al., 1975). In the present study, we have found that endothelial cells of the pulmonary artery of pig are also capable of degrading $(^{125}I)Tyr^8$-bradykinin to yield $(^{125}I)Tyr$-Arg. With 4×10^5 cells in an incubation volume of 5 ml, the reaction proceeds at a rate of about 0.6% (product formation) as a percentage of initial substrate per min. The cells which we have identified as smooth muscle gave a strikingly different result. Even during prolonged incubations, these cells do not form $(^{125}I)Tyr$-Arg, the product expected of kininase II.

Having shown the presence of kininase II in endothelial cell cultures, we proceeded to localize the site of the enzyme by immunofluorescence and immunocytochemistry using both direct and indirect labelling techniques. The immunocytochemical localization of kininase II on endothelial monolayers appears to be essentially similar to that using blocks of lung tissue (Ryan et al., 1975). The marker is localized on the endothelial plasma membranes and associated caveolae as well as on endothelial projections. Fig. 11 shows pig aortic cells in primary culture which had been incubated with anti-kininase II coupled to 8-MP.

The immunofluorescence of clusters of pig pulmonary artery cells after incubation with anti-kininase II-MDPF is illustrated in Figs. 9 and 10. Again, the localization appears to be on endothelial plasma membranes.

Although our results with endothelial cells of aorta indicate that kininase II (angiotensin converting enzyme) is not unique to pulmonary endothelial cells, it is not yet clear whether, among all lung cells, kininase II is unique to or more prevalent in endothelial cells. It is of some interest that cultures of what appear to be smooth muscle cells of the pulmonary artery do not degrade $(^{125}I)Tyr^8$-bradykinin to yield $(^{125}I)Tyr$-Arg. Similarly, these cells do not react with conjugates of antibody to kininase II. However, the lungs contain more than 40 different cell-types. On the other hand, there appears to be little need to invoke cell-

types other than endothelial cells to explain the extremely efficient processing of circulating bradykinin and angiotensin I by
intact lungs. As has been shown previously, lungs perfused with
^{14}C-Pro^2-bradykinin, ^3H-Phe^8-bradykinin, ^{14}C-Leu^{10}-angiotensin I
or ^{14}C-Phe^8-angiotensin I do not take up nor delay the transit of
the radioactivity (Ryan et al., 1968, 1969, 1970a, 1970b, 1971,
1972) even though the metabolism of these compounds is essentially
complete during a single passage.

ACKNOWLEDGEMENTS

    This work was supported in part by grants from the U.S. Public
Health Service (HL 15691 and HL 16407 and contract NO1 HR3-3015),
from the John A. Hartford Foundation, Inc., the Council for Tobacco
Research--U.S.A., Inc., and by an Established Investigatorship
Award to Dr. Una S. Ryan from the American Heart Association and
with funds contributed by Heart Association of Palm Beach County,
Florida.

REFERENCES

Bakhle, Y.S., Nature, 220, 919-921, 1968.

Chiu, A.T., Ryan, J.W., Ryan, U.S. and Dorer, F.E., Biochem. J.,
    in press.

Dorer, F.E., Kahn, J.R., Lentz, K.E., Levine, M. and Skeggs, L.T.,
    Circ. Res., 31, 356-366, 1972.

Dorer, F.E., Kahn, J.R., Lentz, K.E., Levine, M. and Skeggs, L.T.,
    Circ. Res., 36, 824-827, 1974.

Ferreira, S.H. and Vane, J.R., Nature, 215, 1237, 1967.

Gimbrone, M.A., Cotran, R.S. and Folkman, J., J. Cell Biol., 60,
    673-684, 1974.

Jaffe, E.A., Nachman, R.L., Becker, C.G. and Minick, C.R., J.
    Clin. Invest., 52, 2745-2756, 1973.

Kraehenbuhl, J.P., Galardy, R.E. and Jamieson, J.D., J. Exp. Med.,
    139, 208-223, 1974.

Lanzillo, J.J. and Fanburg, B.L., J. Biol. Chem., 249, 2312-2318,
    1974.

Maruyama, Y., Z. Zellforsch. Mikrosk. Anat., 60, 69, 1963.

Ng, K.K.F. and Vane, J.R., Nature, 216, 762-766, 1967.

Nigam, V. and Cantero, A., in Advances in Cancer Research (eds. G. Klein and S. Weinhouse), Vol. 16, Academic Press, New York and London, 1972, pp. 1-96.

Ryan, J.W., Niemeyer, R.S., Goodwin, D.W., Smith, U. and Stewart, J.M., Biochem. J., 125, 921-923, 1971.

Ryan, J.W., Roblero, J. and Stewart, J.M., Biochem. J., 110, 795-797, 1968.

Ryan, J.W., Roblero, J. and Stewart, J.M., Pharmac. Res. Commun., 1, 192, 1969.

Ryan, J.W., Roblero, J. and Stewart, J.M., in Adv. Exp. Med. Biol., (eds. N. Back, F. Sicuteri and M. Rocha e Silva), Vol. 8, Plenum Press, New York, 1970a, pp. 263-272.

Ryan, J.W., Ryan, U.S., Schultz, D.R., Whitaker, C., Chung, A. and Dorer, F.E., Biochem. J., 146, 497-499, 1975.

Ryan, J.W. and Smith, U., in Protides of the Biological Fluids (ed. H. Peeters), Vol. 20, Pergamon Press, Oxford, England, 1973, pp. 379-384.

Ryan, J.W., Smith, U. and Niemeyer, R.S., Science, 176, 64-66, 1972.

Ryan, J.W., Stewart, J.M., Leary, W.P. and Ledingham, J.G., Biochem. J., 120, 221-223, 1970b.

Sander, G.E. and Huggins, C.G., Nature New Biol., 230, 27-29, 1971.

Smith, U. and Ryan, J.W., in Adv. Exp. Med. Biol. (eds. N. Back and F. Sicuteri), Vol. 21, Plenum Press, New York, 1972, pp. 267-276.

Smith, U. and Ryan, J.W., Fed. Proc., 32, 1957-1966, 1973a.

Smith, U., Ryan, J.W. and Smith, D.S., J. Cell Biol., 56, 492-499, 1973b.

Soffer, R.L., Reza, R. and Caldwell, P.R.B., Proc. Nat. Acad. Sci., 71, 1720-1724, 1974.

Stefanini, M., de Martino, C. and Camboni, L., Nature, 216, 173-174, 1967.

HISTAMINE AND KALLIKREIN SYSTEM IN MAN*

Pedata F., Del Bianco P.L., Curradi C., Anselmi B., and Sicuteri F.

Department of Clinical Pharmacology

University of Florence, Italy

Histamine is a well-known pain producing substance; and its acute administration in essential headache provokes or exacerbates the ache; the chronic administration of histamine can improve headache, probably through a sort of desensitization at the level of the nociceptors. Other pain producing substances, such as kinins, can take part in the mechanism of the histamine desensitization; in fact, histamine and the histamine liberator 48/80, when acutely administered, are able to lower the plasma kininogen level in man (1). Interactions between histamine and the kallikrein-kinin system have been shown by other authors (2,3,4,5,6).

In the present study the activity of histamine on plasma prekallikrein and kallikrein inhibitor has been evaluated.

METHOD

23 headache patients were treated for therapeutic purpose with histamine diydrochloridre, in a slow venous infusion of 2,4 mg at a range of 10 mcg per minute for 4 hours. Venous blood was sampled before, half an hour, 1, 2 and 3 hours after the start of the infusion, at the end of the infusion, and 24 hours after the end of the infusion. The prekallikrein and kallikrein inhibitor levels were evaluated according to the Colman and coworkers method (7,8) that is a modification of the Siegelman and coworkers method (9). In the same way, as control, ten headache patients were treated with slow venous infusion of a different vasodilating drug, such as nicotinic acid, at a dose of 400 mcg per minute for a

---

* Sponsored by a grant from the National Research Council, Rome.

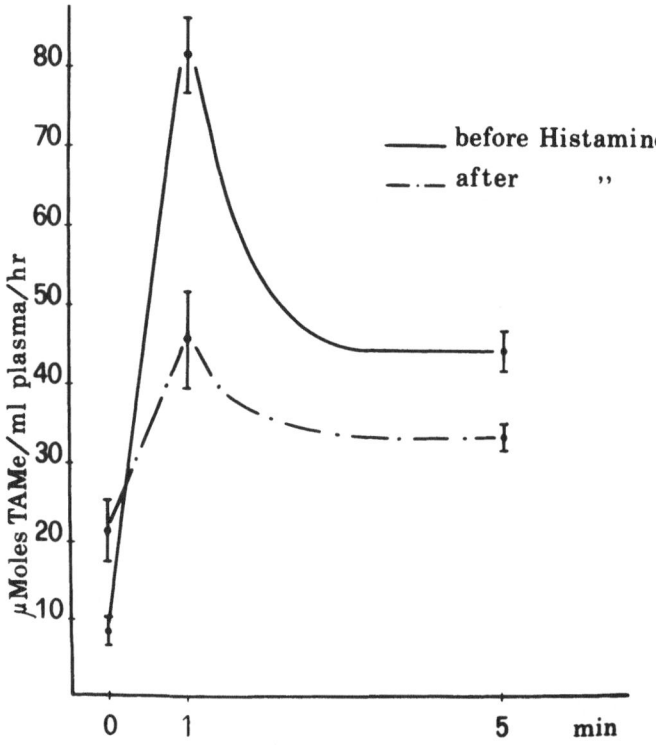

Figure 1. Plasma prekallikrein and kallikrein inhibitor before
          and at the end of histamine infusion (2,4 mg): 23 cases.

total of 0.1 gr in four hours. At the same times already mentioned
for the histamine group, blood was sampled, and the prekallikrein
and kallikrein inhibitor were evaluated.

RESULTS (Fig. 1, 2, 3)

     The final results can be summarized as follows: 1.) The
plasmatic esterase activity at the zero point, that is, before
kaolin, gradually and promptly increases, and its enhancement becomes significant immediately after a half an hour from the start
of the histamine infusion; at the fourth hour, at the end of the
2.4 mg histamine infusion, it reaches the maximum value, and after
24 hours, it returns to the normal level.

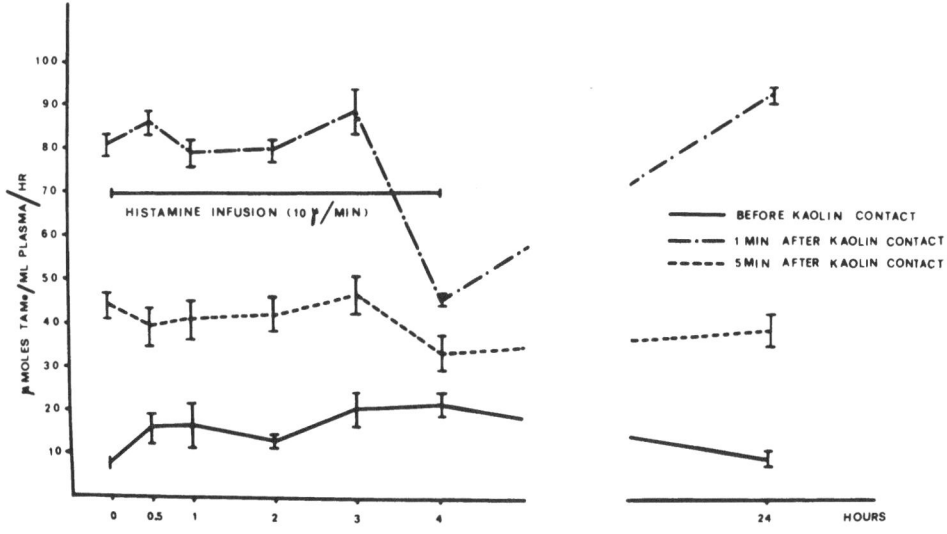

Figure 2.   The change of prekallikrein and kallikrein inhibitor in
            plasma of 23 headache sufferers treated with histamine
            infusion.

2.) The 1 minute kaolin activated esterase, that is prekallikrein,
significantly decreases, only at the end of the infusion: its
decrease is about 67%. It appears completely restored 24 hours
after the infusion. 3.) The 5 minute kaolin activated esterase,
which indicates the kallikrein inhibitor, expressed in inhibiting
unities, only after the first hour of the infusion significantly
increases, and returns to the normal level in all the other
samples. 4.) No important variations were found in the plasma
after the infusion of nicotine acid.

COMMENT

This experiment confirms the relationship between histamine
and the kallikrein system. The most important result is the decrease of the plasmatic prekallikrein following the histamine
administration. This occurs only at the end of infusion and it may
depend upon either the dose of the administered histamine or the
prekallikrein pool.

The significance of the enhancement of the spontaneous esterase
activity is not clear. In fact, this activity is not demonstrated

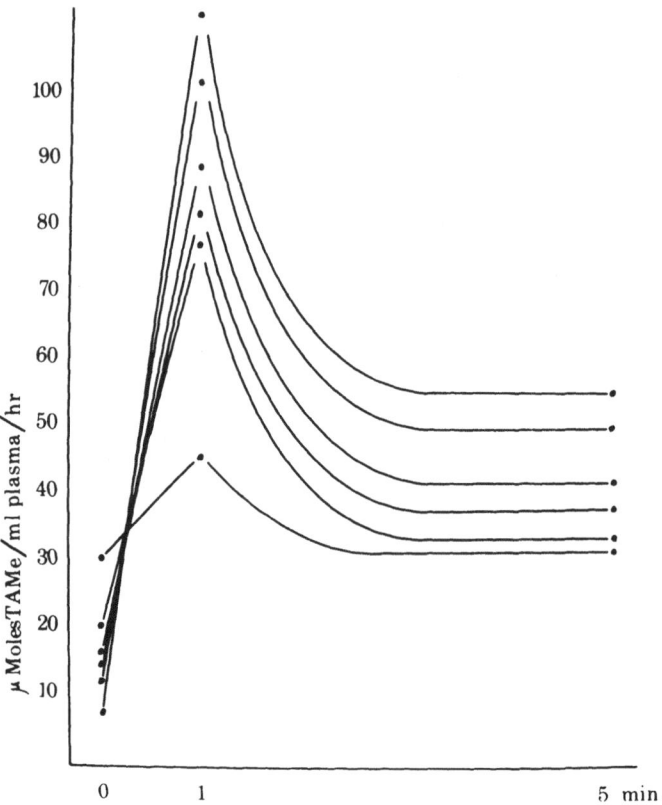

Figure 3. Plasma prekallikrein and kallikrein inhibitor changes
following histamine infusion (10 mcg/min): an exemplary
case: from top to bottom, the values before the histamine infusion, and after 0.3, 0.6, 1.2, 1.8, and 2.4 mcg
of histamine are reported.

to be wholly due to kallikrein. On the other hand, since the
histamine infusion modifies the kallikrein system, the increase of
the spontaneous esterase activity could be due to the activated
kallikrein. Thus, we may think that histamine slowly activates
prekallikrein which initially is completely restored by the
synthesis in liver; subsequently it is gradually consumed, and only
after a certain dose of histamine, the prekallikrein decreases.

The kallikrein inhibitor does not modify following histamine
infusion except for a momentary increase at the first half hour

from the start of the infusion.

The effects of histamine on the kallikrein system do not apparently depend upon a generic aspecific vasodilatating activity of histamine. In fact, the vasodilatation following nicotinic acid does not affect the kallikrein system.

SUMMARY

Histamine infusion modifies the kallikrein system, studied by kaolin contact method, in man. The main modifications are the increase of the spontaneous esterase activity and the prekallikrein lowering. Apparently the histamine administration activates the kallikrein, and consequently a release of kinin can take place.

BIBLIOGRAPHY

1. Periti P., Sicuteri F., Franchi G., and Michelacci S.: Azione dell'istamino-liberatore 48/80 sul bradichininogeno e plasma-chinine del sangue venoso umano dopo somministrazione venosa o endoarteriosa., Boll. Soc. Ital. Biol. Sper., 40, 951, 1964.

2. Zweifach B.W.: Microcirculatory effects of polypeptides., In. "Hypotensive Peptides", pg. 451, Springer Verlag, New York, 1966.

3. Edery, H., and Lewis G.P.: Kinin forming activity and histamine in Lymph after tissue injury., J. Physiol., 169, 568-583, 1963.

4. Erdos E.G., and Johnson A.R.: Interrelationship of histamine release and vasoactive peptides., In "New Aspects of Trasylol Therapy", International Symposium, Sweden, 1973.

5. Mannaioni P.F.: Influence of bradykinin and prostaglandin E_1 on the uptake and release of histamine by murine neoplastic mast-cells in vitro., Bioch. Pharmacology, 19, 1159-1163, Pergamon Press, 1970.

6. Zachariae M., Molmquist J., Oates J.A., and Pettinges W.: Studies on the Mechanism of kinin formation in inflammation., J. Physiol., 190, 81-90, 1967.

7. Colman R.W., Mattler R., and Sherry S.: Studies on the kalli-kreinogen-kallikrein enzyme system on human plasma. II. Evidence relating the kaolin activated arginine esterase to plasma kallikrein., J. Clin. Invest., 48, 23, 1969.

8. Colman, R.W., Mason J.W., and Sherry S.: The kallikreinogen-
    kallikrein enzyme system of human plasma: Assay of components
    and observations in disease states., Annals of Internat.
    Medicine., 71, 763, 1969.

9. Siegelman, A.M., Carlson A.S., and Robertson T.: Investigation
    of serum trypsin and related substances., Arch. Biochem.
    Biophys., 97, 159, 1962.

FURTHER EVIDENCE ON THE SUBCELLULAR SITES OF KININASE II (ANGIOTENSIN CONVERTING ENZYME)

J.W. Ryan, Una S. Ryan, D.R. Schultz, A.R. Day

Papanicolaou Cancer Research Institute and University of Miami School of Medicine, Miami, Florida 33136, U.S.A.

F.E. Dorer

Cleveland Veterans Hospital and Department of Biochemistry, Case Western Reserve, Cleveland, Ohio, 44106, USA

There is an abundant indirect evidence indicating that circulating bradykinin and angiotensin I are metabolized by enzymes situated along the luminal surface of pulmonary endothelial cells (for reviews, see Ryan et al., 1970a, 1972a & b; Smith & Ryan, 1973; Ryan & Ryan, 1975). The metabolism of bradykinin results in loss of biological activity, but the activity of angiotensin I is enhanced, in part by conversion to its lower homolog, angiotensin II. Recently, Dorer et al. (1972, 1974a) have succeeded in isolating an enzyme (angiotensin converting enzyme or kininase II) from pig lung which has the capacity of metabolizing angiotensin I and bradykinin to produce metabolites like those produced by intact lungs: The enzyme converts angiotensin I to angiotensin II by releasing the C-terminal dipeptide, His-Leu, and inactivates bradykinin by releasing the C-terminal dipeptide, Phe-Arg (cf Ryan et al., 1969, 1970a & b, 1971). Furthermore, the enzyme shows the same selectivity of metabolism as was observed with intact lungs: none of the higher homologs of bradykinin is inactivated as fast as is bradykinin itself (Ryan et al., 1970a; Roblero et al., 1973; Dorer et al., 1974b). Inactivation of the homologs appears to vary inversely with size and charge.

We have prepared antibodies to pure preparations of the pig lung enzyme and have begun to use the antibodies to localize the cellular and subcellular site(s) of the enzyme in intact lungs and in pulmonary endothelial cells in culture (see Ryan, U.S., et al., this volume). A preliminary report of our results has been published (Ryan et al., 1975). In our initial studies, we used partially-purified antibody to kininase II conjugated via gluta- raldehyde (Avrameas, 1969) to microperoxidase (11-MP, a heme- undecapeptide of cytochrome c). During the course of the studies, it became evident that the conjugation technique gave rise to the development of complex polymers, some of which might be expected to possess little or no immunoreactivity. Thus, in our subsequent studies, we have attempted to develop less ambiguous means of con- jugating specific antibody (anti-kininase II) to a marker suitable for electron microscopy. Recently, Kraehenbuhl et al. (1974) have described a new conjugation procedure in which antibody is bound to 8-MP (a heme-octapeptide of cytochrome c) using p-formyl- benzoyl-N-OH-succinimide. In addition to its small size (1555 daltons), 8-MP has the advantage of having only one reactive amine. Its peroxidase activity exceeds that of cytochrome c by more than 300-fold. In the present study, we have conjugated 8-MP to anti- kininase II using bis-succinyl succinate. Using the procedure described below, antibody-8-MP conjugates are obtained having a substitution ratio of ~3 (8-MP:antibody).

MATERIALS AND METHODS

Antibodies to pig lung angiotensin converting enzyme (kininase II) were obtained, purified and characterized as described pre- viously (Ryan et al., 1975). In some experiments, the partially- purified antibody was conjugated to 11-MP (obtained from Sigma Chem. Co., St. Louis, Mo., U.S.A.) using glutaraldehyde (Avrameas, 1969). In other experiments, the antibody was conjugated to 8-MP using bis-succinyl succinate in a two-step procedure. Bis-succinyl succinate was synthesized as described by Lindsay (1972), and 8-MP was obtained by chromatography (Bio-Gel P-6) of a tryptic hydroly- sate of 11-MP (Kraehenbuhl et al., 1974). In the two-step conjuga- tion procedure, 8-MP and antibody were used in excess: 8-MP in pyridine was added dropwise to bis-succinyl-succinate in DMSO until the reaction mixture contained 3.2 μmoles of 8-MP and 16 μmoles of bis-succinyl succinate. The 8-MP-succinyl succinate was precipi- tated by adding ether and then was dissolved in DMSO and added to the antibody preparation in phosphate buffered saline (~10 mg of protein/ml). The reaction sequence is shown in Fig. 1.

The material obtained in step II was applied to a Bio-Gel P-300 column (2.5 x 50 cm) to remove N-OH-succinimide released in steps I and II and to remove any unreacted 8-MP and 8-MP-succinyl- 8-MP dimers. The Ab-8-MP conjugate was separated from unconjugated antibody by chromatography on DEAE-cellulose as described by Kraehenbuhl et al. (1974). Unconjugated antibody is eluted in the void volume and the conjugate is eluted with 300 mM KCl.

I.

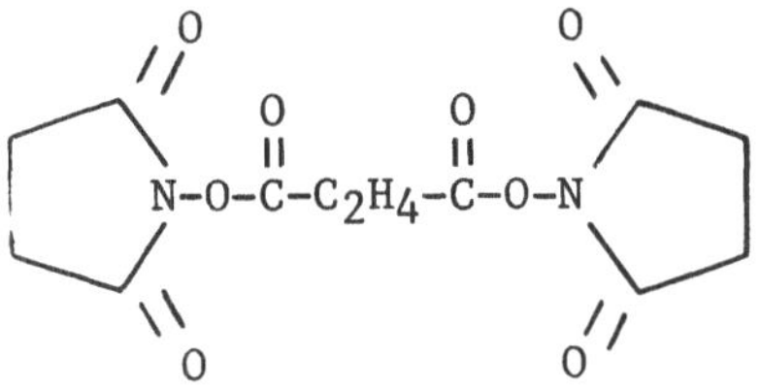

bis-succinyl succinate

I. (chemical reaction) $+$ 8-MP-NH$_2$ $\longrightarrow$ 8-MP-NH-succinyl succinate

II.   8-MP-NH-succinyl succinate + Ab-NH$_2$ 8-MP-NH-succinyl-NH-Ab

Fig. 1. Preparation of anti-kininase II-succinyl-8-MP. See text for details. Bis-succinyl succinate in excess is reacted with the α-amino group of 8-MP (Step 1), and then 8-MP-succinyl succinate is reacted (presumably via ε- and α-amino groups) with the antibody (Step II).

The anti-kininase II-8-MP conjugate has been reacted with blocks of fixed lung tissue, fixed and unfixed endothelial cells in culture and endothelial cells in situ. Prefixed tissue, using glutaraldehyde or picric acid-paraformaldehyde, has been used with and without treatment with sodium borohydride. Borohydride was used to reduce free aldehydes and unstable Schiff bases (Kraehenbuhl et al., 1974). Other details of the tissue preparation and reaction with antibodies have been reported elsewhere (Ryan, U.S., this volume; Ryan et al., 1975).

RESULTS AND DISCUSSION

The purified antibody-8-MP conjugates obtained after chromatography on DEAE-cellulose have a marker:antibody ratio of approx. 3:1. These conjugates retain both immunoreactivity and enzymic activity: 2.6 μg of antibody-8-MP inhibits the enzymic hydrolysis of Hip-His-Leu by 50% when converting enzyme (Fraction G, Dorer et al., 1972) is at a concentration of 3 μg/ml. Similarly, the 8-MP moiety of the conjugate degrades H$_2$O$_2$ (o-dianisidine assay). Two μg of conjugate protein possesses the same peroxidase activity as does 40 ng of free 8-MP.

Fig. 2 shows the immunocytochemical result observed on reaction of the anti-kininase II-8-MP conjugate with pig aortic endothelial cells. The reacted tissue preparation was incubated with

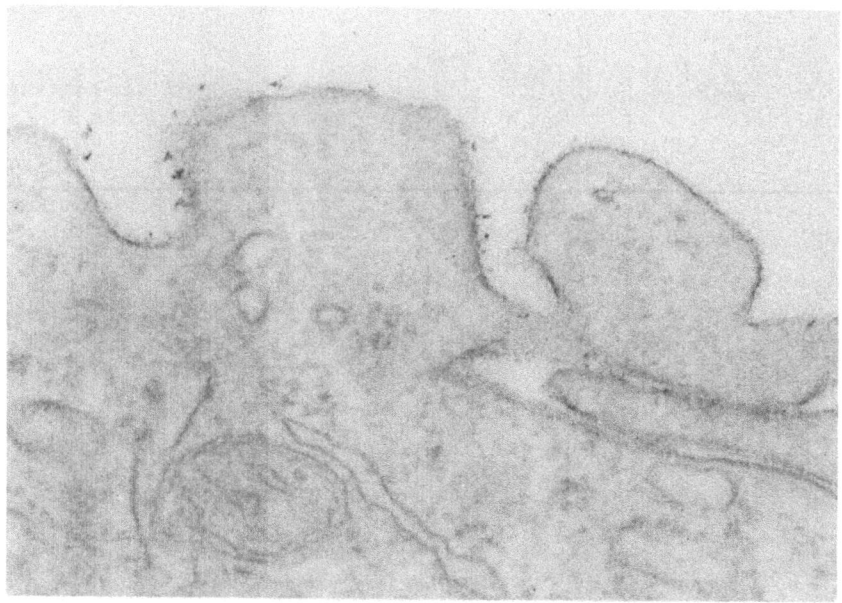

Fig. 2.   Reaction of anti-kininase II-8-MP with pig aortic endothelial cells.   The antibody conjugates were detected after
reaction of the 8-MP moieties with H_2O_2 and diaminobenzidine.
Deposits of oxidized diaminobenzidine are restricted to the plasma
membrane and associated caveolae.

X   97,000

H_2O_2 and 3,3'-diaminobenzidine.   The deposits of oxidized diaminobenzidine are restricted to the plasma membrane and to those
caveolae which communicate with the exterior of the cell.   Fig. 3
shows the results obtained using an anti-kininase II-II-MP conjugate.   In this experiment, we used blocks of rat lung prefixed with
paraformaldehyde-picric acid.   Fig. 3 depicts an endothelial cell
of a capillary at the alveolar-capillary level.   The most prominent
immunocytochemical reactions were evident in capillaries and small
venules.

When our studies were first begun, the use of immunoabsorption
procedures was not feasible because lung kininase II was in short

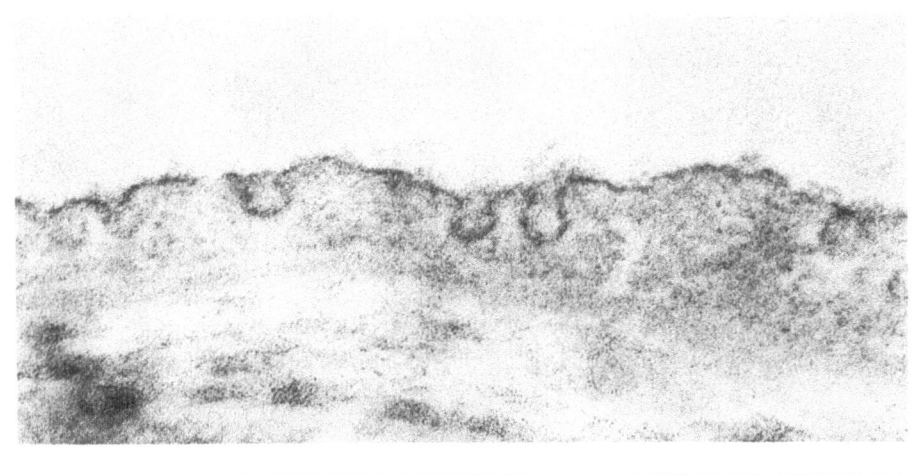

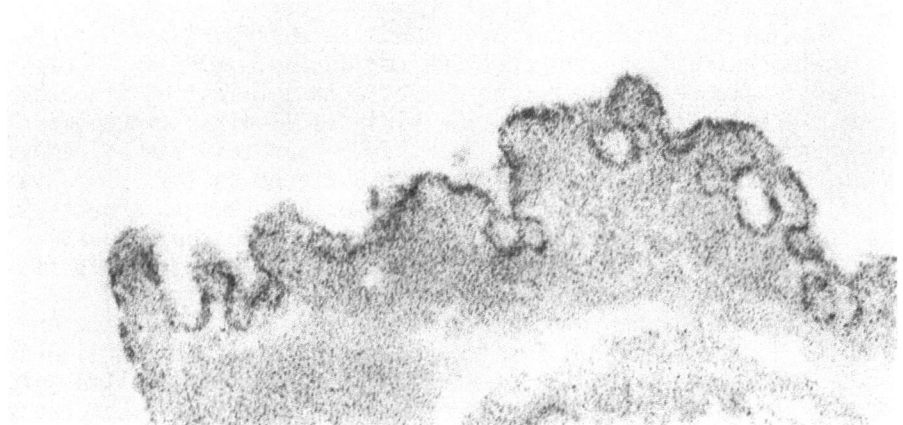

Fig. 3. Reaction of anti-kininase II-II-MP with rat pulmonary endothelial cells in situ. See text for details. (Reproduced by permission of the publishers, Biochem. J., 146, 497, 1975).

(a) X   93,000
(b) X   101,000

supply. As more enzyme became available, it was immobilized on to controlled pore glass beads derivatized with N-OH-succinimide to yield an active ester. The structure of the chain extending from the silanized surface of the glass beads is shown in Fig. 4.

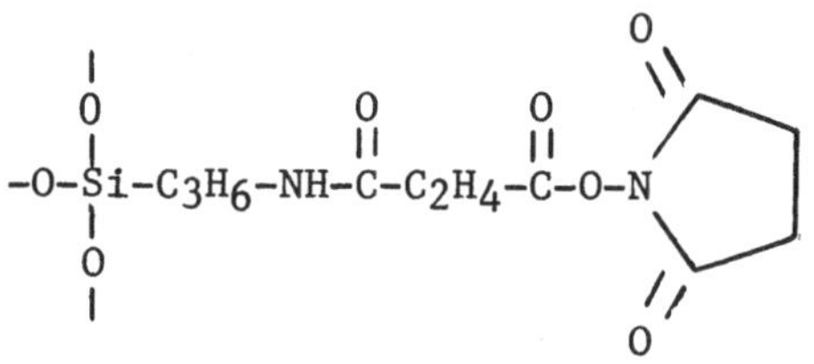

$$-O-\overset{\displaystyle |}{\underset{\displaystyle |}{\overset{\displaystyle O}{\underset{\displaystyle O}{Si}}}}-C_3H_6-NH-\overset{O}{\overset{||}{C}}-C_2H_4-\overset{O}{\overset{||}{C}}-O-N$$

Fig. 4. Side-chain structure of silanized controlled pore glass beads derivatized with N-OH-succinimide. Pig lung angiotensin converting enzyme (kininase II) was immobilized via the active ester. In a subsequent step, unreacted N-OH-succinimide esters were removed by adding glycine methyl ester in excess.

The immunoabsorbent has been used for purifying antibody-8-MP conjugates as well as antibody-MDPF conjugates. MDPF is a compound related to fluorescamine but which has a longer lasting fluorescence (Wiegele et al., 1973). The kininase II-glass immunoabsorbent binds either conjugate, and extraneous protein can be removed by washing exhaustively with phosphate-buffered saline. The highly purified conjugates are then removed by washing the absorbent with progressively higher concentrations of KI, a chaotropic agent (Edgington, 1971). With the present antibody, 2M KI in neutral phosphate buffer suffices. The eluate is dialyzed immediately to remove KI, and the non-diffusible material is used for reaction with the tissue antigen. The immunoabsorption step is particularly convenient for purification of MDPF- or fluorescein-labelled antibody. The elution of the antibody from the immunoabsorbent can be monitored by fluorescence alone. Removal of KI by dialysis proceeds rapidly and the labelled antibody can be used on the day in which the experiment was begun.

The results obtained using highly purified antibody-succinyl-8-MP conjugates were not substantially different from results obtained with antibody coupled to 11-MP via glutaraldehyde. Kininase II (angiotensin converting enzyme) appears to be restricted to the plasma membrane and associated caveolae of endothelial cells, especially those of the pulmonary capillaries and venules. However, it is also evident that the antibody conjugates react with endothelial cells of the aorta and mainstem pulmonary artery, findings consistent with previous biochemical demonstrations of converting enzyme activity in association with these cells (Ryan & Smith, 1973; Ryan, U.S., this volume).

Whether kininase II is unique to or more prevalent in endothelial cells remains to be determined. Preliminary evidence (Ryan, U.S., this volume) indicates that other cells derived from the mainstem pulmonary artery, tentatively identified as smooth muscle cells, do not metabolize (^{125}I)Tyr^8-bradykinin to yield (^{125}I)Tyr-Arg (cf Chiu, et al., 1975). These observations may have implications for cell identification and for studies on subcellular sites of receptors for bradykinin and angiotensin II. Richardson & Beaulnes (1971) have adduced evidence to indicate that receptors for angiotensin II may exist on endothelial cells, and Mauger, et al. (1975) have reported that, in culture, smooth muscle cells of rabbit aorta are extremely insensitive to both angiotensin II and norepinephrine. The latter investigators suggested that the lack of sensitivity might be owing to loss of receptors during culture or to a fault in the excitation or excitation-coupling mechanisms. However, it may well be that the receptors are not present on smooth muscle _in vivo_.

The immunocytochemical results provide further support for our hypothesis that circulating bradykinin and angiotensin I are metabolized by enzymes on the luminal surface of pulmonary endothelial cells. Our results with aorta indicate that its endothelial cells also have kininase II on their surfaces. Endothelial cells from other vascular beds have not been surveyed, but it would not be surprising to find that kininase II is a surface protein common to continuous endothelium. Should this be the case, it would not lessen the importance of the pulmonary vascular bed as the primary site for inactivation of circulating bradykinin and for the formation of angiotensin II. The lung contains one of the largest capillary networks of the body, processes the entire cardiac output and is unique among all organs and tissues in that its venous effluent empties directly into the systemic arterial circulation.

ACKNOWLEDGEMENTS

This work was supported in part by grants from the U.S. Public Health Service (HL 15691 and HL 16407 and contract N01 HR3-3015), from the John A. Hartford Foundation, Inc., the Council for Tobacco Research--U.S.A., Inc., and by an Established Investigatorship Award to Dr. Una S. Ryan from the American Heart Association and with funds contributed by the Heart Association of Palm Beach County, Florida, and the Veterans Administration (Project no. 7963-01).

REFERENCES

Avrameas, S., Immunochemistry, 6, 43, 1969.

Chiu, A.T., Ryan, J.W., Ryan, U.S. and Dorer, F.E., Biochem. J.,
   in press.

Dorer, F.E., Kahn, J.R., Lentz, K.E., Levine, M. and Skeggs, L.T.,
   Circ. Res., 31, 356-366, 1972.

Dorer, F.E., Kahn, J.R., Lentz, K.E., Levine, M. and Skeggs, L.T.,
   Circ. Res., 34, 824-827, 1974a.

Dorer, F.E., Ryan, J.W. and Stewart, J.M., Biochem. J., 141, 915-
   917, 1974b.

Edgington, T.S., J. Immunol., 106, 673-680, 1971.

Kraehenbuhl, J.P., Galardy, R.E. and Jamieson, J.D., J. Exp. Med.,
   139, 208-223, 1974.

Lindsay, D.G., F.E.B.S. Letters, 21, 105, 1972.

Mauger, J.P., Worcel, M., Tassin, J. and Courtois, Y., Nature, 255,
   337-338, 1975.

Richardson, J.B. and Beaulnes, A., J. Cell Biol., 51, 419, 1971.

Roblero, J., Ryan, J.W. and Stewart, J.M., Res. Commun. Chem. Path.
   Pharmac., 6, 207-212, 1973.

Ryan, J.W., Niemeyer, R.S. and Goodwin, D.W., in Adv. Exp. Med.
   Biol. (eds. N. Back and F. Sicuteri), Vol. 21, Plenum Press,
   New York, 1972b, pp. 259-266.

Ryan, J.W., Niemeyer, R.S., Goodwin, D.W., Smith, U. and Stewart,
   J.M., Biochem. J., 125, 921-923, 1971.

Ryan, J.W., Roblero, J. and Stewart, J.M., Pharmac. Res. Commun.,
   1, 192, 1969.

Ryan, J.W., Roblero, J. and Stewart, J.M., in Adv. Exp. Med. Biol.
   (eds. N. Back, F. Sicuteri and M. Rocha e Silva), Vol. 8. Plenum
   Press, New York, 1970a, pp. 263-272.

Ryan, J.W., and Ryan, U.S., Proc. 5th Inter. Davos Symp. on "Aspects
   of Lung Metabolism," (ed. R. de Haller), Academic Press, in
   press.

Ryan, J.W., Ryan, U.S., Schultz, D.R., Whitaker, C., Chung, A. and
    Dorer, F.E., Biochem. J., 146, 497-499, 1975.

Ryan, J.W. and Smith, U., in Protides of the Biological Fluids
    (ed. H. Peeters), Vol. 20, Pergamon Press, Oxford, England, 1973,
    pp. 379-384.

Ryan, J.W., Smith, U. and Niemeyer, R.S., Science, 176, 64-66,
    1972a.

Ryan, J.W., Stewart, J.M., Leary, W.P. and Ledingham, J.G.,
    Biochem. J., 120, 221-223, 1970b.

Smith, U. and Ryan, J.W., Fed. Proc., 32, 1957-1966, 1973.

Wiegele, M., De Barnardo, S., Leimgruber, W., Cleeland, R. and
    Grunberg, E., Biochem. Biophys. Res. Commun., 54, 899-905,
    1973.

THE VASOPEPTIDE KININ SYSTEM IN ACUTE CLINICAL CARDIAC DISEASES

Hashimoto, K.*, Wanka, J.**, Kohn, R.N.,** Wilkens,
H.J., Steger, R., and Back, N.

Dept. of Biochemical Pharmacology, School of Pharmacy,
State University of New York at Buffalo and Department
of Medicine** Buffalo General Hospital, Buffalo, N.Y.

Most deaths in patients with acute myocardial infarction (AMI)
have been due to severe arrhythmia and cardiogenic shock. While
continuous electrocardiographic monitoring and drug treatment have
significantly reduced mortality due to arrhythmia, cardiogenic
shock still remains a major cause of death in patients with AMI.(1).

Even though the major contributing factor to shock is ultimately the myocardial damage per se, metabolic disturbances such
as lactic acidosis, (2) and the release of biochemical mediators
(3-5) must not be ignored. Sicuteri, et al. (6) have postulated
dynamogenic (cardiac insufficiency) and autogenic (kininogenases
from myocardial necrosis) factors to play a role in the etiology
of cardiogenic shock.

Earlier we have reported the occurrence of a marked increase
of kinin levels in coronary sinus blood following experimental
coronary artery ligation in dogs. (7,8). The vasoactive kinin
system was found to be activated also in patients with AMI, with
significant differences showing between survivors and non-survivors
(9). A decrease in kininogen (KGN) and a concomitant increase of
kinin levels in the peripheral blood was observed in the survivors,
accompanied by lowering of the blood pressure, a decrease in total
peripheral resistance, and prolonged circulation time. In the non-
survivors who died of cardiogenic shock or congestive heart

---

* Supported by an International Fellowship from the Eli Lilly Co.,
 Indianapolis, Indiana, and NIH grant #HE-11492

failure, KGN levels also decreased, but kinin levels remained normal.

To investigate further this phenomenon and to identify the biochemical cause(s) responsible for the differences in the kinin levels of AMI survivors and non-survivors, changes in the components of the plasma kinin system were studied in patients who were admitted to the Coronary Care Unit of the Buffalo General Hospital.

Materials and Methods

1. <u>Patient Material</u>. Sixty-one patients admitted to the Coronary Care Unit of the Buffalo General Hospital during December 1974 until March 1975 were included in the study. The patients were divided into 5 groups. Group 1 consisted of 22 patients with AMI (14 male, 8 female). Three of these died of cardiogenic shock. Group 2 consisted of 20 cases of angina pectoris (10 male, 10 female). Five of them were of the intermediate type. Group 3 included 10 patients with congestive heart failure (CHF) without AMI (6 male, 4 female). Group 4 consisted of 5 cases of tachyarrhythmia (4 male, 1 female). Group 5 were 4 cases of Adams-Stokes Syndrome due to heart block (HB). An additional group of five normal subjects served as a control. Underlying diseases of CHF in the patients of group 3 were five cases of hypertensive heart disease, three cases of old myocardial infarction, and one case each of rheumatic valvular disease and of pulmonary embolism. The tachyarrhythmias in group 4 consisted of 3 cases of rapid atrial flutter and 2 cases of transient atrial fibrillation. Group 5 included 3 patients with complete A-V block, and one with sick sinus syndrome.

The mean age for the five groups of patients was as follows: Group 1: 66 (42-85) for the survivors, 60 (48-69) years for the non-survivors; Group 2: 60 (39-93) years; Group 3: 63 (46-86) years; Group 4: 69 (50-85) years; Group 5: 54 (46-67) years.

2. <u>Blood Sampling</u>. From each patient 8 ml of blood was taken from the cubital vein with a vacuum syringe containing 1 ml of 3.8% sodium citrate and 1 ml (10 mg) hexadimethrine bromide. The plasma was separated and stored at -20°C for later assay. In all instances the blood was taken on 3 consecutive days following admission. In 19 survivors with AMI, and one AMI non-survivor who died on the 11th day, additional blood samples were obtained on day 5, 7, and 10. At the time of blood sampling no chest pain was present in the patients of group 1 and 2, with the exception of the 3 non-survivors.

3. <u>Biochemical assays</u>.

a) <u>Prekallikrein (PKK)</u>. The method described by Wilkens and Steger (10) was modified as follows: a) 30% acetone was used to activate prekallikrein to kallikrein; b) after mixing plasma with 30% acetone, the pH was adjusted to 2, stored in the refrigerator overnight, and readjusted to pH 5.3. With this procedure considerably more kallikrein was obtained. Prekallikrein values were expressed in terms of the kinin activity produced upon incubation of the formed kallikrein with 10 mg of standard KGN. Standard KGN was prepared from Human ACD Plasma so that 10 mg yields 200 ng of kinin when incubated for 30 minutes at 37°C with excess bovine trypsin (5 μg).

b) <u>Kininogen (KGN)</u>. Total KGN was assayed according to the method described by Wilkens and Steger (10), and expressed in terms of the kinin produced when 0.05 ml of test plasma was incubated with 50 μg of bovine trypsin for 30 minutes at 37°C. KGN I was assayed and expressed as the amount of kinin released upon incubation of 0.05 ml test plasma with 0.5 mg of purified human plasma kallikrein. Human plasma kallikrein obtained by acetone treatment of ACD Plasma was purified by hydroxylapetite column chromatography, so that 0.5 mg of the material was able to release the maximum amount of kinin from 0.05 ml of normal human plasma. KGN II was calculated as the difference between total KGN and KGN I.

c) <u>Kininase</u>. Kininase activity was assayed according to the method described by Wilkens and Steger (10), and expressed as the volume of plasma needed to destroy 50% of 10^{-6}g of synthetic bradykinin in 10 minutes at 37°C.

The kinin generated or remaining as a result of the above procedures was determined through bioassay, using the isolated perfused virgin rat uterus.

d) <u>Other Parameters</u>. Serum CPK, GOT, and LDH were assayed according to routine laboratory procedures.

RESULTS

1. <u>Changes in components of the kinin system during the first 3 days</u>.

<u>Figure 1</u> shows the changes in PKK levels in the 5 groups. Compared to the values obtained from the 5 normal subjects, PKK levels were markedly decreased in all 5 groups during the initial 3 day observation period. In every group these decreases were statistically significant. In the AMI survivors the lowest mean

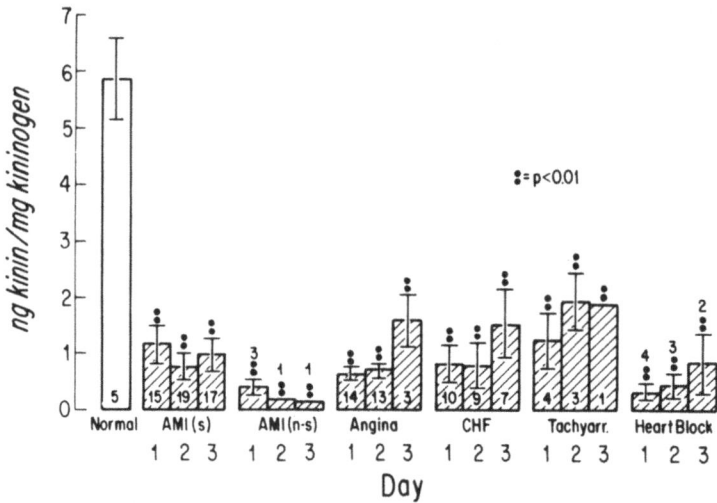

Figure 1. Changes in prekallikrein levels in venous blood in patients with acute myocardial infarction (AMI), angina pectoris (Angina), congestive heart failure (CHF), Tachyarrhythmia (TA), and heart block shown by mean ± SEM. The numbers in or above the columns indicate the number of the samples. (s): survivors, (n-s) non-survivors

value was seen on the 2nd day, whereas the AMI non-survivors showed a further decrease on the 3rd day. These differences between AMI survivors and non-survivors were statistically significant (p<0.05). The patients in the other 4 groups showed a gradual increase in PKK levels on the 2nd and 3rd day. There were no statistically significant differences in the PKK levels between AMI survivors and the patients with angina pectoris, tachyarrhythmia, or heart block throughout the 3-day observation period.

Figure 2 shows the changes in total KGN seen on the first three days in the 5 groups of patients. A significant decrease in total KGN was noted in both survivors and non-survivors of AMI on the first day. A further significant decrease was observed in the one patient who died of cardiogenic shock 11 days after the

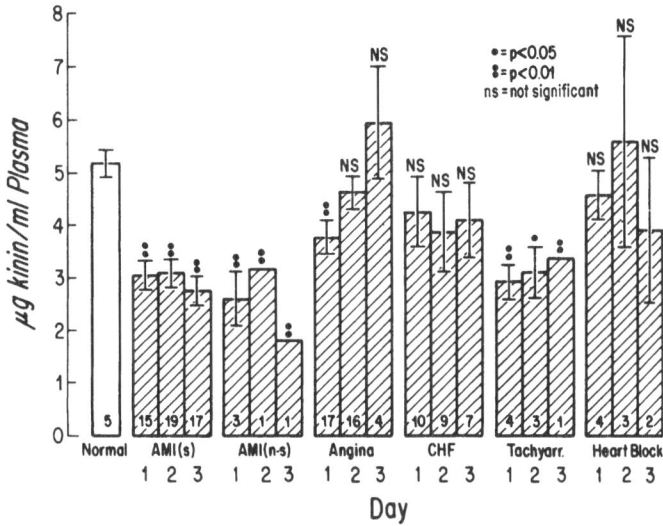

Figure 2.   Changes in total kininogen levels in venous blood
in each group.

onset of AMI. A significantly decreased total KGN was seen on
the 1st day in a patient with angina pectoris, followed by an increase to normal on the 2nd day. Patients with TA likewise showed
significantly low levels of total KGN, whereas patients with HB
exhibited normal levels.

Figure 3 shows the levels of KGN I for the 5 groups of
patients. KGN I was significantly decreased in the patients with
AMI, with a marked difference between survivors and non-survivors
observable on the 3rd day. Other significant decreases in KGN I
were seen in patients with angina pectoris on the third day, in
patients with CHF on the second day, and in patients with HB on
the first day.

Figure 4 shows the levels of KGN II, calculated as the
difference between total KGN and KGN I. The changes seen are
largely identical with those occuring in the level of KGN, since

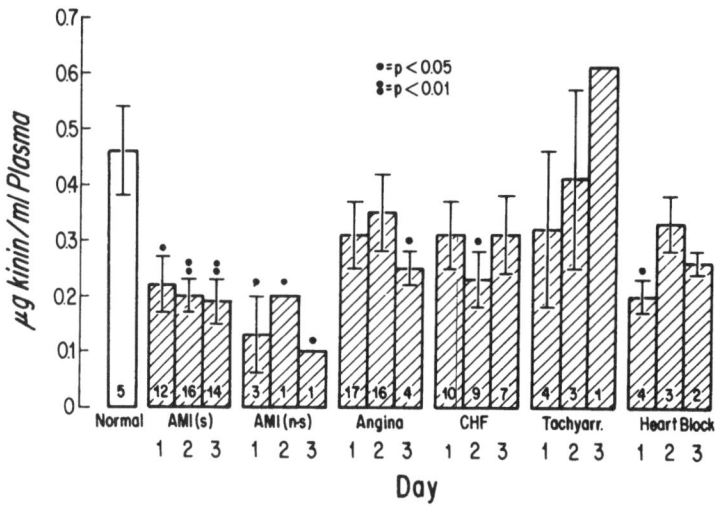

Figure 3.   Changes in kininogen I levels in venous blood in each group.

nearly 90% of the total KGN consisted of KGN II.

Figure 5 shows the level of kininase activity in patients of all 5 groups. A significant difference in kininase activity was observed between AMI survivors and non-survivors. Whereas the AMI survivors showed a marked decrease in kininase activity, this activity remained at its normal high level in patients who subsequently died of cardiogenic shock. In the one patient who died on the 11th day, normal kininase activity was maintained throughout. A significant decrease in kininase activity also occurred in patients with angina pectoris on the 1st and 2nd day, in patients with CHF on the 2nd day, and in patients with TA on the 1st and 3rd day. No significant changes were noted in patients with HB.

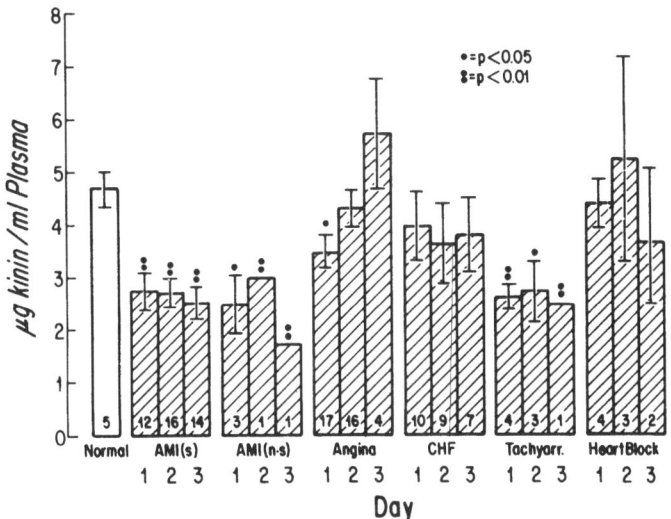

Figure 4.   Changes in kininogen II levels in venous blood in each groups.

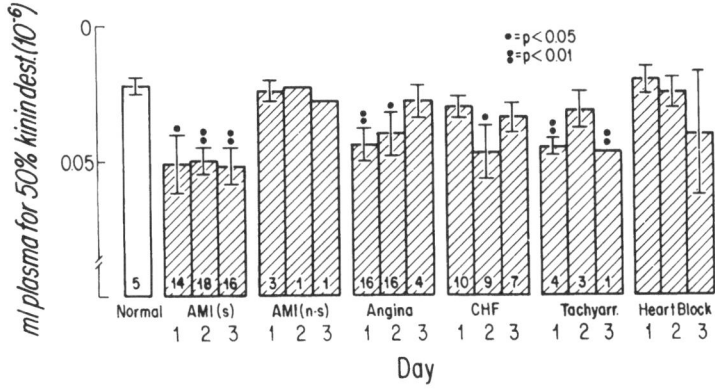

Figure 5.   Changes in kininase activity in venous blood in each group.

2. Changes in components of the kinin system in AMI survivors during 10 day observation period.

Figure 6 shows the changes in PKK levels in the AMI survivors over 10 days. The PKK levels were markedly decreased throughout the entire observation period, with the lowest mean level occurring on the 2nd day.

Figure 7 shows the changes in the total KGN level in the AMI survivors for the 10 days of observation. Total KGN levels were significantly decreased over the entire period, with the lowest levels noted on the 3rd day.

Figure 8 shows the KGN I levels seen in the survivors of AMI, which also were significantly decreased throughout, except for the 7th day. The lowest level was noted on the 10th day.

Figure 9 shows the KGN II levels in AMI survivors over the same 10 day period. The changes observed were essentially similar to the changes in total KGN.

Figure 10 shows the level of kininase activity in the AMI survivors. There was a significant decrease in kininase activity throughout the entire observation period with the lowest level seen on the 7th day.

3. Correlation between components of the kinin system and other parameters.

No significant correlation appeared to exist between the aforementioned changes in components of the kinin system and such laboratory findings as CPK, LDH, and GOT.

DISCUSSION

A decrease in PKK, total KGN, KGN I and KGN II was noted in both survivors and non-survivors of AMI. However, whereas the kininase activity was significantly reduced in the AMI survivors, kininase activity was maintained at its normal high level in the non-survivors. This striking difference in the level of kinin-destroying activity between survivors and non-survivors of AMI appears to be most significant.

While a decrease in KGN levels in patients with AMI has been reported earlier by several authors, (3,4,9,11) there is a discrepancy in the data regarding the level of KGN in the survivors as compared to the level found in non-survivors who died of shock. Sicuteri et al.,(3), and Dzizinski et al. (4), reported that KGN levels were lower in non-survivors than in survivors, whereas

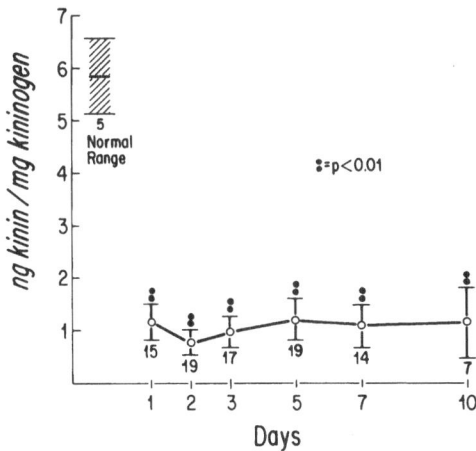

Figure 6.   Changes in prekallikrein levels in venous blood during
10 days observation period in patients with acute myocardial
infarction (AMI) who survived, shown by mean ± SEM.   The numbers
below the columns indicate the number of the samples.

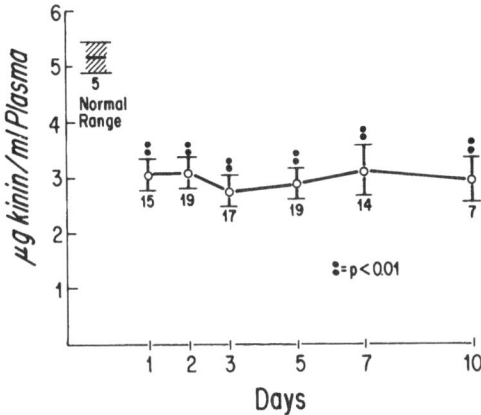

Figure 7.   Changes in total kininogen levels in venous blood
during 10 days observation period in patients with
AMI who survived.

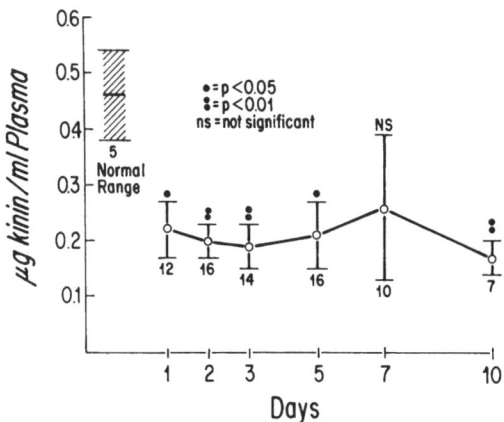

Figure 8.   Changes in kininogen I levels in venous blood
             during 10 days observation period in patients
             with AMI who survived.

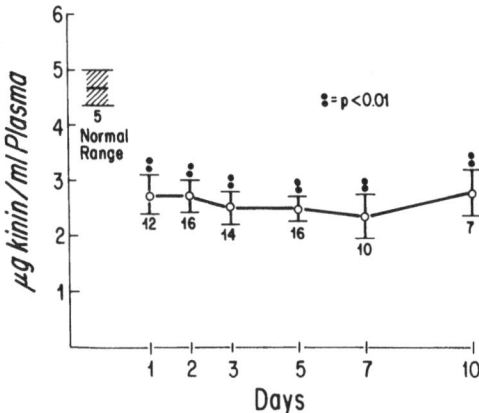

Figure 9.   Changes in kininogen II levels in venous blood
             during 10 days observation period in patients
             with AMI who survived.

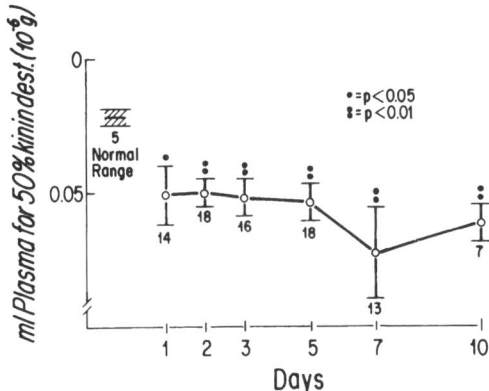

Figure 10.   Changes in kininase activity in venous blood
              during 10 days observation period in patients
              with AMI who survived.

Wiegershausen, et al. (11) as well as our own previous studies (9)
have shown no difference between survivors and non-survivors.   In
the present study we also have noted no difference in the levels
of total KGN, except for one case on the 3rd, 5th and 7th day.

     There are also contradictory reports regarding the correlation
between lowering of blood pressure and decrease in KGN level.
Sicuteri, et al. (3) observed a close relationship between both,
whereas no such relation was noted by Wiegershausen, et al. (11).
In our own study (9), we have observed a significant correlation
between low blood pressure and decreased KGN levels in the AMI
survivors, in contrast to the non-survivors where no such correlation was seen.

     According to the observations of Sicuteri, et al. (6) the
PKK level decreased gradually after the onset of AMI, showing the
lowest level on the 8th day.   These observations differ somewhat
from the findings in our present study, but might be explainable
on the basis of differences in assay techniques.   Concerning the
fact that the changes in KGN I and KGN II levels in our AMI
patients were essentially identical, it needs to be pointed out
that nearly 90% of the total plasma KGN consisted of KGN II.   The
resultant conclusion that changes in the level of KGN II are apt
to play a more dynamic role in AMI than any changes in the level
of KGN I necessarily limits the potential role of plasma kallikrein, which acts only on KGN I to release kinin.   Consequently,
additional enzymes, such as plasmin or trypsin which form kinin
from both KGN I and KGN II, may be involved.

While it is clear that the plasma kinin system is activated in the course of AMI, the pathogenetic significance of this occurrence remains to be elucidated. Pharmacological cardio-vascular responses to kinin include an increase in heart rate, a lowering of the blood pressure due to decreased peripheral resistance, an increase in cardiac output, and coronary vasodi-lation (12). Microscopic observation of the rat mesentary vasculature has revealed kinin-induced dose-dependent dilatation of venules, precapillaries, metarterioles and arterioles (13). Similar effects of kinin were observed in the vasa vasorum of the abdominal aorta (14). In our previous study (9) we had found that AMI survivors had a low cardiac output and increased peripheral vascular resistance on the 1st day. This was followed by a de-crease in peripheral resistance on the 2nd and 3rd day, coincident with an increase in kinin levels in the peripheral blood. On the other hand, in the patients who died of cardiogenic shock, the low cardiac output and the increased peripheral vascular resistance persisted until death. No increase in kinin levels was seen in the non-survivors, which, in light of our findings in the present study, appears to have been due to the maintenance of a normally high kininase activity in these individuals. With respect to the low kininase activity seen in the AMI survivors, it is tempting to speculate that the associated increase in kinin levels in the peripheral blood may have been helpful by reducing the work load of the injured heart. Such a view of kinin in AMI obviously contrasts with reports assigning a detrimental role for the release of kinin in the pathogenesis of various types of experimental shock (15-18). These latter conclusions are based primarily on observed decreases in plasma KGN and on the increased rates of survival obtained with the administration of proteinase inhibitors, such as Trasylol. Trasylol, however, inhibits other actions of proteases other than kinin release. Stock et al. (19) found that Trasylol effectively prevented postischemic edema and significantly reduced the rate of mortality in rat tourniquet shock, whereas carboxypeptidase B reduced neither one. Urbanitz, et al. (20) have presented evidence that the decrease in KGN associated with hemorr-hagic, burn, traumatic, and endotoxin shock are merely the reflection of a decrease in plasma protein. An increase in kininase activity in experimental anaphylactic shock has been reported by Back et al. (18).

Since the patients with angina pectoris in our study have displayed a markedly reduced level of PKK, a transient decrease in total KGN and KGN II, and low kininase activity, it may be concluded in retrospect that the activation of the kinin system seen in the AMI patients was not due necessarily to the myocardial injury alone. A decrease in KGN in patients with angina pectoris, most prominently in its active phase, has been reported by Dzizinskii et al (21). Pitt et al. (22) have observed a decrease in PKK and in factor XII, and an increase in TAME activity in 7 out of 11 patients during anginal attacks provoked by cardiac pacing. These authors felt that release of kinin under the given circumstances represented a hemodynamic adjustment through its coronary vasodilating action. Raab (23) has pointed to the role of catecholamines in angina pectoris, and both Melmon and Cline (24), as well as Roche e Silva (25) have shown the existence of a close relationship between catecholamines and kinin, with either one capable of effecting the release of the other. Consequently, catecholamine release must be considered as a possible activating mechanism of the kinin system in our group of patients. Of the 20 patients studied by us, 5 had the intermediate type of angina pectoris. The activation of the kinin system in these 5 individuals was more prominent than in the 15 others with angina pectoris of effort.

The patients with CHF exhibited a markedly decreased level of PKK, accompanied by significantly decreased levels of KGN I on the 2nd day. Since kininase activity also was significantly reduced on that same day, the plasma kinin level may have been elevated at that time. The hemodynamic changes commonly associated with CHF include a reduction in cardiac output and an increase in systemic as well as pulmonary vascular resistance. In this context it is perhaps revealing that the improvement of symptoms seen in our patients on the 2nd day, following the administration of cardiac glycosides or diuretics, coincided with the time of kinin system activation.

The patients with TA and those with HB exhibited very low levels of PKK, especially on the 1st day. The TA patients had low levels of total KGN and KGN II throughout, whereas the level of KGN I was significantly reduced on the 1st day, followed by an increase thereafter. Kininase activity was within the normal range in the patients with HB, but showed significantly decreased values on the first and third day in the patients with TA. Up to the present there appear to be no reports concerning the role of kinin in cardiac arrhythmia, except for noting an increase in heart rate. Therefore, further studies will be required to elucidate the pathophysiological role of the kallikrein-kinin system in that condition.

REFERENCES

1. Anderson, R.: The relation between metabolic acidosis and cardiac arrhythmias in acute myocardial infarction. Am. Heart J. 76: 1, 1968.
2. Peretz, D.I., Scott, H.M., Duff, J., Dosseter, J.B., MacLean, L.D. and McGregor H.: The significance of lacticacidemia in the shock syndrome. Ann. New York Acad. Sci 119: 1133, 1965.

3. Sicuteri, F., Franchi, G., Del Bianco, P.L. and Del Bene, E.:
    A contribution to the interpretation of shock and pain in
    myocardial infarction. Malattie Cardiovasculari 8: 343, 1967.
4. Dzizinskii, A.A. and Kuimov, A.D.: Blood kinin system in path-
    ogenesis and clinic of ischemic heart disease. Cor. Vasa
    14: 9, 1972.
5. Glenn, T.M., Lefer, A.M., Martin, J.B., Lovett, W.L., Morris,
    J.N., and Wangensteen S.L.: Production of a myocardial
    depressant factor in cardiogenic shock, Am. Heart J. 82: 78,
    1971.
6. Sicuteri, F., Antonini, F.M., Del Bianco, P.L., Franchi, G.
    and Curradi, C.: Prekallikrein and kallikrein inhibitor in
    plasma of patients affected by recent myocardial infarction.
    Advances in Experimental Medicine and Biology (eds. Back, N.
    and Sicuteri, F.) Vol. 21: p. 445 Plenum Press, N.Y. London
    1972.
7. Kimura, E., Hashimoto, K., Furukawa, S. and Hayakawa, H.:
    Changes in bradykinin level in coronary sinus blood after the
    experimental occlusion of a coronary artery. Am. Heart J. 85:
    635, 1973.
8. Hashimoto , K., Furukawa, S., Hirose, M., and Hayakawa, H.:
    Changes in bradykinin level in coronary sinus blood after
    experimental coronary occlusion, and their relationships to
    hemodynamic changes. Singapore Med. J. 14: 356, 1973.
9. Hashimoto, K., Hamamoto, H., Tajima, N., and Kimura, E.:
    Changes in kinin system and hemodynamics in acute stage of
    myocardial infarction. A clinical study. VII World Congress
    of Cardiology, Buenos Aires, 1974.
10. Wilkens, H.J., and Steger, R.: in Screening Methods in
    Pharmacology,(eds. Turner, R.A. and Hebborn, P.) Vol. II
    p. 61 Academic Press Inc. 1971
11. Wiegershausen, B., Hennighausen, G., Klausch, B., Korber, H.G.
    and Hauzeur, F.: Plasma kininogen level in myocardial in-
    farction. Advances in Experimental Medicine and Biology
    (eds. F. Sicuteri, M. Rocha e Silva, & N. Back) Vol. 8
    p. 221 Plenum Press, N.Y. 1970.
12. Reichgot, M.J., and Melmon, K.L.: Bradykinin and the cardio-
    vascular system. Circulation 42: 563, 1970.
13. Altura, B.M., Hershey, S.G., and Altura B.T.: Microcirculatory
    actions of polypeptides and their use in the treatment of ex-
    perimental shock, in Bradykinin and related kinins. Cardio-
    vascular, biochemical and neutral actions. Advances in
    Experimental Medicine and Biology (eds. F. Sicuteri, M. Rocha
    e Silva, & N. Back) Vol. 8, New York, Plenum Press, p. 239,
    1970.
14. Shionoya, S., Nakata, Y., Kamiya, K., Inagaki, A., and Yano, T.
    Influences of bradykinin on the microcirculation. Angiology
    22: 456, 1971.

15. Webster, M.E. and Clark, W.R.: Significance of the callicrein-callidinogen-callidin system in shock. Amer. J. Physiol.: 197: 406, 1959.
16. Brocklehurst, W.E. and Lahiri, S.C.: The production of bradykinin in anaphylaxis. J. Physiol. 160: 15, 1962.
17. Dawson, W., Starr, M.S. and West, G.B.: Inhibition of ana-phylactic shock in the rat by antihistamines and ascorbic acid. Br. J. Pharmac. Chemother. 27: 249, 1966.
18. Back, N., Wilkens, H.J., and Steger, R.: Proteinases and proteinase inhibitors in experimental shock states. Ann. N.Y. Acad. Sci. 146: 691, 1968.
19. Stock, W. and Eigler, F.W.: Indirect evidence against a major role of kinins in tourniquet-shock by use of carboxypeptidase B. in Advances in Experimental Medicine and Biology (eds. Back, N. and Sicuteri, F.) Vol. 8 p. 355 Plenum Press, N.Y. 1970
20. Urbanitz, D., Sailer, R., and Habermann, E.: In vivo investi-gations on the role of the kinin system in tissue injury and shock syndromes, in Advances in Experimental Medicine and Biology (eds. Back, N. and Sicuteri, F.) Vol. 8, p. 343, Plenum Press, N.Y. 1970.
21. Dzizinskii, A.A., and Kuimov, A.D.: Blood kinin system in pathogenesis and clinic of ischemic heart disease. Cor. Vasa 14: 9, 1972.
22. Pitt, B., Mason, J., Conti, C.R., and Colman, R.W.: Activation of the plasma kallikrein system during myocardial ischemia in Advances in Experimental Medicine and Biology (eds. Back, N. and Sicuteri, F.) Vol. 8, p. 403, Plenum Press, N.Y. 1970.
23. Raab, W.: Myocardial metabolism in the pathogenesis and treat-ment of angina pectoris. Cardiologia 22: 291, 1953.
24. Melmon, K.L., and Cline, M.J.: Kinins. Amer. J. Med. 43: 153, 1967.
25. Rocha e Silva, M.: Chemical Mediators of the acute inflammatory reaction. Ann. N.Y. Acad. Sci. 116: 899, 1964.

PLASMATIC PREKALLIKREIN AND KALLIKREIN INHIBITOR IN PREGNANCY, LABOR AND IN NEWBORN*

Branconi, F., Faldi, P., Seravalli, G., Curradi, C.+, DelBianco, P.L.+, Sicuteri, F.+

Department of Obstetrics and Gynaecology, +Department of Clinical Pharmacology
University of Florence, Italy

Previous research has shown that the kininogen-kinin system is affected during pregnancy and labour. In fact, plasmatic kininogen significantly increases in pregnant women while after the espulsive stage of labour, it decreases and returns to the prelabour values at the early hours of puerperium (1,3).

At the end of physiological pregnancy the arterial plasma kininogen level is significantly higher than the venous one; this difference does not occur during gestosis (2).

Moreover difference exists between the plasmatic kininogen of newborns of normal and gestosic mothers.

In the present study prekallikrein and kallikrein inhibitor are evaluated in pregnancy, labour and in the newborn's blood.

METHOD

The plasmatic prekallikrein, and the kallikrein inhibitor have been evaluated, according to the Colman and coworkers method (4) in 15 pregnant women and in their newborn hospitalized in the Department of Obstetrics and Gynaecology. Blood samples were drawn from the mothers' during the last 3 weeks of pregnancy and immediately after the end of the labour. In the newborn the blood was drawn from the umbilical chord at the moment of delivery and from external jugularis vein 24 hours after birth.

* With the help of the National Research Council, Rome.

RESULTS AND COMMENTS (FIGURE 1)

1. No difference exists between the plasmatic prekallikrein and kallikrein inhibitor during pregnancy and that at the end of labour, the values are similar to those reported by other authors (5).

2. In the newborn, very low prekallikrein amounts were found, and its mean value resulted about 19 μmoles TAMe/ml plasma/hour, that is, values extremely lower than those in the normal adult.

3. In the venous blood 24 hours after birth, the prekallikrein is still significantly lower.

4. No kallikrein inhibiting activity is present in the newborn's blood, neither at birth, nor 24 hours after birth.

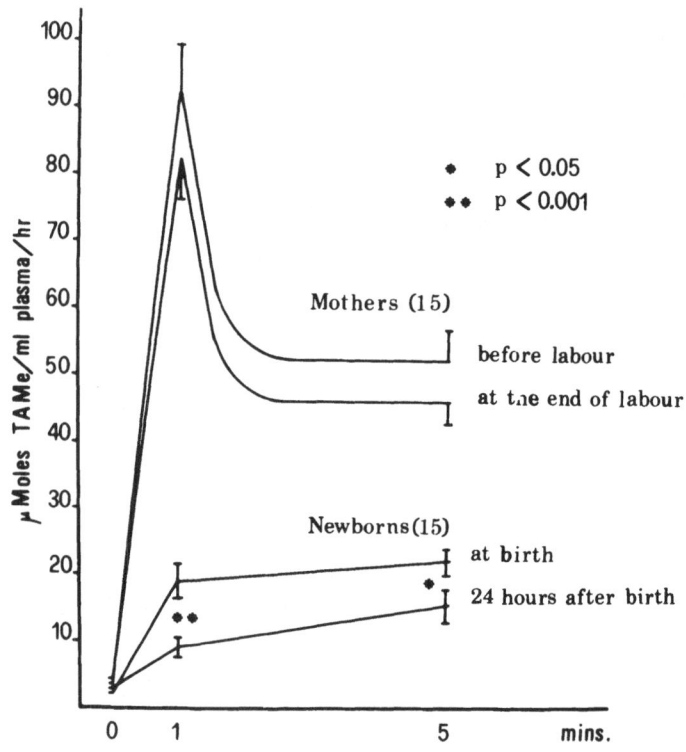

Figure 1. Plasma Prekallikrein and Kallikrein Inhibitor in Mother and Newborn.

In conclusion, the most interesting data resulting from this study, is the very low amount of activatable prekallikrein in the newborn. This is in agreement with the low kininogen level found in the newborn who seems to have an immaturity of the kinin forming enzyme system.

SUMMARY

In order to reveal the possible physiological role of the kallikrein during the stress of birth, the prekallikrein and kallikrein inhibitor were evaluated in 15 pregnant women and in 15 newborns from terminated pregnancies.

The results show a very low level of prekallikrein in the funiculus blood at the moment of birth and a still lower level in venous blood 24 hours after birth.

No important changes resulted in the mother's blood either in pregnancy, nor at the end of the labour.

REFERENCES

1. Periti P., Centaro A., Sicuteri F., Leocani B.: Bradichininogeno ematico durante il parto. Boll. Soc. Ital. Biol. Sperim., 38, 672, 1962.

2. Periti P., Gasparri G.: Bradykininogen in the blood of women during pregnancy, labour and puerperium. In: Hypotensive Peptides, pg. 536, Springer-Verlag, New York, 1966.

3. Severi S., Paradiso M., Periti P.: Fetal distress and Plasma Kininogen in the newborn. Adv. Exp. Med. Biol., 21, 367, 1972.

4. Colman R.W., Mason J.W., Sherry S.: The Kallikreinogen-Kallikrein enzyme system of human plasma: Assay of components and observations in disease states. Annals of Internat. Medicine, 71, 763, 1969.

5. Melmon K.L., Cline M.J., Hughes T., Nies A.S.: Kinins: Possible Mediators of Neonatal Circulatory Changes in Man. J. Clin. Invest., 47, 1295, 1968.

METHIONYL-LYSYL-BRADYKININ: THE KININ RELEASED BY PEPSIN FROM

HUMAN KININOGENS

Jorge A. Guimaraes, Jack V. Pierce, Valdemar Hial and
John J. Pisano

Section on Physiological Chemistry, Laboratory of
Chemistry, National Heart and Lung Institute, National
Institutes of Health, Bethesda, Maryland 20014

Since Croxatto and coworkers (1, 2) first described and named
the hypotensive, leiomyokinetic peptide released from mammalian
serum by pepsin, the identity of pepsitocin has been in question.
Habermann and coworkers (3, 4) reported the isolation of two related peptides from pepsin digests of highly purified bovine
kininogen: MLBK-Ser-Val-Gln[1] (90%) and MLBK-Ser-Val-Gln-Val-Met
(10%). In contrast, Hochstrasser and Werle (5) found Gly (or Ser)-
Arg-MLBK in pepsin digests of bovine plasma Fraction IV-6. Inasmuch as we had in hand appreciable amounts of highly purified
human plasma kininogens (6), we undertook this study of the
identity of pepsitocin.

RESULTS

Kinin Release from Kininogens. Several highly purified human
and bovine kininogen preparations were incubated with pepsin and
trypsin (Table 1). They included two LMW and two HMW forms (6);
LMW kininogen I, with BK at its carboxyl end and LMW kininogen II,
with BK inside the molecule (7); and bovine LMW kininogen (kinin-
ogen-II), kindly provided by Prof. T. Suzuki (8). Both pepsin
and trypsin released kinin rapidly from all of the kininogen
samples, which were stable by themselves at pH 2.0 and 7.0. Kinin
release was judged complete, inasmuch as additional kinin was not
liberated by prolonged incubation or by incubation of the residual
protein in the peptic digest with trypsin after removal of the
kinin by Sephadex G-25 gel filtration.

Characterization of the Peptic Kinin. The peptic digests
were between 9 and 11 times less active than the trypsin digests.
However, incubation of the peptic kinin with human plasma

TABLE 1

BIOASSAY (GUINEA PIG ILEUM) OF THE KININ
RELEASED FROM KININOGENS BY PEPSIN AND TRYPSIN

KININOGENS	TRYPSIN	PEPSIN	TRYPSIN/PEPSIN RATIO
	µg BK equivalents/mg Kininogen		
B2α(a)	14.7	1.50	9.8
B3.2α(a)	14.2	1.55	9.2
B4β(a)	10.9	1.10	9.9
B4γ(a)	11.2	1.05	10.7
Human Kgn I(b)	7.2	0.65	11.1
Human Kgn II(b)	7.2	0.66	10.9
Bovine Kgn II(c)	6.4	0.60	10.7

Between 100 and 200 µg of the kininogens were incubated with 3 µg
of twice crystallized porcine pepsin (Worthington) for 15 minutes
at 37°, pH 2.0 (0.01 N HCl). The solutions were then adjusted to
pH 7.0 with NaOH and diluted to a final volume of 0.5 ml. Between
10 and 20 µg of the same kininogens were incubated with 5 µg of
twice crystallized trypsin for 20 minutes at 37°, pH 7.8 (0.05 M
Tris-Cl) in a final volume of 0.5 ml.

(a) Reference 6.
(b) Reference 7.
(c) Reference 8.

aminopeptidase, an enzyme able to convert LBK, MLBK, and GAMLBK
to BK (9), gave an 8-fold increase in activity with the isolated
guinea pig ileum, as was found also for synthetic MLBK. Incubation
of LBK with aminopeptidase resulted in only a 2- to 3-fold increase
of activity. In a separate experiment, incubation of synthetic
GAMLBK with pepsin gave a 2-fold activity increase. It is un-
likely that this kinin could be formed by pepsin digestion of
kininogen. The peptic kinin was inactivated by carboxypeptidase
B, indicating the BK sequence to be carboxy-terminal.

TABLE 2

COMPARISON OF RETENTION VOLUMES ON AN SP-SEPHADEX
C-25 COLUMN OF THE PEPTIC KININS FROM SEVERAL KININOGENS WITH
BK, LBK AND MLBK BEFORE AND AFTER TREATMENT WITH DAP I

SUBSTRATES	RETENTION VOLUMES OF PEPTIC PEPTIDES	
	BEFORE DAP I	AFTER DAP I
	ml	
Kininogens		
Human B2α	43-57	Not tested
B3.2α	44-58	14-20
B4β	44-59	13-20
B4γ	43-58	Not tested
Bovine LMW II	46-50	13-20
Kinins		
Standard BK	12-20	12-20
LBK	64-78	64-78
MLBK	44-55	12-20

The kininogens, 500 μg each, were incubated with 5 μg porcine pepsin for 20 minutes at pH 2.0, 37°, in a final volume of 1.0 ml.
The incubates were bioassayed, freeze-dried, dissolved in 1.0 ml
of 0.05 M Tris-Cl-0.08 M NaCl buffer, pH 8.0, and applied to a
0.60 x 13.0-cm SP-Sephadex C-25 column equilibrated with the above
pH 8.0 buffer. This buffer was also used to elute the kinins.
An aliquot of 200 μl of each peak was incubated with 20 μg of
DAP I (Schwarz/Mann) dissolved in 1% NaCl. Mercaptoethanol
(2.5 μl/ml)was added to the incubate.

    Further evidence that the peptic kinin is MLBK was obtained
by comparing the chromatographic properties of the two kinins
before and after treatment with DAP I, an enzyme which splits
the dipeptide Met-Lys from MLBK, but does not attack LBK or BK.
The three kinins, BK, LBK, and MLBK - are resolved with highly
reproducible retention volumes on an SP-Sephadex C-25 column
developed by a modification (10) of the method of Sampaio, et al.
(11). When porcine pepsin digests of several kininogens were
applied to the SP-Sephadex column, all gave a single kinin with
the same retention volume found for authentic MLBK. However,
DAP I treatment of these activity peaks gave an 8-fold activity

increase and a retention volume on the standard SP-Sephadex column characteristic of BK (Table 2). The tridecapeptide GAMLBK is not eluted from the column under the conditions employed.

The peptic peptide from 10 mg of human kininogen B3.2α was purified by gel filtration on Sephadex G-25 and Bio-Gel P-4 columns and by CM-Sephadex C-25 chromatography. Amino acid analysis of a sample equivalent to ca 3 nmole of MLBK gave 1.0 Met, 2.2 Arg, 1.9 Phe, 3.3 Pro, 3.9 Gly, 2.2 Lys, and traces of Glu, Leu, Ser, and Thr. Except for the too high yields of Gly and Lys, the analysis is close to that expected for MLBK. Dansylation (12) of another sample gave a product indistinguishable from dansyl-MLBK when compared on a silica gel H thin-layer plate using 4:1:5 n-butanol-acetic acid-water. Upon hydrolysis of the dansyl-peptide in 6 N HCl overnight, dansyl-methionine was detected by high performance liquid chromatography.

DISCUSSION

Met-Lys-bradykinin was discovered by Elliott and Lewis (13), who isolated the peptide from bovine serum which had been acidified to pH 2.0, dialyzed against 0.01 N HCl, and then incubated at pH 7.5, 37° for 6 hours. Since human plasma and presumably bovine plasma contain pepsinogen, its activation during the acid treatment could account for the formation of MLBK.

Our studies with highly purified human kininogens have shown that porcine pepsin is an unexpectedly good kininogenase. Although the maximal rate of kinin release occurs around pH 1.0, half this rate was found at pH 5.0. There is no significant difference in the rates of kinin release from human kininogens B2α, B3.2α, and B4β by pepsin at pH 2.0. A comparison of the kinetic constants of pepsin at pH 2.0 with those obtained using human urinary kallikrein, human plasma kallikrein, trypsin, and plasmin at pH 7.5 showed that pepsin has a higher catalytic activity (k_{cat}/K_m) than trypsin and plasmin when tested with human kininogens B2α and B4β. In fact, the kinetic constants of porcine pepsin are not greatly different from those found for the kallikreins (14).

The results described above favor the hypothesis that the peptic kinin from highly purified human kininogens is identical with MLBK. This conclusion is based on:
1) The 8- to 10-fold increase in activity on the guinea pig ileum after treatment with aminopeptidase and with DAP I.
2) The inactivation by carboxypeptidase B.
3) The identical retention volumes in the analytical SP-Sephadex C-25 chromatography before and after treatment with DAP I.
4) The identical thin-layer chromatographic properties of the dansyl-peptide and the finding of dansyl-methionine in acid hydrolysates

FOOTNOTES

1) Abbreviations used: BK, bradykinin (Arg-Pro-Pro-Gly-Phe-Ser-
Pro-Phe-Arg); LBK, lysyl-bradykinin; MLBK, methionyl-lysyl-brady-
kinin; GAMLBK, glycyl-arginyl-methionyl-lysyl-bradykinin; LMW,
low molecular weight; HMW, high molecular weight; DAP I, dipep-
tidyl aminopeptidase I; Kgn, kininogen.

REFERENCES

1. Croxatto, H., G. Rojas, and L. Barnafi. Bol. Soc. Biol.
   Santiago, 8, 84 (1950).
2. Croxatto, H. In Polypeptides which Stimulate Plain Muscle,
   J.H. Gaddum, ed. Livingstone, Edinburgh & London, p. 92 (1955).
3. Habermann, E. Naunyn-Schmiedebergs Arch. Pharmakol. Exp.
   Pathol. 253, 474, (1966).
4. Habermann, E. In Hypotensive Peptides, E.G. Erdos, N. Back,
   and F. Sicuteri, eds. Springer, New York, p. 116 (1966).
5. Hochstrasser, K. and E. Werle. Hoppe-Seyler's Z. Physiol.
   Chem., 348, 177 (1967).
6. Guimaraes, J.A., R. Chen-Lu, M.E. Webster and J.V. Pierce.
   Fed. Proc. 33, 641 Abs. (1974).
7. Pierce, J.V. and M. E. Webster. In Hypotensive Peptides, Erdos
   et al.eds. Springer, New York, p. 130 (1966).
8. Yano, M., H. Kato, S. Nagasawa and T. Suzuki, J. Biochem.
   (Tokyo), 62, 386 (1967).
9. Guimaraes, J.A., D. R. Borges, E.S. Prado, and J.L. Prado.
   Biochem. Pharmacol. 22, 3157 (1973).
10. Hial, V., to be published.
11. Sampaio, M.U., M.L. Reis, E. Fink, A.C.M. Camargo, and L. J.
    Greene. Life Sci. 16, 796 Abs. (1974).
12. Tamura, Z., T. Nakajima, T. Nakayama, J.J. Pisano, and S.
    Udenfriend. Anal. Biochem. 52, 595 (1973).
13. Elliott, D.F. and G.P. Lewis. Biochem. J. 95, 437 (1965).
14. Guimaraes, J.A., to be published.

OCCURRENCE OF COMPONENTS OF THE KALLIKREIN-KININ SYSTEM IN HUMAN GENITAL TRACT SECRETIONS AND THEIR POSSIBLE FUNCTION IN STIMULATION OF SPERM MOTILITY AND MIGRATION

S. Palm[1], W.B. Schill[2], O. Wallner[3], R. Prinzen[4] and H. Fritz[1]

Institute of Clinical Chemistry & Clinical Biochemistry[1], Dept. of Dermatology [2], First. Dept. of Gynecology & Obstetrics[3] and Gynecological and Ambulatory Veterinary Clinic[4], University of Munich

As an autonomic cell, the spermatozoon is able to self regulate its metabolism. It is therefore an attractive object to study pharmacological actions. The visual sign of an alive sperm cell is its motility. Recent investigations have shown a possible involvement of the kallikrein-kinin system in the regulation of sperm motility and migration (Schill et al., 1974; Leidl et al., 1975; Wallner et al., 1975).

Components of the Kallikrein-Kinin System in Genital Tract Secretions.

It could be demonstrated more recently that constituents of spermatozoa, seminal plasma and midcycle cervical mucus may be involved in kinin liberation and degradation. (Palm et al., 1975a) and thus in the regulation of sperm migration. Various substances, present in human uterus wall may also participate in kinin liberation (Rybak et al., 1974).

The trypsinlike sperm acrosomal proteinase acrosin (Fritz et al.,1974) is highly active in releasing kinins from purified bovine high molecular weight kininogen (Palm et al., 1975b). Obviously, acrosin has the same splitting specificity as trypsin in its action as a kininogenase. If biological aspects of acrosin-regulated mechanisms are discussed, it has to be considered that acrosin inhibitors are present in high excess in the secretions of the male genital tract and even in spermatozoa after ejaculation.

However, the inhibitors are removed druing residence of the sperm
cell in the secretions of the female genital tract. Hence, after
that so-called "capacitation reaction", which sperm undergo in the
female genital fluids, acrosin may act on its physiological substrates, e.g. on kininogens or on the zona pellucida of the ovum.

The presence of kininogen in human seminal plasma and midcycle
cervical mucus was established by immunodiffusion using monospecific antibodies (kindly provided by Dr. J. Pierce from N.I.H.,
Bethesda) directed against human kininogens. In comparison to
blood serum, the kininogen concentrations in both genital fluids
are considerably lower. However, related to the total protein
content, the kininogen levels in blood serum as well as in genital
secretions are comparable.

Kininase activity is much higher in seminal plasma than in
cervical mucus (Palm et al., 1975c). This observation is in
accordance with results of other investigators (Cushman et al.,
1971; Depierre et al., 1974) who found high levels of kininase II
in testis and epididymis as well as in human seminal plasma. The
occurrence of this enzyme, which is identical to the angiotensin I-
converting enzyme, might be an indication to a kinin-angiotensin
antagonism, but this is still a matter of speculation. Besides
kininase II, various enzymes of the seminal plasma are probably
involved in kinin degradation like aminopeptidases and a so-
called chumotrypsin-like enzyme (Syner et al., 1972). Inhibition
studies indicate that the kininase activity in both fluids is
metal-ion-dependent. Partial inhibition by pepstatin demonstrates
the involvement of catheptic kininases, especially in seminal
plasma.

The relation of these biochemical data to biological
functions has to be further elucidated.

Sperm Motility and Migration

Nevertheless, participation of the kallikrein-kinin system
in sperm motility regulation is indicated, since it could be
shown that the highly specific kininogenase, hog pancreatic kallikrein, interferes with sperm motility and sperm migration.

Employing semen samples from patients suffering from asthenozoospermia, sperm motility could be enhanced significantly over
a period of 24 hours (see Fig. 1) in in vitro studies by addition
of a single dose of 1 unit kallikrein (about 0.75 µg of highly
purified kallikrein) per ml.

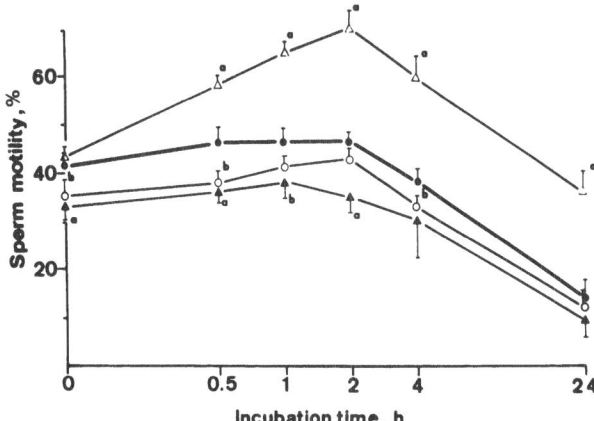

Fig. 1   Stimulation of human sperm motility by 1 unit kalli-
krein/ml (Δ—Δ) in 6 asthenozoospermic ejaculates
over a period of 24 hours at 22°C.
●—● 0.9% NaCl, ▲—▲ denaturated kallikrein, ○—○ 1 KU +
3 KIU/ml Trasylol[R], $a_p < 0.01$, $b_p < 0.05$ (see Schill,
1975a).

Sperm motility was determined microscopically using a method
described by Eliasson (1971). The same effect could be produced
by addition of 0.5 µg bradykinin/ml, but only for about 4 hours.
Previous addition of 0.5 µg pancreatic carboxypeptidase B/ml
abolished the kallikrein or kinin effect. The trypsin-kallikrein
inhibitor from bovine lung (Trasylol[R]) prevented stimulation of
sperm motility by kallikrein. In the presence of serum in a
concentration of 4% (v/v) as presumable kininogen source the
kallikrein effect was enhanced.

Using the capillary tube system according to Kremer, the
migration rate of spermatozoa in ovulatory cervical mucus was
compared to the number of very quick moving spermatozoa (progressive motility). A clear correlation could be found between
both parameters, when semen samples were treated with 1 unit of
hog pancreatic kallikrein (see Fig. 2).

Sperm Metabolism

Fructose is the major sugar in seminal plasma utilized by
spermatozoa. Measurement of fructolysis is therefore a good
index for sperm energy metabolism. Another parameter, oxygen
consumption, may be determined by the Warburg method (Leidl
et al., 1956). As shown recently (Schill, 1975b; Leidl et al.,
1975), the results obtained with both methods indicate an increase

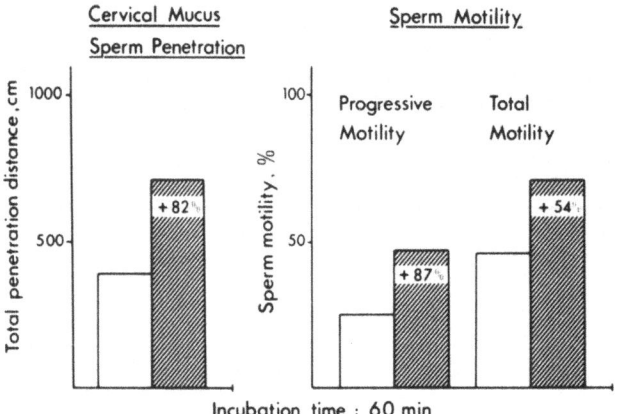

Fig. 2 Effect of kallikrein (1 KU) in human semen (n=14)
       (see Wallner et al.,1975)

in the metabolic turnover of the kallikrein-treated samples.
Studies performed with bull semen showed similar effects. In the
latter case, a statistically significant increase in sperm
motility and oxygen consumption could be only seen at a dose of
100 units kallikrein/ml.

Systemic application of pancreatic kallikrein

     Stuttgen (1973) reported firstly an increase in sperm density
in a few patients with reduced sperm counts subjected to a short-
time treatment with hog pancreatic kallikrein.

     When patients suffering from asthenozoospermia were treated
over a period of 7 weeks three times either by parenteral
application of 40 units hog pancreatic kallikrein or by oral
application of 300 and 600 units daily, a significant improvement
in sperm motility was observed (see Fig. 3).

     In addition, an increase in the total sperm output was ob-
served in patients with reduced sperm count (oligozoospermia)
three months after onset of the kallikrein treatment. This delay
reflects the period of sperm development thus indicating an effect
of kallikrein on spermatogenesis (see Fig. 4).

Possible mode of action

     Human seminal plasma of fertile men contains about 60 µg of
E-prostaglandins (Bydgeman et al., 1970). On the other hand,
in infertile men, who had no apparent other cause for infertility
the prostaglandin levels were found to be only one third as high.

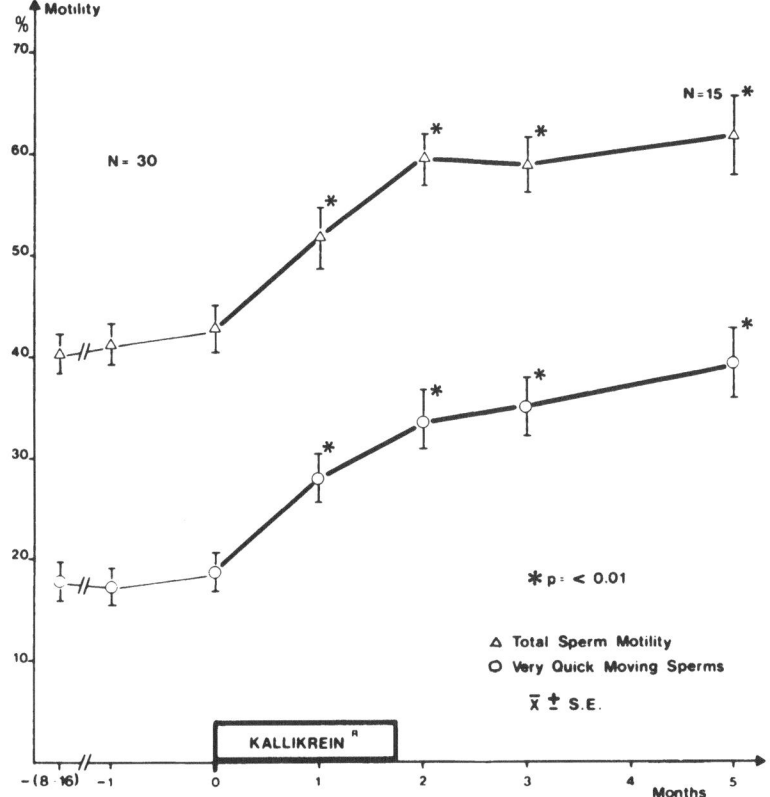

Fig. 3 Treatment of asthenozoospermia with kallikrein and its effect on sperm motility (summarizing parenteral and oral application), see Schill, 1975c.

Results of Eskin et al.,(1973); Hunt et al.,(1975), and our pre-liminary data demonstrate, that sperm motility depends on pro-staglandin action, too. An effect of kinins on prostaglandin synthesis is suggested by various investigators (Vargaftig et al., 1972; Damas et al., 1974; Vane et al., 1975; Terragno et al., 1975). In preliminary experiments with human and bull semen, mefenamate, a potent inhibitor of prostaglandin synthesis (Gryglewski, 1974), was employed in in vitro studies. Remarkably, the described kallikrein-kinin effects on sperm motility and oxygen consumption could be inhibited at a concentration of 0.2 up to 2.0 µg mefenamate per ml. In the presence of mefenamate, stimu-lation could be achieved by further addition of prostaglandins. This excludes a toxic effect of mefenamate. Whether a distinct or an intermediate product, e.g. a biologically highly active

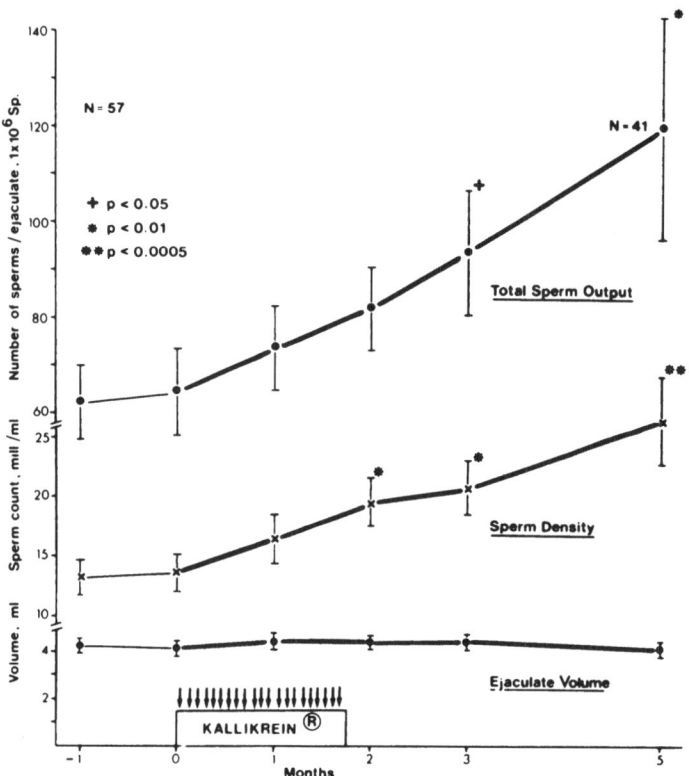

Fig. 4 Treatment of 57 oligozoospermic patients with 3 x 40
       units of kallikrein per week over a period of seven
       weeks (parenteral application).
       ●—●ejaculate volume in ml, ✗—✗ sperm count in mil-
       lions/ml, ○—○ sperm output in millions/ejaculate,
       + p<0.05, * p<0.01, ** p<0.0005 (see Schill,1975a).

endoperoxide (Samuelsson et al., 1974), is the key substance in
the interaction between the kinin and prostaglandin system has to
be further clarified.

     Physiological responses to prostaglandins are apparently
mediated by the activation of the intracellular cyclic nucleotide
system (Kuehl jr., 1974). Tash et al. (1973), showed that there
is a good correlation between motility and the cyclic AMP content
of the sperm cell. In a recent study, the stimulation of sperm
motility by kallikrein was compared to the one induced by caffeine,
an inhibitor of the cyclic AMP inactivating enzyme phosphodieste-
rase. Remarkably, besides the stimulating effect of caffeine as

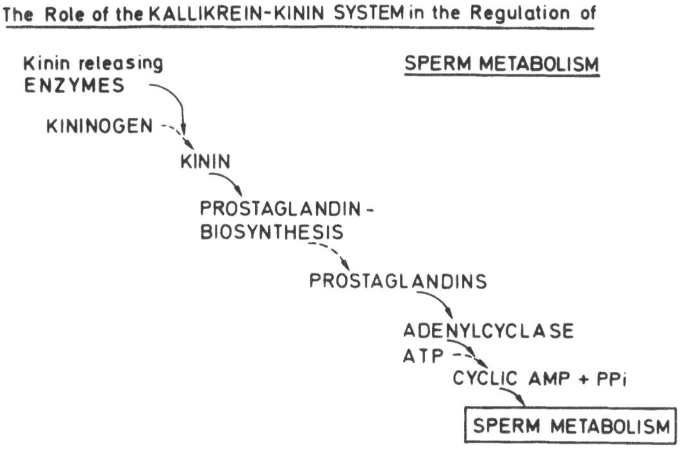

The Role of the KALLIKREIN-KININ SYSTEM in the Regulation of

Kinin releasing   SPERM METABOLISM
ENZYMES

KININOGEN

KININ

PROSTAGLANDIN -
BIOSYNTHESIS

PROSTAGLANDINS

ADENYLCYCLASE
ATP
CYCLIC AMP + PPi

SPERM METABOLISM

Fig. 5

already known (Garbers et al., 1971), the kallikrein-kinin effect
was potentiated over 24 hours when caffeine was present in 5 mM
concentration (Schill, 1975d).

The possible interactions between the kallikrein-kinin system,
the prostaglandin system, and cyclic nucleotides are schematically
illustrated in Figure 5. However, these interrelationships have
to be proven by direct determination of the intermediate metabolites.

Conclusion

The data presented indicate that the kallikrein-kinin system
is involved in spermatogenesis, sperm metabolism and sperm migration. By which mode of action the various components of this
system are related to biological functions in the male and female
reproductive tract has to be further clarified. However, the
observed in vitro and in vivo effects of hog pancreatic kallikrein on spermatozoal viability and sperm count inplicate mechanisms
regulated by biologically active peptides, especially the kinins,
which are released during enzymatic cleavage of kininogens (Han
et al., 1975). There is some evidence, that the physiological
responses to kininogenases like hog pancreatic kallikrein are
mediated by the activation of specific mediators, e.g. prostaglandins and cyclic nucleotides.

Acknowledgement: We gratefully acknowledge the support of this
work by Professor Dr. J. Zander, First Department of Gynecology
and Obstetrics, University of Munich, by the "Deutsche Forschungs-
gemeinschaft", Sonderforschungsbereich 51, Munich, and by the
WHO, Geneva.

LITERATURE

Bydgeman, M., Fredericsson, B., Svanbork, K., Samuelsson, B.: Fert.
    Ster. 21, 622-629 (1970)
Cushman, D.W., Cheung, H.S.: Biochim. Biophys. Acta 250, 261-265
    (1971)
Damas, J., Deby, C., Lecomte, J.: C.R. Soc. Biol. 168, 375 (1974)
Depierre, D., Roth, M.: Experientia 30, 686 (1974)
Eliasson, R.: Andrologie 3, 49-64 (1971)
Eskin, B.A., Facog, S.A., Sepic, R., Slate, W.G.: Obst. and Gyn.
    41, 3, 436-439 (1973)
Fritz, H., Schleuning, W.-D., Schill, W.-B.: Bayer Symposium V,
    "Proteinase Inhibitors", ed. by H. Fritz, H. Tschesche, E.
    Truscheit, and L.J. Greene, Springer Verlag, Berlin-Heidelberg
    New York, 118-127 (1974)
Garbers, D.L., First, N.L., Sullivan, J.J., Lardy, H.A.: Biol.
    Reprod. 5, 336-339 (1971)
Gryglewski, R.J.: Prostaglandin Synthetase Inhibitors, ed. by
    H. J. Robinson and J.R. Vane, Raven Press, New York,
    33-52 (1974)
Han, Y.N., Komyia, M., Iwanaga, S., Suzuki, T.: J. Biochem. 77,
    55-68 (1975)
Hunt, W.L., Zaneveld, L.J.D.: Conference Proceedings of the Inter-
    national Conference of Andrology in Detroit, April 24-26, ed.
    by E.S.E. Hafez, abs. no 31 (1975)
Kuehl, Jr.: Prostaglandins and Cyclic AMP, ed. by H. Kahn and
    W.E.M. Lands, Academic Press, Inc., New York and London,
    223-225 (1973)
Leidl, W., Russe, M.: Zuchthygiene und Haustierbesamung 6, 117-119
    (1956)
Leidl, W., Prinzen, R., Schill, W.-B., Fritz, H.: Kininogenases-
    Kallikrein, 2nd Symposium on Physiological Properties and
    Pharmacological Rational - Reproduction, ed. by G.L. Haberland
    and J.W. Rohen, Schattauer Verlag, Stuttgart-New York, in
    press (1975)
Palm, S., Fritz, H.: Kininogenases-Kallikrein, 2nd Symposium on
    Physiological Properties and Pharmacological Rational-
    Reproduction, ed. by G.L. Haberland and J.W. Rohen, Schattauer
    Verlag, Stuttgart-New York, in press (1975a)
Palm, S., Fritz, H.: to be published (1975b)
Palm. S., Fritz, H.: in preparation (1975c)
Rybak, M., Rybakova, B., Koutsky, J.: Physiol. bohemoslov. 23 467-473
    (1974)
Samuelsson, B., Hamberg, M.: Prostaglandin Synthetase Inhibitors,
    ed. by H. J. Robinson and J.R. Vane, Raven Press, New York,
    107-119 (1974)
Schill, W.-B., Braun-Falco, O., Haberland, G.L.: Int. J. Fert.
    19, 163-167 (1974)

Schill, W.-B.: Kininogenases-Kallikrein, 2nd Symposium on Physiological Properties and Pharmacological Rational - Reproduction, ed. by G.L. Haberland and J.W. Rohen, Schattauer Verlag, Stuttgart-New York, in press (1975a)

Schill, W.-B.: andrologia 7, 105-107 (1975b)

Schill, W.-B.: Int. J. Fert. 20, 61-63 (1975c)

Schill, W.-B.: Advances of Andrology (ed. by C. Schirren), Fortschritte der Fertilitatsforschung III, Grosse Verlag, Berlin-Chicago, in press (1975d)

Stuttgen, G.: Kininogenases-Kallikrein, 1st Symposium on Physiological Properties and Pharmacological Rational, ed. by G.L. Haberland and J.W. Rohen, Schattauer Verlag, Stuttgart-New York, 189-193 (1973)

Syner, F.N., Moghissi, K.S.: Biology of Mammalian Fertilization and Implantation, ed. by K.S. Moghissi and E.S.E. Hafez, Charles C. Thomas Publisher, Springfield, Illinois, 3-18 (1972)

Terragno, N.A., Terragno, A., Jennings, D.S., McGiff, J.C.: Conference Proceedings of the 22nd Annual Meeting of the Society for Gynecologic Investigation in San Antonio, abs. no. 23 (1975)

Vane, J.R., Ferreira, S.H.: Conference abstracts of the International Conference on Chemistry and Biology of the Kallikrein-Kinin System in Health and Disease, Life Sciences 16, 804-805 (1975)

Vargaftig, B.B., Dao Hai, N.: J. Pharm. Pharmac., 24, 159-161 (1972)

Wallner, O., Schill, W.-B., Grosser, A., Fritz, H.: Kininogenases-Kallikrein, 2nd Symposium on Physiological Properties and Pharmacological Rational - Reproduction, ed. by G. L. Haberland and J.W. Rohen, Schattauer Verlag, Stuttgart-New York, in press (1975)

AN ACTIVE KALLIKREIN-α_2-MACROGLOBULIN COMPLEX GENERATED BY TREATMENT OF HUMAN PLASMA WITH ACETONE

W. Vogt

Max-Planck-Institut für experimentelle Medizin
Department of Biochemical Pharmacology
D-34 Gottingen, Hermann-Rein-Str. 3, Germany

Earlier functional studies on endogenous kinin formation in human plasma suggested that depending on the mode of treatment of the plasma, different kininogenases are activated predominantly: kininogenase I, activated by e.g. acid or acetone, acting on kininogen I; kininogenase II, activated by contact of plasma with glass, quartz etc., acting on kininogen II (Vogt, 1966). The existance of two kininogens, differing in molecular weight and affinity to plasma kallikrein, has meanwhile been well established. Kininogen II, highly sensitive to contact activated kininogenase(s), can be equated with high molecular weight kininogen (HMW-K), whereas kininogen I corresponds to low molecular weight kininogen (LMW-K) (Habal and Movat, 1972; Seidel, 1973; Habal et al., 1974). The existence of two kininogenases has been questioned however, since by fractionation of plasma other investigators found only one kinin-forming enzyme, plasma kallikrein - apart from the weakly active plasmin. Wendel et al. (1972) purified the contact-activated kininogenase (II) and found that it was not distinguishable in molecular size and isoelectric point from plasma kallikrein. The enzyme acted predominantly but not exclusively, on HMW-K (kininogen II). An attempt was therefore made to purify the acetone-activated enzyme (kininogenase I by the original definition) and to see whether it differs in its properties from the contact-activated enzyme.

CHROMATOGRAPHY OF ACETONE-ACTIVATED PLASMA

Human citrate plasma was treated with one fifth its volume of acetone, for 4 hrs at room temperature. It was then dialyzed

for 20-30 hrs against isotonic phosphate buffer pH 7.3 and subsequently passed through a column of Sephadex G-200 with the same
buffer. The peak of esterolytic activity (substrate: benzoyl-
arginine-ethylester) was found in the macromolecular fraction (SI),
it coincided with the distribution of α_2-macroglobulin (α2M). The
latter protein was assayed by radial immunodiffusion. SI also
contained kinin-forming activity. In most experiments no extra
peak of esterase activity could be detected in the globulin
fraction where plasma kallikrein would be expected to elute.
Only on rechromatography of the globulin fraction did esterase
activity become apparent in the globulin region as a small peak
(SII) separate from the much larger peak of SI. SII had com-
parably little esterolytic but substantial kinin-forming activity.

The ratio between SI and SII varied according to the treatment
of the plasma with acetone: when the incubation was performed at
about 4° and was prolonged to 20-24 hrs, SII was virtually absent,
not even detectable after rechromatography, and all esterase and
kinin-forming activity was concentrated in SI. In contrast, when
the time of treatment comprised just the 4 hrs at room temperature
omitting the overnight dialysis, considerable kinin-forming
activity was found in SII, even then accompanied by relatively
little esterolytic activity.

Chromatography of acetone-activated plasma on DEAE cellulose
gave corresponding results. Fractionation was started with 0.02 M
phosphate buffer pH 8.0 followed by a NaCl gradient. Depending
on the time of treatment with acetone comparatively little or no
esterase was found in the excluded protein peak which contains
plasma kallikrein if present. The bulk of esterolytic and kinin-
ogenolytic activity eluted at higher ionic strength. This peak
again coincided with α2M. Chromatography of the Sephadex fractions
SI and SII on DEAE cellulose showed that SII corresponds to the
non-absorbed DEAE fraction and SI to the one eluting later from
DEAE cellulose.

IDENTIFICATION OF SI AND SII

The major enzyme of SII is certainly plasma kallikrein. It
has the same elution characteristics in DEAE cellulose and Sephadex
chromatographies, it is a potent kininogenase which releases
kinin from HMW-K better than from LMW-K; in immunodiffusion against
anti-kallikrein serum it gives a precipitation line which fuses
with that of purified plasma kallikrein. The anti-kallikrein
serum was kindly provided by Dr. Henry Movat, Toronto, and was
made monospecific by absorption with Fletcher factor-deficient
serum.

The main fraction, SI, was further purified by rechromatography on DEAE cellulose followed by fractionation on CM cellulose,
SP-Sephadex and isoelectric focussing. The final product moved
more anodically than plasma kallikrein in immunoelectrophoresis
and gave a single, identical precipitation line with anti-α2M
serum and anti-whole human serum. Attempts to separate the
enzymic activity from α2M failed. These results indicated that
SI contained a complex of α2M with an esterase, probably plasma
kallikrein. An α2M complex is further indicated by the fact that
esterase and kinin-froming activities of SI were not inhibited
by addition of α2M; the esterase was also resistant to soybean
trypsin inhibitor. Acetone treatment of human plasma from which
α2M had been selectively eliminated by absorption with anti-α2M
γ-globulins did not lead to generation of SI activity, but SII
appeared instead. That the complex contains plasma kallikrein is
indicated by the finding that neither SI nor SII were generated
by acetone treatment of Fletcher factor-deficient plasma which
lacks prekallikrein (Wuepper, 1972). SI did not react with anti-
kallikrein serum. This is, however, not at variance with the
conclusion that SI is a kallikrein-α2M complex, since Bagdasarian
et al. (1974) found that binding of plasma kallikrein to α2M buries
its antigenic sites so that their reactivity with antibodies is
largely lost. Further, indirect support for the presence of
plasma kallikrein in the α2M complex is given by the observation
that by acetone treatment human plasma loses its reactivity with
anti-kallikrein serum, but preserves it when α2M had been eliminated
before the treatment.

FUNCTIONAL PROPERTIES OF THE α2M-Kallikrein
COMPLEX, SI

In agreement with other reports (Harpel, 1970; McConnell,
1972) the α2M-bound kallikrein is still a potent esterase but a
weakly active kininogenase only, compared with the free enzyme.
Like free kallikrein it cleaves kinin from HMW-K at a higher rate
than from LMW-K. At a concentration of 180 mU/ml the kallikrein-
α2M complex released 0.4 μg bradykinin equivalents from LMW-K and
1.4 μg from HMW-K in 30 min at 37°. Under the same conditions free
kallikrein (110 mU/ml) released 4.4 μg bradykinin equivalents from
LMW-K, and 11 μg from HMW-K. In whole plasma the relative effi-
ciencies of free and α2M-bound kallikrein are different. Due to
the rapid reaction with plasma inhibitors free kallikrein stops
releasing kinin soon after its addition; in contrast, the α2M
complex slowly continues releasing kinin, for hours and thus
eventually is more efficient than free kallikrein.

Under natural conditions of kallikrein activation in plasma
(e.g. contact activation) the free enzyme's activity is mainly
restricted to the highly susceptible HMW-K, whereas LMW-K escapes

from cleavage because of the short half-life of free kallikrein.
Part of the enzyme will be bound by completely inactivating inhibitors, e.g. C$\overline{1}$ inhibitor; however, a fraction will become bound
to α2M (Harpel, 1970) and this complex may then continue to release
kinin at a slow rate and may act on the LMW-K which was not
attacked by the free enzyme. In fact, slow kinin-release in glass-
activated plasma, subsequent to the original burst, was observed
in our experiments. Thus the α2M-kallikrein complex, found as
the major enzyme in acetone-activated plasma, is not an enzyme
specific for LMW-K as was originally expected; it is, however,
a kinin-releasing agent potentially capable of utilizing LMW-K in
plasma after HMW-K has been consumed by free plasma kallikrein
and this has been inactivated. Insofar the α2M-kallikrein complex
differs functionally from free kallikrein and corresponds to the
kininogenase I which was earlier postulated.

REFERENCES

Bagdasarian, A., Lahiri, B., Talamo, R.C., Wong, P., Colman, R.W.:
     Immunochemical studies of plasma kallikrein. J.Clin.Invest.
     54, 1444 (1974).
Habal, F.M., Movat, H.Z.: Kininogens of human plasma. Res. Comm.
     Chem. Path. Pharmacol. 4, 477 (1972).
Habal, F.M., Movat, H.Z., Burrowed, C.E.: Isolation of two functio-
     nally different kininogens from human plasma - Separation
     from proteinase inhibitors and interaction with plasma kalli-
     krein. Biochem. Pharmacol. 23, 2291 (1974).
Harpel, P.C.: Human plasma α2-macroglobulin. An inhibitor of
     plasma kallikrein. J. exp. Med. 132, 329 (1970).
McConnell, D.J.: Inhibitors of kallikrein in human plasma. J. Clin.
     Invest. 51, 1611 (1972).
Seidel, G: Two functionally different kininogens in human plasma.
     Agents and Actions 3, 12 (1973).
Vogt, W.: Demonstration of the presence of two separate kinin-
     forming systems in human and other plasma. In: Hypotensive
     peptides, p. 185, ed. by E.G. Erdos, N. Back and F. Sicuteri,
     Berlin-Heidelberg-New York: Springer 1966.
Wendel, U., Vogt, W., Seidel, G.: Purification and some properties
     of a kininogenase from human plasma activated by surface
     contact. Hoppe-Seylers Z. physiol. Chem. 353, 1591 (1972).
Wuepper, K.D.: Biochemistry and biology of components of the plasma
     kinin-forming system. In: Inflammation mechanism and control,
     p. 93, ed. by I.H. Lepow and P.A. Ward. Academic Press, New
     York, 1972.

ACTIVATION OF SURFACE-BOUND HAGEMAN FACTOR: PRE-EMINENT ROLE OF

HIGH MOLECULAR WEIGHT KININOGEN AND EVIDENCE FOR A NEW FACTOR

Marion E. Webster, Jorge A. Guimaraes, Allen P. Kaplan
Robert W. Colman* and Jack V. Pierce

Laboratory of Chemistry, National Heart and Lung Inst.,
Bethesda, Md. 20014; Laboratory of Clinical Investigation,
National Institute of Allergy and Infectious Diseases,
Bethesda, Md. 20014; and Coagulation Unit, Hematology-
Oncology Section, Department of Medicine, University of
Pennsylvania, Philadelphia, Pa. 19104, U.S.A.

Hageman factor (factor XII) is present in plasma as an inactive precursor and is thought to be activated by contact with negatively charged surfaces of particles or macromolecules (1). The activated factor XII then acts directly on its three substrates, factor XI (PTA)(2), prekallikrein (3,4) and plasminogen proactivator (5), thus initiating the plasma proteolytic systems responsible for coagulation, kinin formation and fibrinolysis (Fig. 1).

In the past few years, evidence has accumulated indicating that this scheme is oversimplified. Studies with purified Hageman factor and its substrates (6-9) have suggested that previously unidentified factor(s) are required for activation of factor XII on a negative surface. In addition, plasma of patients with Fletcher trait (10) which lack prekallikrein (11) showed profound abnormalities in the rate of Hageman factor-dependent coagulation, fibrinolysis and kinin generation (11,12). However, prekallikrein by itself does not correct the defect found with the purified components (6-9). Recently, four patients have been described (13-18) who exhibit a new coagulation defect which can be corrected by high molecular weight (150,000-200,000) kininogen but not by low molecular weight (70,000-80,000) kininogen (16,17). High molecular

---

*
Supported in part by grant HL 16642 from the National Institutes
of Health

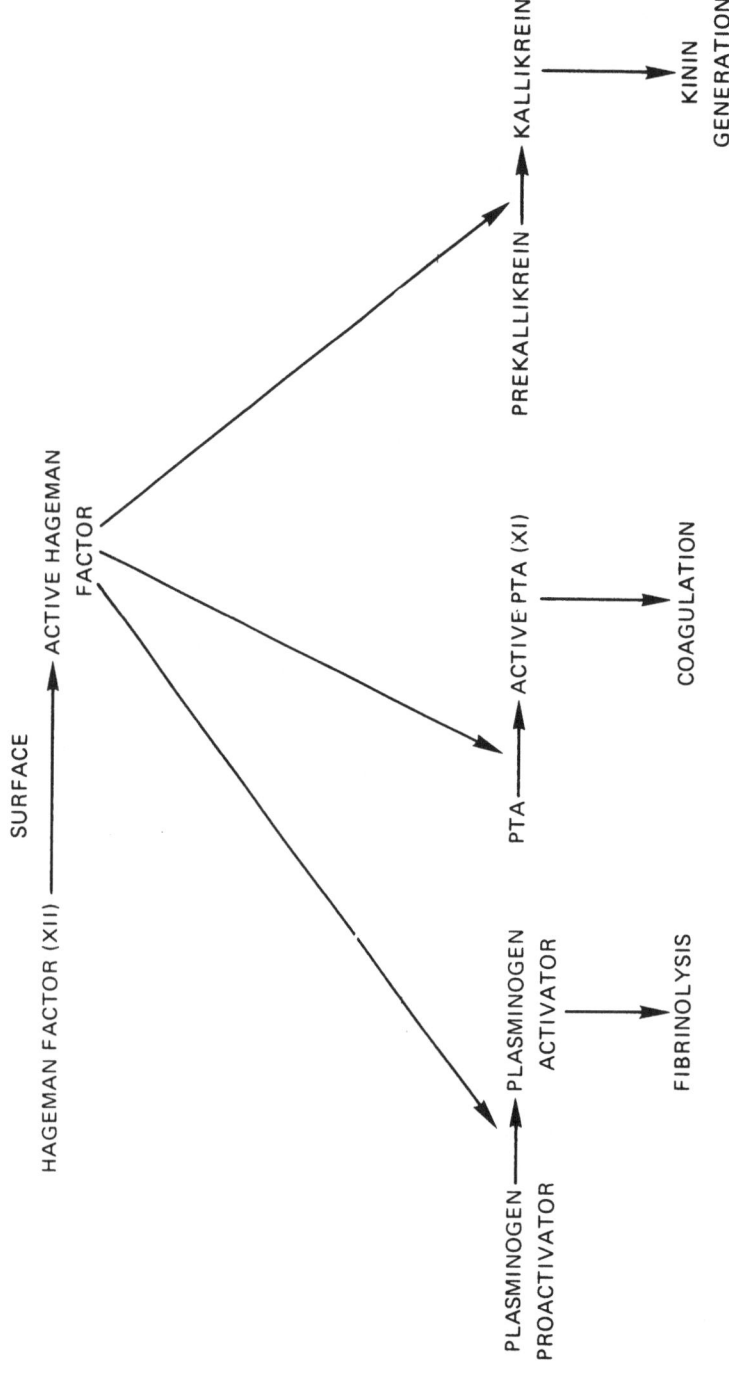

Fig. 1.   Earlier scheme for the activation of Hageman factor
(factor XII)

weight kininogen represents approximately 20% of the total kininogen content of human plasma and is the preferred substrate for
plasma kallikrein (19).

This report provides evidence for the pre-eminent role of
high molecular weight kininogen and that a new factor is required
for the normal rate of activation of Hageman factor on a negative
surface.

METHODS AND MATERIALS

Determination of active Hageman factor. Hageman factor and
its activators were adsorbed to supercel and the bound active
Hageman factor quantitated by measuring the amount of kallikrein
it generates from purified prekallikrein. The supercel (5 mg)
was washed with buffer by suspending it in 0.5 ml of 0.04 M Tris-
0.15 M NaCl, pH 8.0, separating it by centrifugation and resus-
pending it in chilled buffer. The fractions to be assayed for
active Hageman factor or for activators of Hageman factor were
added to the washed supercel and incubated at room temperature
for 10 min (final volume 1.0 ml). The adsorbed supercel was
washed three times with 0.5 ml chilled buffer, resuspended in 0.5
ml buffer and stored in an ice bath until assayed. The active
Hageman factor on the supercel was measured as previously described (20) by adding 20 µl of the suspension to a mixture of
20 µl prekallikrein (containing 0.015 TU (TAME esterase units) or
15,500 cpm if fully activated) and 10 µl {^{3}H}-TAME (o-tosyl-L-
arginine methyl ester) (0.047 nC, 280 mC/mole) was added for an
additional 30 min at room temperature. All samples were run in
duplicate both in the presence and absence of prekallikrein.
Results are reported in cpm generated in the 20 µl aliquot
corrected for cpm in the absence of prekallikrein (usually 600-
950 cpm).

Crude Hageman factor was prepared as previously described
by Ratnoff and Davie (21). Citrated human plasma was stirred
with 1/10 volume of aluminum hydroxide gel (Amphogel, Wyeth Lab.
Inc., Philadelphia, Pa.) for 10 min at room temperature. The
precipitate was removed by centrifugation (5 min at 500 x g) and
the supernatant plasma stirred for 10 min with Celite 512 (7.5 mg/
ml), which had been previously washed with 0.15 M NaCl. The
supernatant plasma was separated by centrifugation and stored in
liquid nitrogen. Highly purified unactivated Hageman factor was
a gift from Dr. C.G. Cochrane, Scripps Clinic and Research
Foundation, La Jolla, Ca.

Plasma deficient in high molecular weight kininogen was
obtained from Ms. Williams (15,17). Plasmas deficient in

prekallikrein (Fletcher) and in Hageman factor were kindly supplied
by Dr. C. F. Abildgaard, University of California (Davis) and
Dr. P. G. Iatridis, Indiana University School of Medicine, respectively. Partially purified plasma prekallikrein (20) was used
in most experiments and was found to be functionally pure when
compared with highly purified prekallikrein (ca 70 TU/A_{280})
(Pierce, unpublished).

RESULTS

Activation of Crude Hageman Factor.   We reported earlier (6,
7) that addition of human plasma to supercel formed active Hageman
factor which was completely adsorbed to the supercel. However,
when the same quantity of crude Hageman factor was adsorbed no
active Hageman factor was formed. As shown in Fig. 2A, 5 μl of
the crude Hageman factor alone generated only 800 cpm. The
addition of as little as 2 μl of Hageman deficient plasma
resulted in the generation of 5,500 cpm. Maximal activation of
the adsorbed Hageman factor occurred with 10 μl of Hageman factor
deficient plasma. The quantity of active Hageman factor found
was similar to that formed when 5 μl of plasma is adsorbed to
supercel (7).

Activation of Crude Hageman Factor by Prekallikrein. The
first activator to be investigated was prekallikrein. As shown
in Fig. 2B, 5 μl of Fletcher trait (prekallikrein deficient)
plasma generated only 200 cpm when adsorbed to supercel. However,
if prekallikrein equivalent to that amount found in normal plasma
was added, normal levels of activated Hageman factor were found
(7,000-9,000 cpm). The arrow in this panel and in panel C denotes
the amount of prekallikrein and/or high molecular weight kininogen
found in 10 μl of the Hageman factor deficient plasma.

Although prekallikrein could readily activate the Hageman
factor in Fletcher trait plasma, these same quantities of prekallikrein when mixed with crude Hageman factor gave only a partial
activation (2,000 cpm). Even the addition of kallikrein in amounts
greater than that normally found in plasma failed to fully activate
the crude Hageman factor.

Activation of Crude Hageman Factor by High Molecular Weight
Kininogen. As shown in Fig. 2C, Williams trait (high molecular
weight kininogen deficient) plasma, like Hageman deficient and
Fletcher trait (prekallikrein deficient) plasma, did not form
active Hageman factor when adsorbed to supercel. Of the multiple
forms of human plasma kininogen previously isolated (22,23) only
those kininogens which exhibited a low Km with plasma kallikrein
corrected the defect found in Williams trait plasma (Table 1).

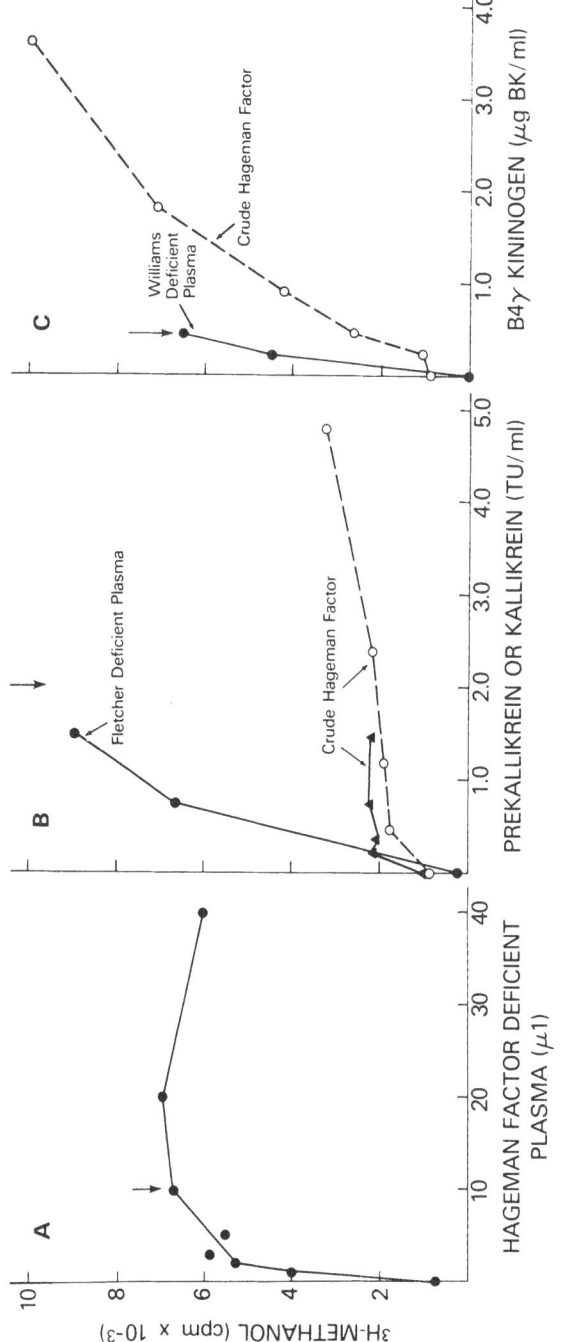

Fig. 2. Activators of Hageman factor. (A) Crude Hageman factor (5 μl) was mixed with indicated amounts of Hageman factor deficient plasma and then adsorbed to supercel. (B) Fletcher trait (prekalli-krein deficient) plasma (5 μl) was mixed with indicated amounts of prekallikrein (●————●) or crude Hageman factor (5 μl) was mixed with prekallikrein (▲————▲) or kallikrein (o————o). (C) Williams trait (high molecular weight kininogen deficient) plasma (5 μl) (●————●) or crude Hageman factor (5 μl) (o————o) were mixed with indicated amounts of B4γ kininogen. Arrows in panel B and C repre-sent the amount of prekallikrein or high molecular weight kininogen found in 10 μl Hageman factor deficient plasma.

TABLE I.   Correction of defect in Williams trait plasma by human
           kininogens.

Kininogens (500 ng)	Apparent Molecular Weight*	Bradykinin released (ug/A_{280})		Formation of Active Hageman factor (cpm ^{3}H-methanol)
		Trypsin	Plasma Kallikrein	
B1α	79,000	13.2	< 1	< 1
B2α	77,000	21.8	< 1	95
B2β	150,000	15.6	< 1	< 1
B3.1α	84,000	9.7	< 1	139
B3.1β	158,000	10.3	< 1	63
B3.2α	73,000	19.6	< 1	< 1
B3.2β	150,000	16.8	< 1	6
B4α	80,000	10.6	3.3	633
B4β	150,000	14.2	8.3	6051
B4γ	225,000	15.2	11.9	6435

*Estimated by gel filtration.

TABLE II.   Plasma components as activators of Hageman factor adsorbed
            to supercel.

Plasma Component			Formation of Active Hageman factor	
Prekallikrein (TU/ml)	Kallikrein (TU/ml)	B4γ kininogen (μg BK/ml)	Crude Hageman factor (5 μl)	Pure Hageman factor (520 ng)
			923	164
0.76			2268	130
	4.8		3235	656
	2.4		2112	164
		0.45	4222	1074
		3.6	9911	10326
0.76		0.45	6197	4577
0.38		0.45	5626	2218
	2.4	0.45	7018	3568
	1.2	0.45	5790	2114
Hageman factor deficient plasma (10 μl)			7725	8792

A mixture of Williams trait plasma with B4γ kininogen in amounts equivalent to those in plasma (Fig. 1C) led to the generation of active Hageman factor. However, these levels of kininogen added to crude Hageman factor yielded only partial activation. When the amount of kininogen was increased to about eight times that found in normal plasma more active Hageman factor was generated than was found with Hageman factor deficient plasma (Fig. 1A). In fact, 13,000 cpm could be generated from this crude Hageman factor, if the amount of kininogen was increased to 20 to 40 times that found in plasma.

It was found also that the ability of B4 kininogen to form active Hageman factor was independent of the kinin moiety. As shown in Fig. 3, when B4 kininogen was incubated with plasma kallikrein (given in mTU on the abscissa) for two hours at room temperature, increasing levels of kallikrein gave increasing amounts of kinin. However, all of the incubation mixtures were equally active in their ability to activate Hageman factor. Further, the kinin-free kininogen separated by Sephadex G-25 filtration was fully capable of forming active Hageman factor from crude inactive Hageman factor.

Activation of Crude and Highly Purified Hageman Factor by Combinations of Prekallikrein (or Kallikrein) and B4 Kininogen. The ability of various combinations of prekallikrein and B4 kininogen to activate both crude and pure Hageman factor is given in Table 2. Prekallikrein, kallikrein or B4 kininogen, when mixed individually with crude Hageman factor and then adsorbed to supercel, gave only partial activation, except when B4 kininogen was present in an amount 8 times that found in normal plasma (3.6 ug vs 0.45 ug BK equiv./ml). The addition of both prekallikrein (or kallikrein) and B4 kininogen to crude Hageman factor resulted in the formation of normal levels of active Hageman factor, or at least in levels which approached those formed by the combination of Hageman factor deficient plasma and crude Hageman factor. However, when these same activators were mixed individually with highly purified Hageman factor, they were much less effective in forming active Hageman factor; although again, an excess of B4 kininogen gave activation which was even better than that achieved with Hageman factor deficient plasma. The addition of both prekallikrein (or kallikrein) and B4 kininogen to the purified Hageman factor yielded increased levels of active Hageman factor, but these levels were significantly less than those formed from crude Hageman factor.

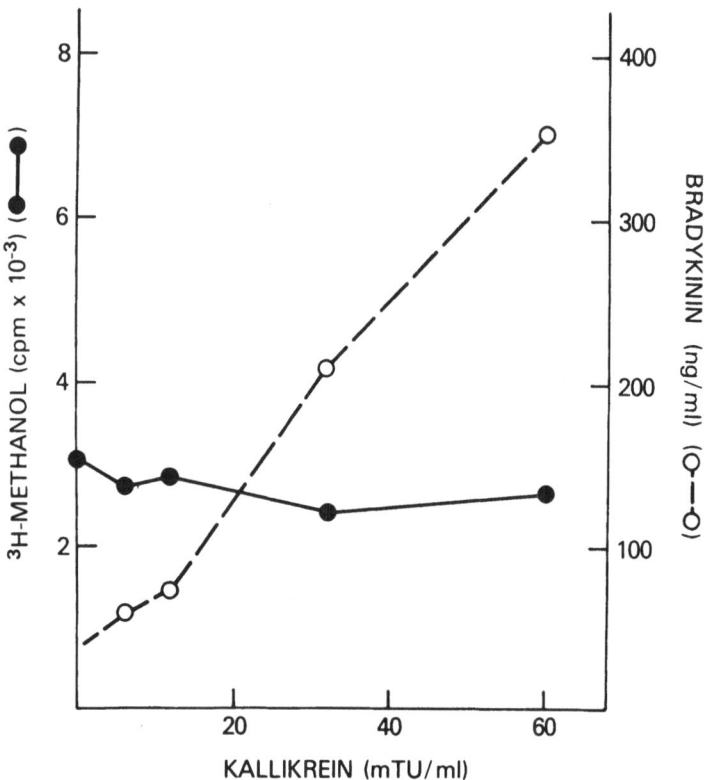

Fig. 3. Kallikrein does not alter the potency of B4 kininogen to
activate Hageman factor. B4γ kininogen was incubated with indicated
amounts of kallikrein for two hours at room temperature. The bradykinin released (o-----o) was determined by bioassay on the guinea
pig ileum. Also the ability of the mixtures to activate crude Hageman factor was measured (●———●).

DISCUSSION

Two distinct means have been proposed through which Hageman factor is activated: that occuring by contact with negatively charged particles and that caused by enzymatic attack. The first has been called solid phase and the latter fluid phase or enzymatic activation. Both of these mechanisms have been recently reviewed (1, 24). Studies from several laboratories (12, 25, 26) have shown that kallikrein in solution (liquid phase activation) acts on Hageman factor to activate it and/or form fragments which are still capable of activating prekallikrein.

Solid phase activation is thought to occur by inducing conformational changes in the molecule during adsorption to the negatively charged surface, and, indeed, such changes have been reported utilizing circular dichroism (27). However, it is evident that surface activation of Hageman factor also involves enzymatic attack. Earlier studies with Fletcher trait (prekallikrein deficient) plasma (7,9,11,12) clearly indicated that prekallikrein is essential for the normal rate of activation of Hageman factor on a negative surface and kallikrein corrects this defect only if kaolin is present (9,24). In the present study both pre-kallikrein and/or kallikrein were capable of partially activating crude Hageman factor, although they were less effective in the activation of highly purified Hageman factor. This inability of kallikrein to yield significant activation of highly purified Hageman factor bound to a surface suggested to us that other factors were required.

High molecular weight kininogen appeared to provide an answer to this problem. Plasma from patients deficient in this kininogen failed to form active Hageman factor (13-18, 28) and in the present studies this kininogen was necessary for the activation of both crude and purified Hageman factor. However, when it was present in amounts similar to that found in the normal plasma, only a partial activation occurred and, even in the presence of pre-kallikrein (or kallikrein), less active Hageman factor was gene-rated than could be formed with Hageman factor deficient plasma or with an excess of kininogen. These data suggest that still other factor(s) may be involved.

Fig. 4 illustrates our present concept of the solid phase activation of Hageman factor. As is shown, Hageman factor, pre-kallikrein and B4 (high molecular weight) kininogen are firmly bound to the negative surface. High molecular weight kininogen is required for the activation of a small amount of Hageman factor and this active Hageman factor in turn activates prekallikrein to kallikrein which in turn acts on the B4 kininogen to release a kinin-free protein, bradykinin and perhaps histidine rich peptides

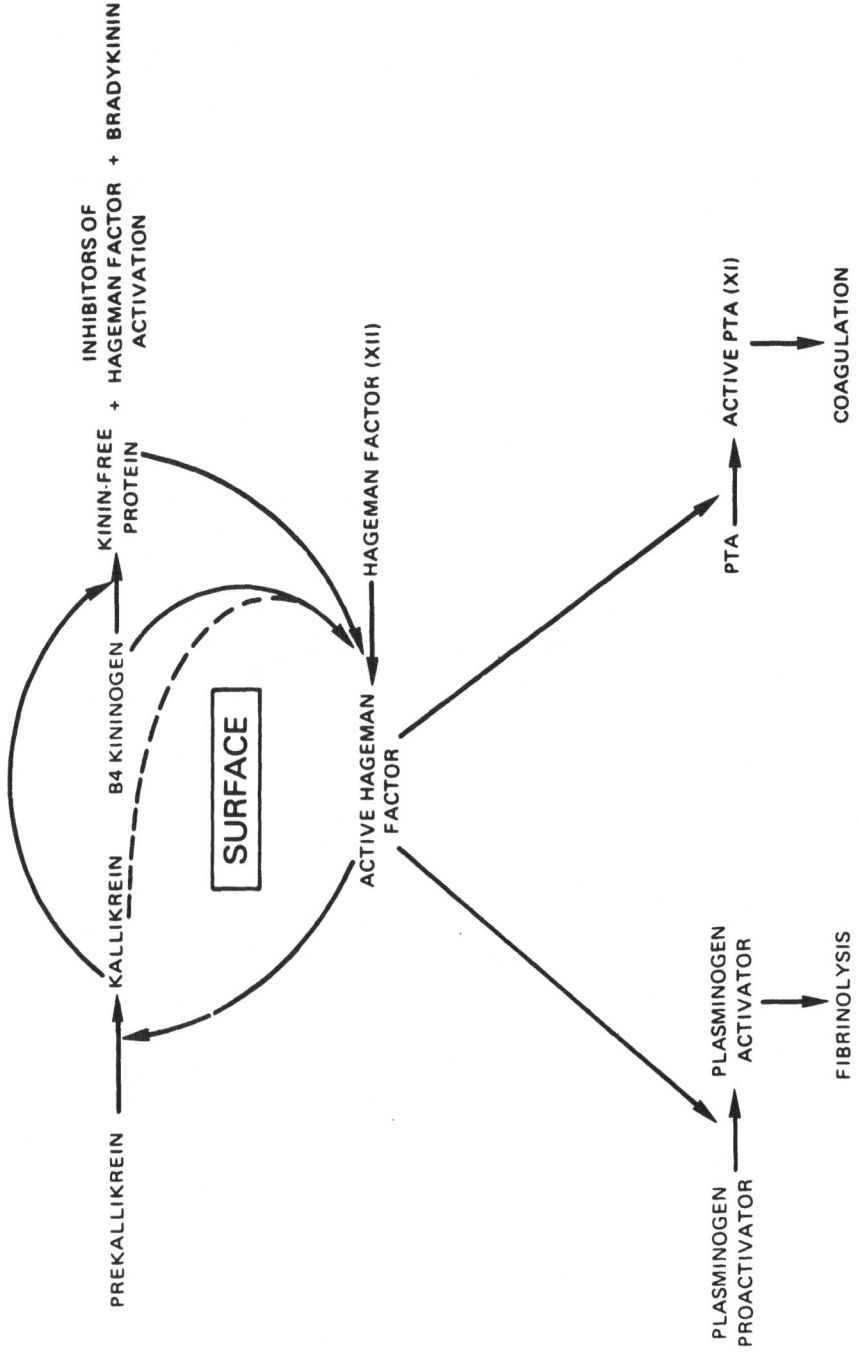

Fig. 4.   Proposed scheme for solid phase activation of Hageman factor.

which have been shown to be released from bovine kininogen (29)
and which inhibit the activation of Hageman factor. The action of
kallikrein is represented by a dotted line, since kallikrein did
not activate highly purified surface-bound Hageman factor in the
absence of kininogen, yet enhances the activation once kininogen
is present. It is unclear whether this effect is upon the Hageman
factor or upon the kininogen. However, since the kinin-free
protein from kininogen was no more active than the intact molecule
and since kallikrein can form active Hageman factor in the fluid
phase, an interaction with surface bound Hageman factor is likely.

Although both prekallikrein and B4 kininogen are essential
to the formation of an active Hageman factor with proteolytic
activity capable of activating prekallikrein, PTA or plasminogen
activator still additional factor(s) may be required. This
possibility is shown by the data in Table II which demonstrate
that both prekallikrein and the kininogen, at levels similar to
those found in plasma, are much less effective in the formation
of an active Hageman factor from pure than from crude Hageman
factor. Similarly, the combination of these factors, while fully
activating crude Hageman factor, only partially activates pure
Hageman factor. Crude Hageman factor, therefore, may contain the
missing factor(s) as may the highly purified kininogen used in
these studies.

Whether the kininogen acts enzymatically to cleave a bond on
the adsorbed Hageman factor and thus expose an active site or
whether it facilitates exposure of the active site or augments
the function of the active site remains to be determined. Nevertheless the present evidence clearly places the plasma kallikrein-
kinin system in the intrinsic clotting pathway. Even though prekallikrein and B4 kininogens have not as yet been assigned the
appropriate clotting numerals, it is now clear that the coagulation
and kinin systems are intimately conjoined. Also, the release of
bradykinin from B4 kininogen by plasma kallikrein may be analogous
to the release of biologically active fragments C3a and C5a (30)
during activation of complement. Other biologically active fragments are released elsewhere in the clotting system as fibrino-
peptides not only potentiate the action of bradykinin on smooth
muscle (31) but are chemotactic (32) as are kallikrein and the
plasminogen activator (33-35). The necessity for two different
types of kininogens in most mammalian plasma may now begin to be
appreciated. Kininogens with great affinity for plasma kallikrein
could readily be exhausted during clot formation leaving intact
kininogens capable of releasing a kinin with glandular kallikreins.

REFERENCES

1. Cochrane, C.G., S.D. Revak, R. Ulevitch, A. Johnston and D. Morrison. Hageman factor: characterization and mechanism of activation. In: Chemistry and Biology of the Kallikrein-Kinin System in Health and Disease, (Ed. J.J. Pisano and K.F. Austen) U.S. Gov. Printing Office: Washington, D.C., 1976

2. Ratnoff, O.D., E.W. Davie and D.L. Mallett. Studies on the action of Hageman factor: evidence that activated Hageman factor in turn activates plasma thromboplastin antecedent. J. Clin. Invest. 40, 803, 1961.

3. Nagasawa, S., H. Takahashi, M. Koida and T. Suzuki. Partial purification of bovine plasma kallikreinogen, its activation by the Hageman factor. Biochem. Biophys. Res. Comm. 32, 644, 1968.

4. Kaplan, A.P. and K. F. Austen. A prealbumin activator of Pre-kallikrein. J. Immunol. 105, 802, 1970.

5. Kaplan, A.P. and K.F. Austen. The fibrinolytic pathway of human plasma: isolation and characterization of the plasminogen activator. J. Exp. Med. 136, 1378, 1972.

6. Webster, M.E. and J.V. Pierce. Activators of Hageman factor (factor XII): identification and relationship to kallikrein-kinin system. Fed. Proc. 32, 845 (Abs.), 1973.

7. Webster, M.E. and S. Oh-ishi. Activation of Hageman factor (factor XII): requirement for activators other than prekallikrein. In: Chemistry and Biology of the Kallikrein-Kinin System in Health and Disease, (Ed. J.J. Pisano and K.F. Austen.) Fogarty Int. Center Proc. 27, U.S. Gov. Printing Office: Washington, D.C., 1976.

8. Schiffman, S. and P. Lee. Preparation, characterization and activation of a highly purified factor XI: evidence that a hitherto unrecognized plasma activity participates in the interaction of factors XI and XII. Brit. J. Haemat. 27, 101, 1974.

9. Saito, H., O.D. Ratnoff and V.H. Donaldson. Defective activation of clotting, fibrinolytic and permeability enhancing systems in human Fletcher trait plasma. Circ. Res. 34, 641, 1974.

10. Hathaway, W.E., L.P. Belhansen and H.S. Hathaway. Evidence for a new plasma thromboplastin factor. I. Case report, coagulation studies and physico-chemical properties. Blood, 26, 521, 1965.

11. Wuepper, K.D. Prekallikrein deficiency in man. J. Exp. Med. 138, 1345, 1973.

12. Weiss, A.S., J.I. Gallin and A.P. Kaplan. Fletcher factor deficiency: abnormalities of coagulation, fibrinolysis, chemotactic activity and kinin generation attributable to absence of prekallikrein. J. Clin. Invest. 53, 622, 1973.

13. Saito, H. and O.D. Ratnoff. Fitzgerald trait: an asymptomatic disorder with impaired blood coagulation, fibrinolysis, kinin generation and generation of PF/Dil. In: Chemistry and Biology of the Kallikrein-Kinin System in Health and Disease, (ed. J.J. Pisano and K.F. Austen) Fogarty Int. Center Proc. 27. U.S. Gov. Printing Office: Washington, D.C., 1976.

14. Saito, H., O.D. Ratnoff, R. Waldmann and J.P. Abraham. Fitzgerald trait. Deficiency of a hitherto unrecognized agent, Fitgerald factor, participating in surface-mediated reactions of clotting, fibrinolysis, generation of kinins, and the property of diluted plasma enhancing vascular permeability PF/dil). J. Clin. Invest. 55, 1082, 1975.

15. Colman, R.W., A. Bagdasarian, R.C. Talamo and A.P. Kaplan. Williams trait: combined deficiency of plasma plasminogen proactivator and kininogen. In: Chemistry and Biology of the Kallikrein-Kinin System in Health and Disease, (Ed. J.J. Pisano and K.F. Austen.) Fogarty Int. Center Proc. 27. U.S. Gov. Printing Office: Washington, D.C., 1976.

16. Wuepper, K.D., D.R. Miller and M.J. Lacombe. Flaujeac trait: deficiency of kininogen in man. Fed. Proc. 34, 859 (Abs.), 1975.

17. Colman, R.W., A. Bagdasarian, R.C. Talamo, C.F. Scott, M. Seavey, J.A. Guimaraes, J.V. Pierce and A.P. Kaplan. Williams trait: human kininogen deficiency with diminished levels of plasminogen proactivator and prekallikrein associated with abnormalities of the Hageman factor dependent pathways. J. Clin. Inv. (In press), 1975.

18. Donaldson, V.H., H.I. Glueck and M.A. Miller. Kininogen deficiency and defective surface activation of blood coagulation and fibrinolysis in a kindred with Fitzgerald trait. Fifth Cong. of Int. Soc. of Thromb. and Hemo. (Abs.)(in press).

19. Jacobsen, S. and M. Kriz. Some data on two purified kininogens from human plasma. Br. J. Pharmac. Chemother. 29, 25, 1967.

20. Webster, M.E., V.H. Beaven, Y. Nagai, S. Oh-ishi and J.V. Pierce. Interaction of Hageman factor, prekallikrein and plasmin. Life Sciences 13, 1201, 1973.

21. Ratnoff, O.D. and E.W. Davie. The purification of activated Hageman factor (activate Factor XII). Biochemistry 1, 967, 1962.

22. Guimaraes, J.A., R. Chen Lu, M. E. Webster and J. V. Pierce. Multiple forms of human plasma kininogen. Fed. Proc. 33, 641 (Abs.), 1974.

23. Pierce, J.V. and J.A. Guimaraes. Further characterization of highly purified human plasma kininogens. In: Chemistry and Biology of the Kallikrein-Kinin System in Health and Disease, (Ed. J.J. Pisano and K.F. Austen) Fogarty Int. Center Proc. 27. U.S. Gov. Printing Office: Washington, D.C., 1976.

24. Kaplan, A.P., H.L. Meier, L.D. Yecies and L.W. Heck. Hageman factor and its substrates: the role of factor XI (PTA), prekallikrein and plasminogen proactivator in coagulation, fibrinolysis and kinin-generation. In: Chemistry and Biology of the Kallikrein-Kinin System in Health and Disease,(Ed. J.J. Pisano and K.F. Austen.) Fogarty Int. Center Proc. 27 U.S. Gov. Printing Office: Washington, D.C., 1976.

25. Cochrane, C.G., S.D. Revak and K.D. Wuepper. Activation of Hageman factor in solid and fluid phases. J. Exp. Med. 138, 1564, 1973.

26. Bagdasarian, A., B. Lahiri and R.W. Colman. Origin of the high molecular weight activator of prekallikrein. J. Biol. Chem. 248, 7742, 1973.

27. McMillin, C.R., H. Saito, O.D. Ratnoff and A.G. Walton. The secondary structure of human Hageman factor (Factor XII) and its alteration by activating agents. J. Clin. Invest. 54, 1312, 1974.

28. Schiffmann, S., P. Leeand, R. Waldmann. Identity of contact activation cofactor and Fitzgerald factor. Thromb. Res. 6, 451, 1975.

29. Iwanaga, S., M. Komiya, Y. N. Han, S. Oh-ishi, M. Katori and T. Suzuki. Amino acid sequence of a fragment (histidine-rich peptide) released from bovine high molecular

weight kininogen by plasma kallikrein and its biological
activity. In: Chemistry and Biology of the Kallikrein-Kinin
System in Health and Disease, (Ed. J.J. Pisano and K.F.
Austen) Fogarty Int. Center Proc. 27. U.S. Gov. Printing
Office: Washington, D.C., 1976.

30. Ruddy, S. Chemistry and biologic activity of the complement
    system. Transpl. Proc. 6, 1, 1974.

31. Gladner, J.A. Potentiation of the effect of bradykinin. In:
    Hypotensive Peptides, (Ed. E.G. Erdos, N. Back and F. Sicu-
    teri.) Springer-Verlag: New York, p. 344, 1966.

32. Kay, A.B., D.S. Pepper and R. McKenzie. The identification
    of fibrinopeptide B as a chemotactic agent derived from
    human fibrinogen. Brit. J. Haemt. 27, 669, 1974.

33. Kaplan, A.P., A.B. Kay and F.K. Austen. A prealbumin activa-
    tor of prekallikrein, III. Appearance of chemotactic activity
    for human neutrophils by the conversion of human prekalli-
    krein to kallikrein. J. Exp. Med. 135, 81, 1972.

34. Kaplan, A.P., Goetzl, E.J. and K.F. Austen. The fibrinolytic
    pathway of human plasma II. Generation of chemotactic
    activity by activation of plasminogen proactivator. J. Clin.
    Invest. 52, 2591, 1973.

35. Gallin, J.I. and A.P. Kaplan. Mononuclear cell chemotactic
    activity of kallikrein and plasminogen activator and its
    inhibition by Cl inhibitor and α_2-macroglobulin. J. Immunol.
    113, 1928, 1974.

CARDIOVASCULAR AND RESPIRATORY REFLEXES ELICITED BY BRADYKININ ACTING ON RECEPTOR SITES (K & P) IN THE MUSCULAR CIRCULATORY AREA

G. Tallarida, F. Baldoni, G. Peruzzi, A. Semprini and M. Sangiorgi

Instituto di I Clinica Medica and Cattedra di I Semeiotica Medica
University of Rome, Rome, Italy

It is well known that there are sensory receptors in the heart and lungs which, excited by chemical agents, cause inhibitory reflexes consisting of fall in arterial blood pressure and heart rate accompanied by changes in respiratory movements (Dawes and Comroe, 1954; Linden, 1973). There is also agreement that peripheral blood vessels are supplied with sensory nerve fibres, subserving pain-sensibility, peculiarly sensitive to stimuli of chemical kind. The stimulation of these algoceptive afferents in the muscular circulatory area induces a series of excitatory reflex responses consisting of behavioral agitation, vocalization, rise in blood pressure, tachycardia and hypertachypnea (Moore et al. 1934; Lim, 1960; Guzman et al. 1962).

In the course of our research work on peripheral vascular chemoreception we observed that bradykinin, injected into the femoral artery of rabbits, causes two types of cardiocirculatory reflex effects which occur without loss of continuity. The first-type effects are more precocious and of prevalently inhibitory nature. The second-type effects appear later and are of exclusively excitatory nature (Tallarida et al. 1973, 1974). These findings led us to consider the hypothesis that bradykinin, introduced into the hindlimb circulatory bed, activates two functionally distinct kinds of peripheral sensory receptors.

Such a possibility appeared very interesting, bradykinin being a physiological polypeptide and evidence accumulating that reflexes elicited by muscle afferent fibres play a roll, as a peripheral link, in the cardiovascular and respiratory responses to muscular

exercise (Paterson, 1928; Comroe and Schmidt, 1943; Donald et al.
1967; Coote et al 1971; McCloskey and Mitchell, 1972; Clement et
al. 1973).

In order to provide further elements to characterize such a
double type of peripheral chemoreception we analyzed the reflex
responses of systemic blood pressure, hindlimb vascular resistance,
cardiac activity and breathing evoked in rabbits by injecting into
the femoral artery bradykinin and several substances of physiological significance.

METHODS

The experiments were carried out in rabbits of both sexes,
either conscious or anesthetized with sodium pentobarbital (30-
40 mg/kg i.v.). In conscious animals the preparation was performed
in local procainic anesthesia.

Studies were concerned with reflex changes in systemic blood
pressure, hindlimb vascular resistance, cardiac rate and respiratory
activity induced by injecting into the femoral artery bradykinin
(BRS-640 Sandoz) and the following substances: serotonin, nicotine,
adenosine and adenosin-triphosphate, adrenalin, noradrenalin,
angiotensin, vasopressin, oxytocin, isotonic potassium chloride,
hypertonic sodium chloride, hypertonic glucose and buffer solutions
of sodium phosphates at pH 7 and 6.

Repeated intra-arterial injections were made by means of a
polyethylene loop with a central segment of silicone rubber (thus
insuring the supply of blood to the limb). The marginal vein of
the ear was cannulated with a thin polyethylene tube to perform
intravenous injections. Systemic blood pressure was measured by
cannulating the common carotid or the axillary artery and was
recorded by a rotating kymograph. Hindlimb vascular resistance
was studied by perfusing the external iliac artery (opposite to
the femoral artery injected with the test substances) at constant
flow with a peristaltic pump using autologous blood drawn from the
ipsilateral common iliac artery. A heat-exchanger and a reservoir
bottle were interposed in the perfusion line. The perfusion
pressure was measured via a T-tube down-stream from the pump just
proximal to the point of insertion of the inflow cannula in the
external iliac artery and was recorded on a rotating kymograph.
The pump speed was adjusted to give an initial perfusion pressure
similar to the systemic arterial pressure. It was established that
the output of the pump used did not vary between a perfusion pressure of 30 to 180 mm Hg. Hence any variation in perfusion
pressure was considered as an index of change in vascular resistance. This series of experiments was performed on anesthetized,

immobilized (with Flaxedil) and artificially ventilated animals with denervated carotid sinuses and aortic arch. Cardiac activity was investigated by electrocardiogram. Breathing was recorded via a tracheal cannula connected to a Brodie tambour (Palmer).

The effects on the reflex responses induced by pharmacological autonomic blockades and by sectioning the somatic nerves of the limb or by cutting the carotid sinus and aortic nerves were also investigated.

In some experiments the skin, under deep general anesthesia, was completely removed from the limb. In others a "delay circuit" was inserted in the inferior vena cava, so that drugs injected into the femoral artery did not reach the systemic circulation for 30 to 60 seconds.

RESULTS

As we have already stated microdoses of bradykinin (100-250 ng) injected into the femoral artery of conscious rabbits elicit, after a latent period of about 7 seconds, two types of reflex effects displayed in succession. The first-type effects, prevailingly inhibitory in nature, appear earlier and are represented by arterial pressure fall, bradycardia and hyper-tachypnea, sometimes preceeded by fleeting apnea. The second-type effects, clearly excitatory in nature, appear later and consist of hypertension, tachycardia, hyper-tachypnea and behavioral manifestations typical of the "alarm reaction" to pain (Fig. 1). In some cases the excitatory second-type (Fig. 1), while in others the inhibitory first-type (Fig. 2), responses predominate.

All these effects are reflex in nature; in fact they are not obtained injecting the same small doses of substance intravenously and are not provokable after sectioning the somatic nerves (femoral and sciatic) of the limb where injection of bradykinin was made.

By injecting the artery with gradually increased doses of bradykinin it is sometimes possible to dissociate the two types of reflex responses in the sense that with minimal quantities only the first-type responses are obtained; as the doses are increased the second-type responses become manifest. A more evident dissociation of two reflex effects can be obtained with general anesthesia. In the anesthetized animals the second-type effects are greatly inhibited while the first-type predominate with a conspicuously potentiated fall in arterial pressure (Fig. 3). These effects in the anesthetized animals occur unchanged and with the same latency (7 sec.) also after the insertion of a "delay circuit" into the inferior vena cava, but they are not obtained when the somatic nerves of the intra-arterially injected limb are previously sectioned.

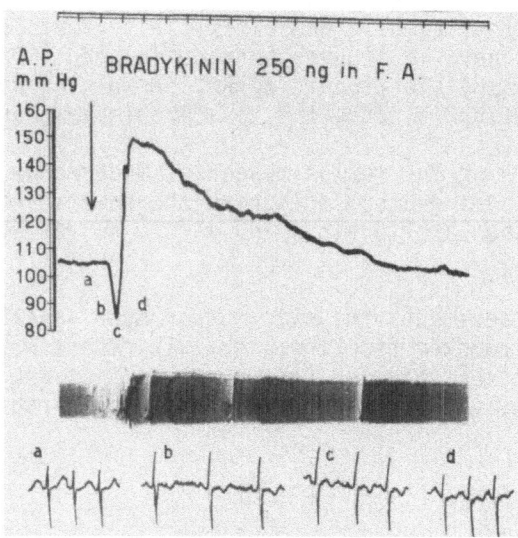

Figure 1. Non-anesthetized rabbit. A microdose of bradykinin
(250 ng) injected into the femoral artery (F.A.) causes initially
a rapid hypotensive effect with bradycardia (first-type effects)
and, subsequently, a more prolonged hypertensive effect with
tachycardia, hyperventilation and behavioral agitation (second-
type effects). Time: 1 div. = 10 sec.

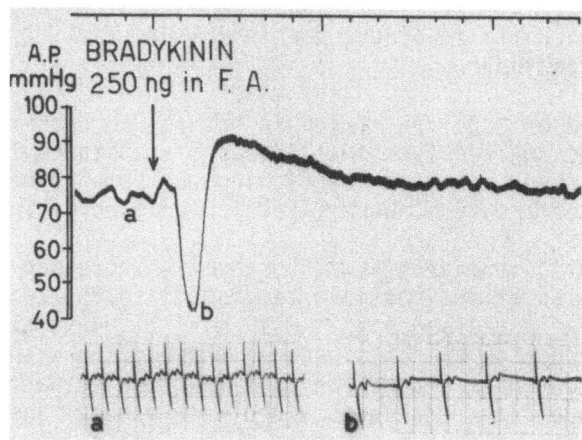

Figure 2. Non-anesthetized rabbit. Intra-arterial injection of
bradykinin (250 ng). In this case the inhibitory first-type effects,
hypotension and bradycardia, clearly predominate.

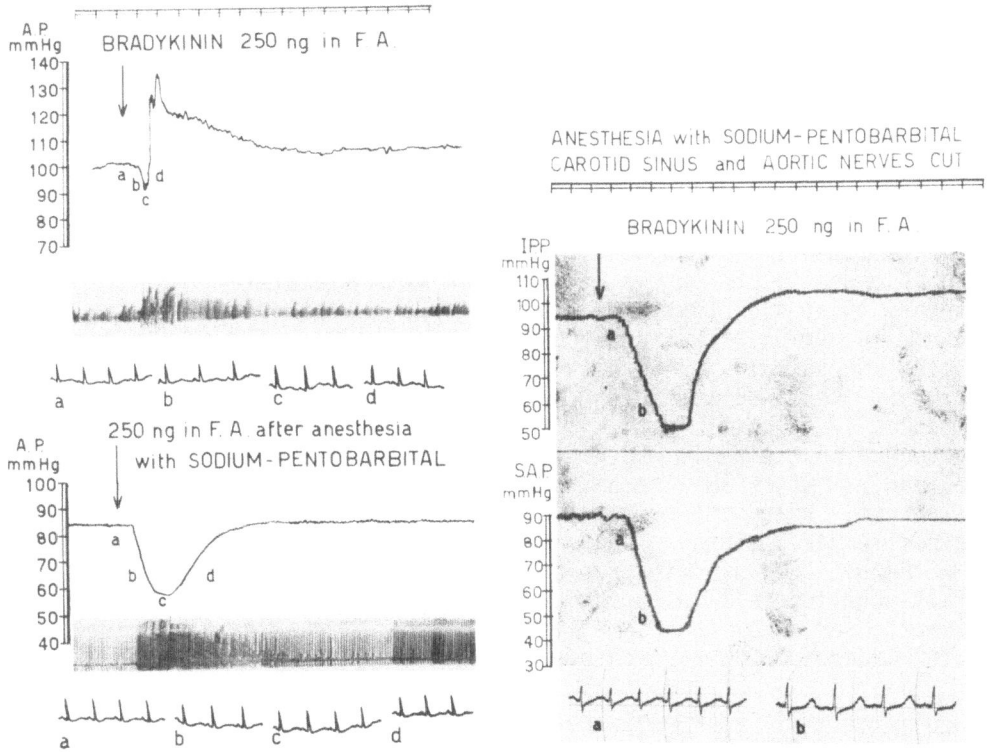

Figure 3. Cardiocirculatory and respiratory reflex responses to intra-arterial injection of bradykinin (250 ng) before and after general anesthesia with sodium pentobarbital. Anesthesia completely inhibits the second-type excitatory effects. The first-type responses remain conserved; bradycardia is slightly reduced but an evident respiratory effect persists. The depressor response is conspicuously potentiated.

Figure 4. Anesthetized, immobilized and artificially ventilated rabbit with carotid sinuses and aortic arch denervated. The injection of bradykinin into the femoral artery causes, concomitantly with the systemic depressor effect, an evident fall in the vascular resistance of the contralateral hindlimb perfused at contant flow.
IPP: external iliac artery perfusion pressure
SAP: systemic arterial pressure.

The circulatory and respiratory responses were not at all inhibited by the removal of the skin from that limb intra-arterially injected with bradykinin. Both types of reflex responses were not affected by sectioning the carotid sinus and aortic nerves; in the anesthetized animals the depressor response was greater after this had been done.

An evident reflex fall in the hindlimb vascular resistance of anesthetized, immobilized and artificially ventialed rabbits with both carotid sinus and aortic nerves cut, was constantly observed in response to bradykinin given into the contralateral femoral artery (Fig. 4). The onset and the maximum of this fall in the hindlimb perfusion pressure coincided with the onset and the maximum point of the fall in systemic blood pressure even if a "delay circuit" was inserted in the inferior vena cava. Both because of the "delay circuit" in the inferior vena cava, and of the hindlimb autoperfusion circuit, such hindlimb vasodilatation occurred evidently before the intra-arterially injected bradykinin could eventually reach the systemic circulation or the autoperfused hindlimb vasculature. The reflex nature of this vasodilatation in the perfused hindlimb was unequivocally indicated also by the fact that the fall in perfusion pressure did not occur when the somatic nerves of the contralateral limb, intra-arterially injected with bradykinin, were previously sectioned.

Both types of reflex responses to bradykinin were not inhibited by atropine sulfate (1-2 ng/kg i.v.) but bradycardia was considerably reduced. Propranolol pre-treatment (2 mg/kg i.v.) did not alter the general picture of reflex changes except for a slight reduction of pressor effect and bradycardia. After administration of phentolamine (1-2 mg/kg i.v.) or phenoxybenzamine (1-3 mg/kg i.v.) all the reflex changes in systemic blood pressure and in hindlimb vascular resistance were greatly inhibited. The cardiac and respiratory changes were not significantly influenced by the α-adrenergic blockade.

The intra-arterial injection of Potassium chloride (0,5 ml 1% KCl) causes, in the conscious rabbit, reflex responses analogous to those caused by bradykinin; that is, pressure fall, bradycardia and hyperventilation, followed by hypertension, tachycardia, hyper-tachypnea and agitation (Fig. 5). The latent period is much shorter (2 or 3 sec.) but the threshold dose is much more elevated (about 10,000 times more, ranging from 1 to 3 mg of potassium ions). As in the case of bradykinin, denervation of the limb completely abolishes all reflex manifestations; general anesthesia abolishes only the second-type responses and consistently increases the first-type reflexes (Fig. 5). These latter responses are maintained, with the same latent period, even after insertion of a "delay

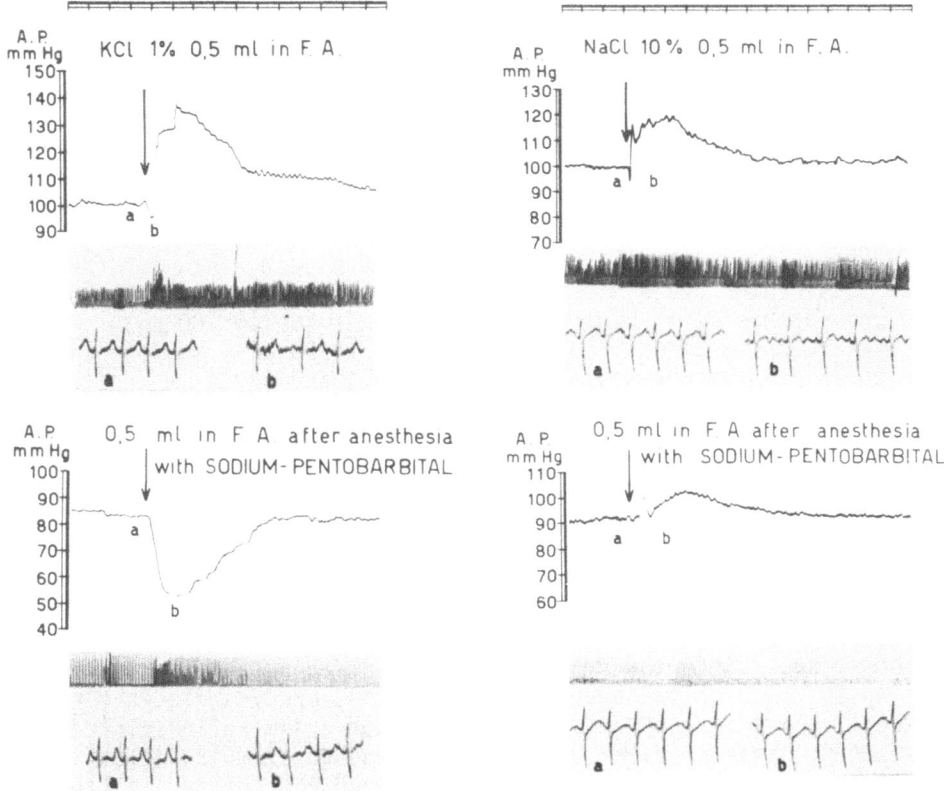

Figure 5. The intra-arterial injection of KCl causes, in the unanesthetized rabbit, reflex responses analogous to those caused by bradykinin (first and second-type responses). The anesthesia abolishes only the second-type responses. The hypotensive effect (first-type response) is enormously potentiated.

Figure 6. The intra-arterial injection of hypertonic solution (NaCl 10%) immediately causes (latent period: 2-3 sec.) only second-type reflex responses (hypertension, hyperventilation, agitation). At the peak of the pressor effect there is a transitory decrease in cardiac rate due to the activation of carotid sinus and aortic baroreceptors. The anesthesia greatly inhibits any reflex responses to the hypertonic solution. Note that in this case (as opposed to that found injecting bradykinin or KCl) no hypotensive effect is manifest.

circuit" into the inferior vena cava and are further enhanced by
denervation of the carotid sinuses and aortic arch. In the
anesthetized animals the intra-arterial injection of KCl, analo-
gously with bradykinin, elicits a marked reflex vasodilatation
in the autoperfused contralateral hindlimb. The effects of autonomic
blockades on the reflex changes caused by intra-arterially injected
KCl were closely similar to those induced on the reflex responses
to bradykinin.

No reflex response is obtained by introducing into the femoral
artery even high doses of serotonin (up to 250 µg), nicotine (up to
100 µg), adenosine and adenosin-triphosphate (up to 100 µg),
adrenalin (up to 20 µg), noradrenalin (up to 20 µg), angiotensin
(up to 20 µg), vasopressin (up to 0.5 I.U.) and oxytocin (up to
0.5 I.U.).

The intra-arterial injections of typical, strong, algesic
agents as hypertonic solutions (0.5-1.0 ml 10% NaCl or 40% glucose)
or acid solutions (0.5 ml sodium phosphate buffers at pH 6 or lower)
immediately cause, in conscious rabbits, with a latent period of
about 2-3 seconds, only second-type excitatory responses: hypertension, hyperventilation and somatic reactions characteristic of
an intense pain, never preceeded by evident first-type inhibitor
effects, thus differing from bradykinin and potassium ions (Fig. 6).
During the rise of the blood pressure slight bradycardia is generally
present. In this case bradycardia does not arise reflexly from
receptors in the hindlimb but is likely due to stimulation of
central baroreceptors since it was abolished and shifted to tachycardia by denervation of the carotid sinuses and aortic arch.

All the excitatory responses are abolished by denervation of
the limb, intra-arterially injected with algesic agents, and are
greatly inhibited by general anesthesia (Fig. 6). Particularly
after anesthesia clear first-type effects are never observed. The
second-type effects, strongly inhibited in the deeply anesthetized
animals, become very evident after elimination of the buffer
reflexes from carotid sinuses and aortic arch (Fig. 7). In this
case the pressor response is constantly associated with slight
tachycardia and with reflex hindlimb vasoconstriction (Fig. 8).
Even after the insertion of a "delay circuit" in the inferior vena
cava the fundamental picture and latency of the reflex excitatory
effects elicited by intra-arterial injections of hypertonic or
acid solutions remained unchanged. Particularly the onset and
peak of the rise in the hindlimb perfusion pressure coincided with
the onset and peak of the systemic hypertension effect. The pressor
effect and the rise in hindlimb vascular resistance are greatly
inhibited by alpha-adrenergic blocking agents (Phentolamine and
phenoxybenzamine).

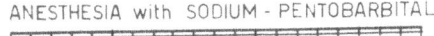

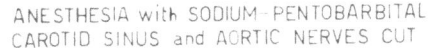

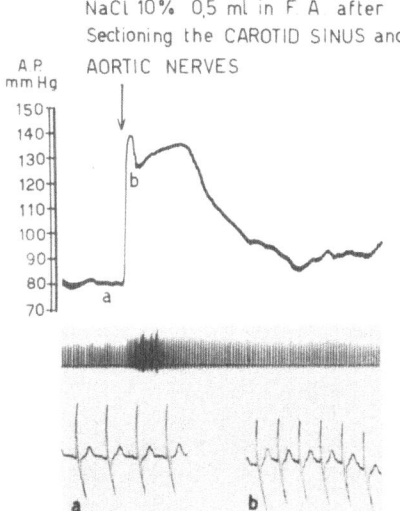

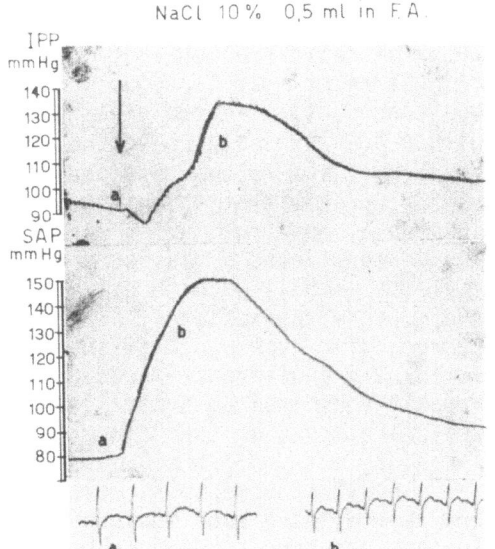

Figure 7. Anesthetized rabbit. Sectioning and carotid sinus and aortic nerves potentiates the reflex responses (second-type effects) to the hypertonic solution given into the femoral artery. After elimination of the main central baroreceptors the pressor response is constantly associated with tachycardia.

Figure 8. Anesthetized, immobilized and artificially ventilated rabbit with carotid sinuses and aortic arch denervated. The injection of hypertonic solution into the femoral artery simultaneously induces a pressor response in the systemic circulation and an evident vasoconstriction in the hindlimb perfused at constant flow.
IPP: external iliac artery perfusion pressure
SAP: systemic arterial pressure

CONSIDERATIONS

The above findings seem to suggest the presence of more than one type of chemosensitive receptor site in the area of distribution of the femoral artery. In fact the two different and opposite types of reflex responses elicited by injecting bradykinin into the femoral artery may reasonably be explained by admitting that the substance activates two distinct kinds of sensory receptors. Those with a low threshold cause the first-type reflexes (hypotension, hindlimb vasodilation, bradycardia, hyperventilation) earlier to appear, predominantly inhibitory, induced by minimal quantities of substance, conserved after general anesthesia and which as a group may be considered a "Jarisch-Bezold" type reflex and do not seem strictly associated with pain. Those with a higher threshold cause the second-type reflexes (hypertension, hindlimb vasoconstriction, tachycardia, hyperventilation and agitation) later to appear, predominantly excitatory, induced by higher quantities of substance, greatly inhibited by general anesthesia and which present the typical picture of the "alarm reaction" to pain.

The first receptors, selectively sensitive to microdoses of bradykinin, have been indicated as K-receptors (from Kinin); the second receptors showing properties of pain receptors, have been indicated as P-receptors (from Pain).

As we have seen, analogous to bradykinin, potassium ions are also capable of causing both first and second-type responses, whereas acid and hypertonic solutions induce univocal second-type responses. Thus, potassium ions, as is the case for bradykinin, stimulate both K and P-receptors, while acid or hypertonic solutions mainly excite P-receptors.

Both sensory receptors are present in the muscular circulatory area; in fact, completely removing the skin from the limb does not inhibit either type of reflex response.

The efferent pathways of these reflexes are mediated by both cholinergic and adrenergic nerves. Bradycardia is essentially a vagal effect. The depressor response and hindlimb vasodilatation are mainly caused by a withdrawal of sympathetic vasoconstrictor tone. The pressor response and hindlimb vasoconstriction are clearly due to activation of alpha-adrenergic receptors.

The afferent pathways of K and P chemoreception pass through somatic nerves as indicated by the fact that sectioning femoral and sciatic nerves abolishes both reflex responses.

It is known that electrical stimulation of the central end of the somatic nerves causes either a pressor or depressor effect; weak stimulation or stimulation at low frequencies generally causes a depressor effect while a pressor effect is produced by increasing either strength or frequency of stimulation. On the basis of electrophysiological investigations it has been suggested that different afferent nerve fibres are involved in the two responses (Hunt, 1895; Gordon, 1943; De Molina et al. 1953; Laporte et al. 1960; Skoglund, 1960; Joansson, 1962; Clement et al. 1973). The depressor effects would be provoked by activation of group III (Aγ and Aδ) afferent fibres; while the pressor ones would be elicited by stimulation of both group III and IV afferent fibres (partly Aδ, but mainly "post δ " group of the finest myelinated A and non-myelinated C fibres).

It is not possible at present to relate with certainty the pharmacologically phypthesized K and P sensitive receptors in the muscular circulatory area to the electrophysiologically identified types of muscle afferent fibres. From the electrophysiological point of view, K-sensory receptors might belong to the depressor subgroup III afferent fibres, while P-sensory receptors might be connected to the pressor subgroup III and possible group IV afferent fibres.

Since in the conscious animals electrical stimulation of the somatic afferents constantly evokes only pressor reflexes while anesthesia or removal of suprabulbar structures are necessary for the appearance of the depressor reflexes, the question arised whether such hypotensive effects are normal responses of the vasomotor centre or experimental artifacts. In this respect it is of interest to the evidence reported here that opposite cardiovascular reflexes analogous to those elicited by graded electrical stimulation of muscle afferents can also be obtained either in conscious or in anesthetized animals by chemical stimuli.

Our finding that anesthesia is not a necessary condition for producing reflex inhibitory responses supports the idea that not only pressor but also depressor reflexes from somatic afferents have to be considered "normal" functions of the bulbar vasomotor centre. In the conscious animals the inhibitory first-type reflexes may be greatly concealed by the successive more intense excitatory second-type responses. In the anesthetized animals the response of the cardiovascular centers to mixed afferent inflow (inhibitory and excitatory) is biased toward inhibition so that the depressor reflexes become overactive and fully predominate. In other words the potentiation of the inhibitory responses after anesthesia seem to be caused by a depression of central transmission of impulses from P-sensory receptors in such a way as to favour the inhibitory inflow. If the stimulus evokes a pure excitatory afferent inflow, the anesthesia cannot reverse but only reduce the univocal excitatory responses. This latter effect can be partly hindered by sectioning the carotid sinus and aortic buffer nerves.

The question of whether both these different kinds of chemo-receptors belong to the nerve system subserving the noci-algoceptive function or whether the different properties we have identified (threshold, latency, type of stimuli, type of response) correspond to different physiological purposes remains to be answered.

The main function of the P-receptors at high threshold, sti-mulated by higher doses of bradykinin and by strong algesic agents, is apparently noci-algoception. These receptors should be identified with those commonly referred to as chemosensitive pain receptors or algoceptors. They do not have the role of receiving one specific type of chemical information, but are destined to transmit one type of message (nociception) and are, in fact, activated by many chemical stimuli that reach a sufficient intensity to constitute a probable injury to the organism. The acid and hypertonic solutions we utilized, which do not represent any physiologic condition, behave, in fact, as pure harmful and algesic stimuli; they do not affect the K-receptor system but activate only the P-receptors capable of specifically evoking pain and the concomitant defense responses which constitute the so-called "alarm reaction". Activation of the P-receptors in the muscular area might also occur during the non-physiological muscular work such as sustained, isometric or tetanic muscular contractions.

Since we do not know the location of the K-sensory receptors and the normal stimulus to these fibres, we can only speculate as to whether they play a role in cardiocirculatory and respiratory regulation. In this case we are dealing with low threshold nerve endings selectively activated by microdoses of a physiologic peptide (bradykinin) but not activated by powerful algesic agents such as acid and hypertonic solutions. In reality the stimulation of K-receptors does not appear to clearly evoke the pain sensation; in fact when the first-type reflexes appear the unanesthetized animal does not demonstrate any pain perception behavior. Only subsequently, after about 2-3 seconds, when the inhibitory effects are already fully manifest, does the agitation supervene, indicating the appearance of pain, and simultaneously second-type reflexes interrupt and substitute the first-type responses. On the other hand, bradykinin, injected into the femoral artery in very small quantities (in some cases even 10-25 ng were capable of causing a reflex depressor response), once diluted in the total blood volume of the limb, must reach the periphery at such a low concentration which hardly represents a harmful factor to the tissues. Therefore the primary function of the K-receptors may be that of collecting some informtion on the metabolic state of the tissue; that is, they should be essentially metabolic receptors.   Activation of the K-receptor system could occur, by changes in their chemical environment, during dynamic muscular exercise and might be competing, as a moderator factor, with the concomitant increase in the sympathetic activity.

This investigation was supported in part by a Research Grant #115/7569 74.00278/04 from the Consiglio Nazionale delle Ricerche (C.N.R.), Italy.
Dr. Sangiorgi is the supervisor of the research program on the circulatory control mechanisms accepted by the Medical and Biological Sciences Committee of the C.N.R.

REFERENCES

Clement D.L., Pelletier C.L., Schepherd J.T.: Role of muscular contraction in the reflex vascular responses to stimulation of muscle afferents in the dog. Circulation Res. 33, 386, 1973.

Comroe J.H. jr., Schmidt C.F.: Reflexes from the limbs as a factor in the hyperpnea of muscular exercise. Amer. J. Physiol. 138, 536, 1943.

Coote J.H., Hilton S.M., Perez-Gonzales J.F.: The reflex nature of the pressor response to muscular exercise. J. Physiol. (London). 215, 789, 1971.

Dawes G.S., Comroe J.H.: Chemoreflexes from the heart and lungs. Physiol. Rev. 34, 167, 1954.

De Molina F., Achard O., Wyss O.: Respiratory and vasomotor responses to stimulation of afferent fibres in somatic nerves. Helv. Physiol. Pharmacol. Acta. 11, 1, 1953.

Donald K.K., Lind A.R., McNicol G.W., Humphreys P.H., Taylor S.H., Staunton H.P.: Cardiovascular responses to sustained (static) contractions. Circulation Res. 20/21 (Suppl. I), 15, 1967.

Gordon, G.: The mechanism of the vasomotor reflexes produced by stimulating mammalian sensory nerves. J. Physiol. (London) 102, 95, 1943.

Guzman F., Braun C., Lim R.K.S.: Visceral pain and the pseudoaffective response to intra-arterial injection of bradykinin and other algesic agents. Arch. int. Pharmacodyn. 136, 353, 1962.

Hunt R.: The fall of blood pressure resulting from the stimulation of afferent nerves. J. Physiol. (London). 18, 381, 1895.

Joansson B.: Circulatory responses to stimulation of somatic afferents with special reference to depressor effects from muscle nerves. Acta Physiol. Scand. 57 (Suppl. 198), 1, 1962.

Laporte Y., Bessou P., Bouisset S.: Action reflexe des differents types de fibres afferentes d'origine musculaire sur la pression sanguigne. Arch. Ital. Biol. 98, 206, 1960.

Lim R.K.S.: Visceral receptors and visceral pain. Ann. N.Y. Acad. Sci. 86, 73, 1960.

Linden R.J.: Function of cardiac receptors. Circulation. 48, 463, 1973.

McCloskey D.I., Mitchell J.H.: Reflex cardiovascular and respiratory responses originating in exercising muscle. J. Physiol. (London) 224, 173, 1972.

Moore R.M., Moore R.E., Singleton A.O.: Experiments on the chemical stimulation of pain-endings associated with small blood-vessels. Amer. J. Physiol. 107, 594, 1934.

Paterson W.D.: Circulatory and respiratory changes in response to muscular exercise in man. J. Physiol. (London). 66, 323, 1928.

Skoglund C.R.: Vasomotor reflexes from muscle. Acta Physiol. Scand. 50, 311, 1960.

Tallarida G., Baldoni F., Peruzzi G., Sangiorgi M.: Risposte cardio-circolatorie e respiratorie riflesse determinate dall'iniezione di bradichinina nei distretti circolatori femorale e carotideo. Boll. Soc. Ital. Biol. Sper. 49, 79, 1973.

Tallarida G., Baldoni F., Peruzzi G.: Ricerche sulla regolazione neuro-umorale della circolazione. Studio delle risposte riflesse cardiovascolari e respiratorie determinate dalla stimolazione di chemocettori sensibili all bradichinina nel distretto circolatorio femorale. Boll. Soc. Ital. Cardiol. 19, 61, 1974.

LEUKOKININS - CLINICAL ENTITIES OF NEOPLASIA?

Lowell M. Greenbaum

Department of Pharmacology, Columbia University

New York, New York 10032

Leukokinins are high molecular weight polypeptides which our laboratory first described. They are potent pharmacological mediators released by an acid protease found in white cells and neoplastic cells. The name leukokinin is derived from leuko - or white cells, the initial source of the enzyme. However, they were also found in L-1210 cells, a human leukemia-derived tumor as well as other tumor cells. Since these polypeptides resembled bradykinin in their pharmacological properties the class of peptides were named leukokinins.

Several reviews of the initial experiments leading to their discovery and isolation have been published (1 - 3). Four different leukokinins have been isolated and their amino acid content determined (Table 1). Leukokinins-PMN and M were isolated following incubation of rabbit polymorphonuclear leukocyte and macrophage enzymes with a human preparation of leukokininogen. Leukokinins-A and H were isolated from murine ascites and human ascites fluids which develop as a result of neoplastic disease.

Ascites fluid accumulation represents a significant problem in the treatment of human ovarian carcinoma since usual chemotherapeutic measures fail in many cases to reduce the enormous quantities (liters) of fluid which develop in these patients. The finding in our laboratory (4 - 7) that a) such ascites fluids contain leukokinin-forming enzymes as well as substrate and b) that quantities of leukokinin may be generated by activity of the acid protease contained in the fluid, led to our hypothesis that leukokinins were important permeability mediators which are released and involved in ascites fluid accumulation. We further demonstrated (6) that Pepstatin,

TABLE 1

AMINO ACID RESIDUES OF LEUKOKININS

Amino Acid	PMN	M	A	H
Alanine	1	2	1	1
Arginine	2	3	4	2
Aspartic acid	1	1	1	0
Cystine ½	0	0	0	0
Glutamic acid	1	2	1	2
Glycine	2	2	0	0
Histidine	1	1	1	0
Isoleucine	0	0	0	0
Leucine	1	1	1	3
Lysine	2	3	3	1
Methionine	0	0	0	0
Phenylalanine	1	1	1	1
Proline	3	3	3	2
Serine	2	2	1	2
Threonine	1	1	1	4
Tyrosine	2	1	1	2
Valine	1	2	1	4
Total A.A.	21	25	20	24

The abbreviations represent the source of enzyme
which catalyzed the formation of peptide. PMN-
polymorphonuclear leukocyte (rabbit), M-alveolar
macrophage (rabbit), A-ascites fluid, mastocytoma
(mouse), H-ascites fluid, ovarian carcinoma (human).

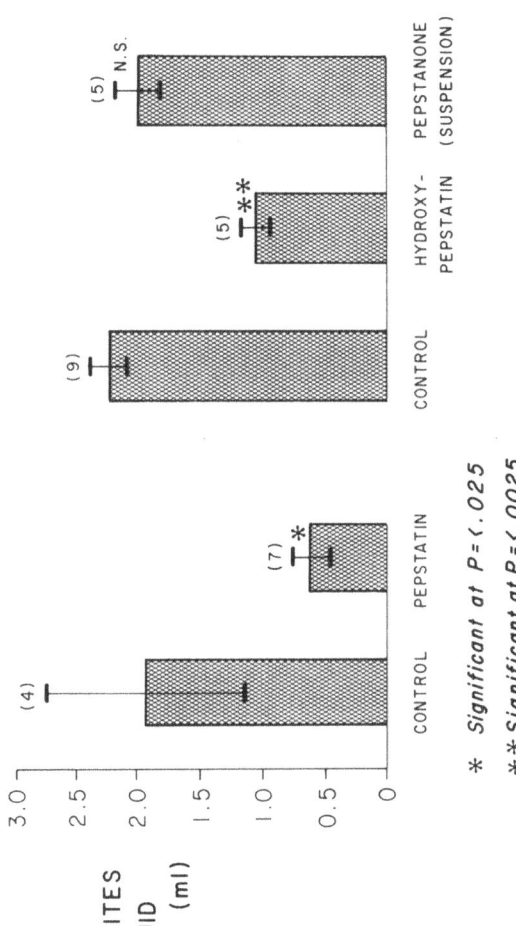

Figure 1. Comparison of Pepstatin and its analogues in reducing ascites fluid accumulation in mice carrying a mastocytoma tumor. Four days following cell inoculation, animals were treated with a total dose of 80 mg/kg of agent. Controls received saline. On the 8th day following inoculation, ascites fluid was measured (6). Pepstatin and hydroxypepstatin significantly prevented ascites fluid accumulation.

a rather specific acid protease and leukokinin-forming enzyme inhibitor could retard ascites fluid accumulation when administered to mice in vivo (Figure 1).

This finding that Pepstatin and its analogues are potent inhibitors of ascites fluid accumulation opens up a new concept in the treatment of pathological fluid accumulation especially since this class of drugs are relatively low in toxicity as compared to usual chemotherapeutic agents.

Studies are now proceeding to determine if the use of such drugs in humans would be appropriate.

REFERENCES

1. Greenbaum, L.M. Leukocyte Kininogenases and Leukokinins from Normal and Malignant Cells. Am. J. Pathol. 68: 613-623, 1972.

2. Greenbaum, L.M. Cellular Kininogenases and Leukokinins. Int'l. Conf. on Chem. and Biol. of the Kallekrein-Kinin System in Health Disease. 1974, in press.

3. Greenbaum, L.M., Grebow, P., Johnston, M., Prakash, A. and Semente, G. Pepstatin, An Inhibitor of Leukokinin Formation and Ascitic Fluid Accumulation. Cancer Res. 35: 706-710, 1975.

4. Greenbaum, L.M., Prakash, A., Semente, G. and Johnston, M. The Leukokinin System; Its Role in Fluid Accumulation in Malignancy and Inflammation. In: Agents and Actions, 3:332-334, 1973. ed: Birkhauser Verlag Basel.

5. Johnston, M. and Greenbaum, L.M. Leokokinin-Forming System in the Ascitic Fluid of a Murine Mastocytoma. Biochem. Pharmacol. 22: 1386-1389, 1973.

6. Spragg, J. The Plasma Kinin-Forming System. In: Mediators of Inflammation. ed.: Weissman, J. Plenum Press, 1974.

7. Greenbaum, L.M. Cathepsin D-generated, Pharmacologically Active Peptides (Leukokinins) and Their Role in Ascites Fluid Accumulation. Cold Spring Harbor Laboratory Symposium on Proteases and Biological Control, 223, 1975.

ACTION OF U.V. RAYS ON THE EXPERIMENTAL CUTANEOUS INFLAMMATION INDUCED BY CANTHARIDIN

R. Galletti, L. Matassi, P. Chiarini, F. Corti

Dept. of Medicine

University of Florence, Italy

In previous researches in man, it was demonstrated that hista-mine injected i.v. in microdoses (40 µg) reactivates a decreasing cutaneous inflammation. It is well known that the experimental inflammation induced on the skin by application of cantharidin presents the following characteristics (Fig. 1): 1.) development of exudate; 2.) sensation of pain that starts about 10 hours after the application of the stimulus; 3.) halo of hyperemia corresponding to primary hyperalgesia; 4.) a larger area of secondary hyper-algesia. After 48 hours all these elements are strongly reduced: this shows how inflammation is fading. In this phase an intrave-nous histamine administration is followed by a new increase of blister exudate, hyperemic halo and secondary hyperalgesia. A short-lasting burning pain in the blister also arises. At the same time, the kininogen level in the blister exudate increased.

In regards to the interpretation of these phenomena, we advance the hypothesis that the histamine injected in the general circulation acts specifically on the microvessels of the blister base, previously sensitized by inflammation, thus inducing the activation of the polypeptides. Pain receptors are consequently excited and we have burning pain.

Another experiment whose interpretation could possibly be the same was executed. Instead of injecting histamine intravenously, we induced a cutaneous erythema by means of U.V. (2990 - 3200Å) irradiation. Sondergaard and Greaves (1970), in fact, with a peculiar technique of cutaneous perfusion, demonstrated that, 8 hours after irradiation, an increase of histamine and kinin concentration is observed in the perfusate. 16 - 24 hours after

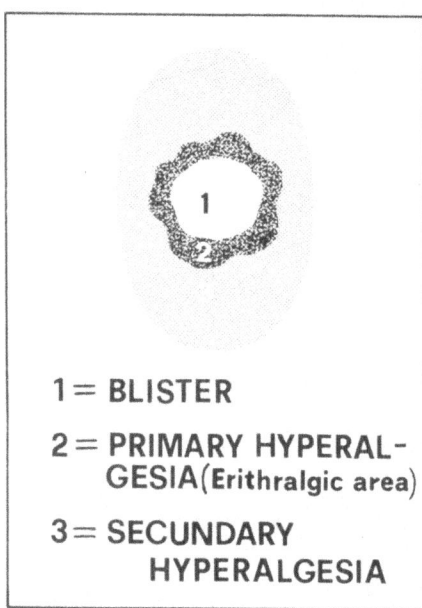

Fig. 1 - Picture of the experimental cutaneous inflammation induced
         by cantharidin on the arm.

8ᵃh a	24ᵃh b	48ᵃh c	after u.v. d irradiation
PAIN	NO PAIN	NO PAIN	PAIN

Fig. 2 - Behaviour of the experimental cutaneous inflammation in-
         duced by cantharidin on the arm before (a-b-c) and after
         U.V. erythema of the back (d).

irradiation a substance, described as U.V.S., apt to induce contractions in the guinea pig ileum and uterus, is present in the perfusate.

This substance, treated with specific antagonists, resulted differently from histamine and kinins, showing instead, the character of a fatty acid extractable with ethyl-acetic acid.

In our experiments, 8 - 10 hours after U.V. irradiation we observed the signs of the reactivation of the cantharidin blister, including the pain sensation (Fig. 2).

As the time elapsed after the tissue damage and after the histamine injection is the same, we propose the same pathophysiological mechanism for the two phenomena.

We assume from our experiments, therefore, the significance of a non specific reactivation of inflammation; a condition common to many clinical states.

KALLIKREINOGEN-KALLIKREIN SYSTEM DURING MUSCULAR WORK IN PATIENTS

WITH INTERMITTENT CLAUDICATION: INFLUENCE OF TAURINE TREATMENT

Franchi G., Fanciullacci M., Curradi C., Nuzzaci G.,

Monetti, M.G. and Caternolo M.
Department of Clinical Pharmacology
University of Florence, Italy

In 1964, Sicuteri and coworkers observed that the muscular work carried out during a local artificially induced ischemia in an arm provoked a lowering of the plasmatic kininogen of the venous blood drawn from the antecubital vein, 5-10 minutes after the end of the exercise. Immediately after stopping the muscular work in ischemia, the kininogen levels were nearly unmodified (6).

Subsequently, we also demonstrated that only local ischemia was able to induce a decrease of the kininogen in the venous blood drawn at the end of the ischemia. This kininogen decrease was on the order of 54%. In the same experiment, we demonstrated that cortison and the sulphurated aminoacid, taurine - a naturally occurring substance - if previously administered, were able to inhibit the fall of kininogen by ischemia (Fig.1). Trasylol also partially blocked the kininogen decrease from ischemia (1). In these studies, kininogen was determined with the Diniz and coworkers method (3).

In a previous study, we pointed out the efficacious therapeutic effect of taurine in patients with angina pectoris (5). These findings prompted the present study. In fact, our aim was to observe whether changes of the plasmatic kinin system at the general level after muscular exercise in the vascular district affected could be found in patients with chronic ischemia in the legs from arterial occlusive disease.

Moreover, we observed if the treatment of these patients with taurine induced a clinical improvement of the arterial disease, and if this therapy was able to provoke modifications of the prekallikrein-kallikrein system in basic conditions, and after muscular work. Therefore, 15 male patients all ranging in age from 50 to 72 were included in this study; they were affected by typical intermittent claudication from arterial occlusive disease, and were examined at the Center for the Study of Angiologic Diseases of our University. Every patient carried out muscular work with an ergometer EM 369 Elena-Schonauder. The muscular exercise started with 300 Kpm for 3 minutes, and increased every 3 minutes by 300 Kpm: the patient stopped spontaneously when the pain in the limbs did not allow the continuation of the work.

A sample of venous blood was drawn from every patient from the antecubital vein for evaluation of the pre-kallikrein-kallikrein system, before, immediately after, and 10 minutes after the exercise. This evaluation is done according to the Colman and coworkers method (2); this method allows the determination of the spontaneous (at the zero point) esterase activity, of the amount of the prekallikrein activity of the physiological kallikrein inhibitor showed by plasma kaolin contact for 5 minutes.

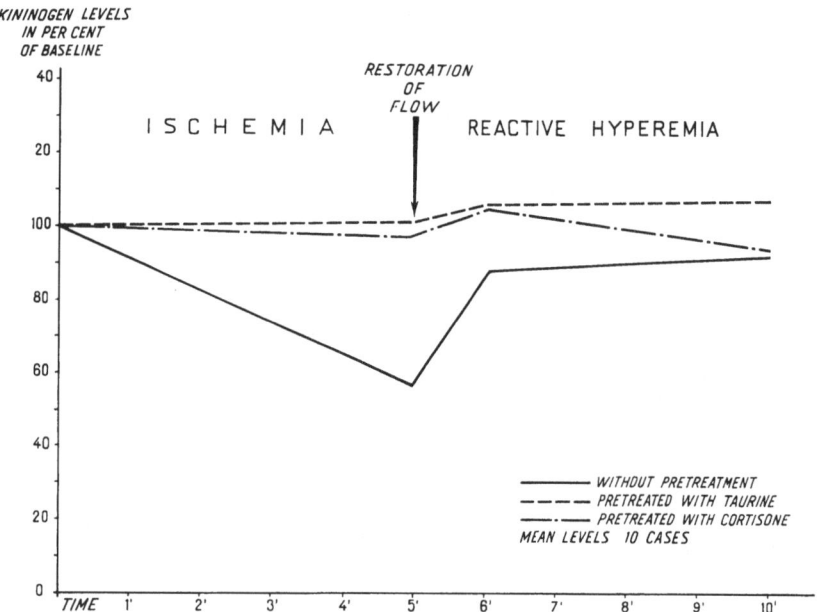

Fig. 1. The decrease in plasma kininogen levels in baseline percent during ischemia and the return to the initial levels in reactive hyperemia (mean of 10 normal subjects).
This phenomenon is inhibited by pretreatment with taurine and cortisone (from: Bavazzano et al., Bradykinin and Related Kinins, Plenum Press).

Every patient repeatedly carried out the exercise four times, that is, after a period of 20-30 days of washout, after 15 days of placebo treatment, and respectively after 1 and 2 months of taurine treatment at the dosage of 3 gm/day by oral administration.

Obviously, all the patients were followed from a clinical point of view during all of the treatment period.

The clinical results demonstrated that in 11 out of 15 patients an increase of 20-30% in the course prior to the appearance of the leg pain was registered. The evaluation of the muscular work with the ergometer demonstrated an increase after taurine treatment, but not of statistical significance. (Fig. 2).

The behaviour of the kallikreinogen-kallikrein system without taurine treatment showed a slight increase of the spontaneous esterase activity (at the zero point) at the end of the muscular work. This increase corresponds to a decrease in the same esterase activity at 1 minute which also lasts 10 minutes after the exercise.

After taurine treatment, the esterase activity is unmodified following the muscular work (Fig. 3). However, this decrease observed without treatment does not have a definite statistical significance, but, seems interesting that after taurine, no change is observed.

These data are only in part in agreement with our findings after muscular work in ischemia, or after ischemia in a limb. This difference can be referred to the different methods respectively used for the plasmatic kininogen and prekallikrein-kallikrein system determination.

WORK ‹ Kpm ›

cases	Before	After
15	1953 ± 259	2103 ± 322

Fig. 2.   After taurine treatment (3 gm/day/2 months), an increase of the muscular work evaluated with the ergometer is demonstrated, even if not statistically significant.

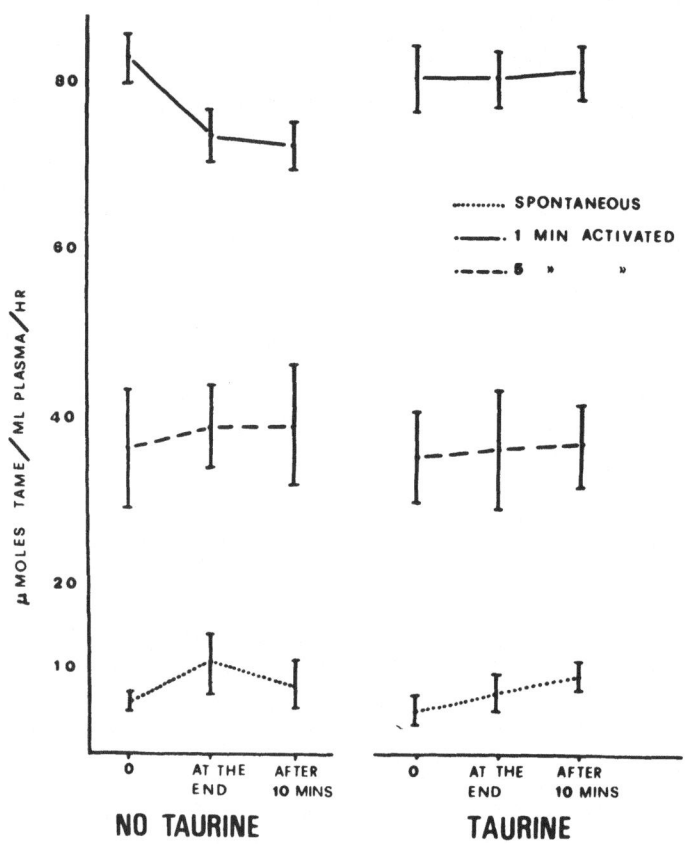

Fig. 3. On the left, the study before taurine is represented, and
         on the right, that after taurine. From the bottom to the
         top, the mean esterase activity of the 15 cases of plasma
         samples is represented at the zero point, after 1 minute,
         and after 5 minutes. The first point (0) represents the
         esterase activity in the basic condition; the second point,
         the esterase activity at the end of the work; and the third
         point, that after 10 minutes.

        On the other hand, we think that it may be a question of
different conditions of the experiments. In fact, the marked
kininogen fall was observed after an intense ischemia in a limited
circulatory district in the venous blood of the same limb. On
the contrary, in the present experiment, the changes in the prekallikrein-kallikrein system were investigated at the general
level after work in a circulatory district in relatively chronic
ischemia. Therefore, it is logical to suppose that even if local

changes of the prekallikrein-kallikrein system are present, these are not evident at the general level. However, on the whole, and in light of the facts previously observed, some conclusions can be drawn. Muscular work in the ischemic condition produces a fall of the local plasmatic kininogen level, and an activation of the pre-kallikrein-kallikrein system at the general level. An aminoacid without any vasoactive action, and with only metabolic activity possesses a therapeutic action in intermittent claudication, and the capability to block the activation of the prekallikrein-kallikrein system by muscular work. These findings can suggest another mechanism besides the other known metabolic mechanisms of taurine action (4). This mechanism consists in the inter-ference on the activation of the prekallikrein-kallikrein system.

BIBLIOGRAPHY

1. Bavazzano A., Sidell N., Michelacci S., and Sicuteri F.: Local ischemia as a kininogen depressant: effect of cortisone taurine as a kallikrein inhibitor., In: Vasopeptides: Chemistry, Pharma-cology, and Pathophysiology. N. Back and F. Sicuteri, Ed., Plenum Press, New York, 1970, p. 377.

2. Colman, R.W., Mason, J.W., and Sherry S.: The kallikreinogen-kallikrein enzyme system of human plasma: An assay of components and observations in disease states. Ann. Int. Med., 71, 4, 1969.

3. Diniz, C.R., Carvalho, J.F., Ryan, J., and Rocha e Silva, M.: A micro-method for the determination of bradykinin in blood plasma. Nature, Lond., 192, 1194, 1961.

4. Jacobsen, J.G., and Smith, L.H.: Biochemistry and physiology of taurine and taurine derivatives. Physiol. Rev. 48, 424, 1968.

5. Sicuteri, F., Franchi, G.C., Fanciullacci, M., Giotti, A., and Guidotti, A.: Sull'azione antianginosa di un aminoacido solforato non coronaro dilatatore., Clin. Ter., 49, 205, 1969.

6. Sicuteri, F., Periti, P., Fanciullacci, M., and Santini, D.: Bradichininogeno dopo lavoro muscolare in ischemia nell'uomo., Boll. Soc. Ital. Biol. Sper., 40, 955, 1964.

URINARY EXCRETION OF KALLIKREIN FOLLOWING MYOCARDIAL INFARCTION

Del Bianco,P.L., Curradi,C., De Saint Pierre,G.*,
Nava, G., and Sicuteri, F.

Department of Clinical Pharmacology, University of
Florence, Italy
* Santa Maria Nuova Hospital, Florence, Italy

Several years ago, the implication of the kallikrein-kinin
system was hypothesized in the pathogenesis of pain and shock
during myocardial infarction (1). This hypothesis was then confirmed by our first observation that demonstrated a significant
decrease of the plasmatic kininogen level in infarcted patients
in the first few days of the disease (2). Furthermore, our
experiences (3,4) and those of other authors (5,6) confirmed
these first observations.

In support of this hypothesis, we subsequently found that
the prekallikrein and kallikrein inhibitor significantly decreased
during myocardial infarction, and that the minimum values resulted
on the ninth day of the disease (7).

The evaluation of urinary kallikrein has recently been proposed
in the study of some pathological situations in which one can pre-
sume the existence of an altered kidney function, such as essential
or secondary hypertension. That is, the renal kallikrein activity
could be in relationship to the regulatory mechanism of renal
perfusion, and therefore, to the homeostatic arterial pressure
mechanisms. Thus, a study of the urinary kallikrein levels in
subjects struck by collapse and shock following myocardial
infarction seemed particularly interesting.

METHODS

The daily urinary kallikrein level was evaluated in thirteen
infarcted patients during the first ten days of the disease,
according to the Porcelli and Croxatto method, modified by Porcelli
(8). This method consists of the measurement of the optical
absorbance provoked by the urinary esterase activity on the specific kallikrein substrate, BAEe. The urinary kallikrein excretion
in thirteen normotensive subjects was evaluated as the control.

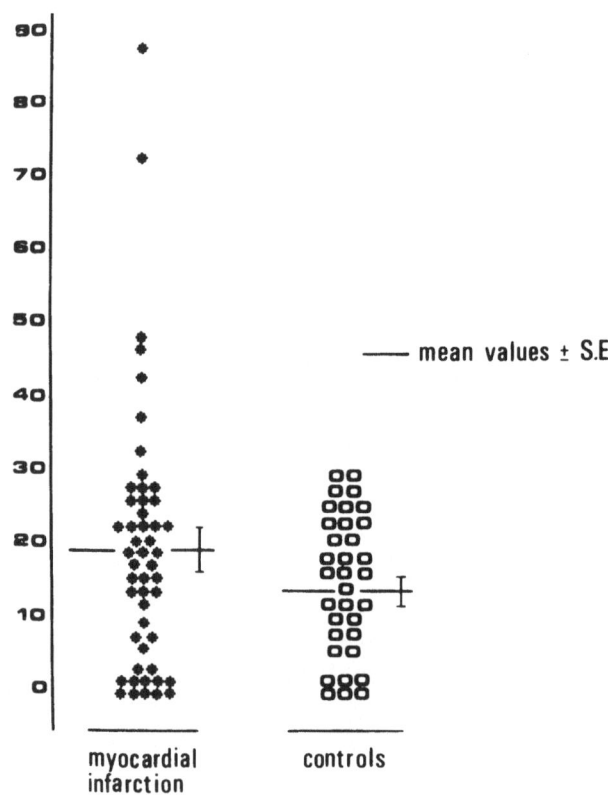

Figure 1. Daily Urinary Kallikrein in 13 infarcted patients and
           in 13 normal subjects. The mean value of the two
           groups differs only slightly. Variability from the
           mean values is more frequent in the infarcted patients
           than in the normal subjects.

RESULTS AND COMMENT

The urinary kallikrein mean level in the normal subjects resulted on 14,2 ± 1,17 unities/24 hours. The urinary kallikrein mean level of the infarcted patients resulted on 19,5 ± 2,25 unities/24 hours, and thus it differs slightly from that of the normal subjects (Fig. 1). But the analysis of the single case indicates that there are some samples in the two groups that vary more or less from the mean values, and this variability is surely more frequent in the infarcted group than in the control group. If we take as parameter the frequency with which the urinary kallikrein varies in the same subject more than 10 unities per day, in respect to the maximum value found, a significant difference between the two groups exists (Fig. 2).

	CHANGES	NO CHANGES	
CONTROLS	8	37	45
INFARCTED SUBJECTS	22	23	45
	30	60	90

$$\chi^2 = \frac{N\left(|AD-BC| - N/2\right)^2}{(A+B)\,(C+D)\,(A+C)\,(B+D)} = 8,45 \qquad P < 0,01$$

Figure 2.   Daily Urinary Kallikrein of normal and infarcted patients. A distribution of the varying samples (changes > 10 kallikrein unities per day)

In conclusion, our previous findings demonstrate that during myocardial infarction, the plasmatic kininogen, prekallikrein and kallikrein inhibitor significantly decrease, and this is probably due to their consumption. This suggests that the kinin release has an important role in the pathogenesis of pain and shock following myocardial infarction.

Our present preliminary studies on urinary kallikrein do not give the same homogeneous results, and honestly we cannot tell if these variations of urinary kallikrein have an exact pathogenetical significance. It is not impossible to establish whether such oscillations are due to the influence of drugs, or whether they depend upon the disease: however, they do not seem to be correlated with the changes of the plasma kininogen, kallikreinogen, and kallikrein inhibitor, be it because the plasmatic and urinary modifications do not correspond as far as time intervals are concerned, be it because plasmatic kallikrein seems to be completely independent in origin and function from renal kallikrein.

SUMMARY

Kinin has been hypothesized to be involved in the mechanism of the precordialgia, collapse, and shock in myocardial infarction. In spontaneous and experimental animal infarction, the long-lasting lowering of plasma kininogen is perhaps the expression of kinin release from the plasma precursor. More recently, a durable reduction of plasma prekallikrein and of the plasma inhibitor of kallikrein, both evaluated with the kaolin contact method, has been demonstrated to support the implication of the kinin system in the course of myocardial infarction. In the present study, the daily urinary excretion of kallikrein, according to the Porcelli and Croxatto method, has been studied in a group of patients with acute myocardial infarction and in a group of control patients. Differences between the two groups have been observed. They consist mainly in strong daily oscillations in the amount of urinary kallikrein excretion during the 24 hour period in the group of patients with myocardial infaction. At this moment, however, it is not possible to give a definite interpretation of these results.

BIBLIOGRAPHY

1. Sicuteri F.: "La mediazione chimica del dolore coronarico" Mal. Cardiovasc., suppl. 2e, 37, 1964.

2. Sicuteri F., Franchi G., Del Bianco P.L., and Fanciullaci M.: "Some physiological and pathological roles of kininogen and kinin", in Proc. Int. Symp. "Hypotensive Peptides", Springer Verlag, ed., 525, 1966.

3. Sicuteri F., Franchi G., Del Bianco P.L., and Del Bene E.:
    "A contribution to the interpretation of shock and pain in
    myocardial infarction", Mal. Cardiovasc., 8, 3, 1967.

4. Sicuteri F., Del Bianco P.L., and Fanciullacci M.: "Kinins
    in the pathogenesis of cardiogenic shock and pain", Adv.
    Exp. Med. Biol., 9, 315, 1970.

5. Massion W.H., Blumel G., and Peschl L.: "The role of plasma
    kinin system in cardiogenic shock and related conditions",
    Proc. Int. Symp. "Proteases and Antiproteases in Cardio-
    angiology", Vietri Sul Mare, Italy 1969, F.K. Schattauer
    Verlag, Stuttgart, N.Y., 81, 1969.

6. Kimura E.: "Changes of Kinin system and hemodynamics in acute
    stage of myocardial infarction", Proc. Int. Symp. on "Trasylol
    and Experimental Myocardial Infarction", Dusseldorf, January,
    1975. (in press).

7. Sicuteri F., Antonini F.M., Del Bianco P.L., Franchi G.C.,
    and Curradi C.: "Prekallikrein and kallikrein inhibitor in
    plasma of patients affected by recent myocardial infarction",
    Adv. Exp. Med. Biol., 21, 445, 1972.

8. Porcelli G.: "Progress on urinary kallikrein tests". "Kinin
    75" Int. Symp., Florence, Italy, 1975. (in press).

RAISED PLASMA KININOGEN LEVELS IN RHEUMATOID PATIENTS - RESPONSE TO THERAPY WITH NONSTEROIDAL ANTI-INFLAMMATORY DRUGS

I. J. Zeitlin*, J.N. Sharma*, P.M. Brooks+ and W.C. Dick+

*Dept. of Pharmacology, University of Strathclyde, Glasgow

+Centre for Rheumatic Diseases, Royal Infirmary, Glasgow

In the aetiology of rheumatoid arthritis there is some evidence to implicate the formation of kinins in synovial fluid (Melmon, Webster, Goldfinger & Seegmiller, 1967; Keele & Eisen, 1970). The relationship between synovial kinin levels and clinical symptoms is, however, inconsistent (Keele & Eisen, 1970; Webster & Maling, 1970). In the systemic circulation no abnormalities in the kinin system have previously been described in this disease. We have recently reported some preliminary findings concerning changes in plasma kininogen levels in rheumatoid patients (Brooks, Dick, Sharma & Zeitlin, 1974; Zietlin, Sharma, Brooks & Dick, In Press). When patients with active rheumatoid arthritis received no treatment for 48 hours, their mean venous kininogen levels rose to more than twice the level found in eleven healthy volunteers or in five non-inflamed convalescent fracture patients. When the rheumatoid patients were put back on indomethacin therapy for one week, their mean plasma kininogen level fell to nearly half of the untreated value and lay within the healthy control range.

We have now examined the time course of the kininogen and plasma protein changes produced by indomethacin and report that aspirin produces similar changes. Some of these results were reported at the Symposium in Future Trends in Inflammation (Paris, 1975).

METHODS

Fifteen patients with seropositive rheumatoid arthritis (age range 26 - 74 years) consented to take part in the study. Four male and 8 female patients were involved in the indomethacin study,

335

6 female patients took part in the aspirin study.

At the start of each test, therapy was stopped for 48 hours and replaced by placebo indistinguishable from the drug to be used in the test. At the end of 48 hours of placebo, blood was sampled from an arm vein for the estimation of plasma kininogen, plasma proteins, PCV and plasma drug levels. Clinical assessment was carried out by a single blind observer. The activity of the disease was monitored by measuring joint diameter, grip strength, an articular index of joint tenderness produced by squeezing or manipulating some 26 joints and a pain index based on the patients own assessment on a 0 - 4 scale (Lee, Webb, Anderson & Buchanan, 1973; Ritchie, Boyle, McInnes, Jasani, Dalakos, Greiveson, Buchanan, 1973). The patients then commenced therapy with the test drug.

Six patients were given oral indomethacin, 50 mg thrice daily for seven days followed by one further day on placebo. In three of these patients and in an additional three the effect was determined of a single 50 mg dose of indomethacin on the biochemical parameters. A further six patients received 975 mg of enteric coated aspirin, four times a day for one week.

Plasma kininogen levels were measured using the method of Brocklehurst and Zeitlin (1967) involving ethanolic precipitation of the kininogen protein which was ultimately activated using trypsin. Bradykinin-like activity was assayed using the isolated oestrus rat uterus. Kininogen concentrations are stated as microgrammes bradykinin equivalent per ml. of plasma (µg Bk Eq per ml) giving mean and standard deviation.

Indomethacin was measured fluorimetrically after extraction from plasma (Emori, Champion, Bluestone, Paulus, 1973).

Plasma proteins were measured using cellulose acetate electrophoresis and scanning densitometry.

Statistical significance of differences was tested using the paired t-test and the Mann-Whitney 'U'-test for small numbers.

RESULTS

Plasma Kininogen Levels in Untreated Rheumatoids

In fifteen rheumatoid patients after 48 hours of placebo administration, the mean venous plasma kininogen concentration was 10.6 ± 1.7 µg Bk Eq per ml. This was almost twice ($P<0.01$) the mean control value found in seven healthy volunteers (5.6 ± 1.2 µg Bk Eq per ml).

Table 1: Sequential study of the effect of indomethacin on plasma kininogen and proteins in rheumatoid patients. The table shows the effect of placebo treatment for 48 hrs., followed by treatment for one week with oral indomethacin (50 mg thrice daily) and a final 24 hrs. on placebo. Statistical significance at P 0.05 and P 0.01 respectively of differences from placebo period is indicated by one and two stars. Two patients did not complete the trial.

Parameter	Placebo for 48 hrs.	After start of therapy			Placebo for 24 hrs.
		1 Hr	24 Hrs	1 Week	
Plasma Kininogen (μg Bk Eq/ml)	10.9 ± 1.0	7.0 ± 1.3 **	6.1 ± 0.8 **	5.9 ± 0.4	9.2 ± 1.3
Total Protein g%	7.9 ± 0.5	7.5 ± 0.9	7.5 ± 0.6 *	7.7 ± 0.6	7.6 ± 0.4
α_2-Globulin g%	0.9 ± 0.10	0.78 ± 0.08 **	0.73 ± 0.12 **	0.83 ± 0.17	0.98 ± 0.17
Albumin g%	3.8 ± 0.3	3.7 ± 0.3	3.7 ± 0.2	3.8 ± 0.2	3.7 ± 0.3
N	6	6	6	4	4

Effects of Indomethacin

By 1 hour after first taking indomethacin, the mean kininogen level had fallen to 65% of the placebo level (P < 0.01) (Table 1). After 24 hours the level had fallen only another 9% to 56% of the initial level. After 7 days of drug treatment, the indomethacin was once again replaced by placebo and a further 24 hours on placebo caused the mean plasma kininogen to rise again to 9.2 ± 1.3 µg Bk Eq per ml, some 64% above the level found in healthy volunteers.

The speed of the initial fall in plasma kininogen level was noteworthy and in a further study in 6 patients the mean kininogen level had fallen significantly (P < 0.05) by 10% only 15 minutes after taking the drug. By 30 minutes, the level had fallen by 34%. Throughout the study the mean haematocrit value was not significantly changed (P > 0.05). Table 1 also shows plasma protein levels in these patients. Albumin was unchanged throughout the 8 days regardless of the presence or absence of therapy. The mean total protein fell slightly during the test, but the maximum fall was only 6% at 24 hours following onset of therapy. The mean α_2-globulin level however, was greatly raised at 0.92 ± 0.10g per cent at the start of the test and fell by 15% (P < 0.01) one hour after ingesting indomethacin and had fallen maximally by 21% (P < 0.01) at 2 hrs.

Of the clinical parameters used to follow the severity of the disease, the joint diameter and grip strength were unaltered by the change from placebo to drug or back again. However, the two forms of pain assessment were dramatically altered by indomethacin therapy. Twenty four hours after starting therapy, both the articular index and the pain index had fallen in every patient, the mean values dropping to half the placebo levels. Twenty four hours after resumption of placebo, the values had returned in every case to their original high levels.

Effects of Aspirin

Table 2 shows plasma kininogen levels in six rheumatoid patients after placebo therapy for 48 hours and then one week after commencing aspirin therapy (975 mg 4 times daily). The plasma kininogen level fell in every case, the mean value falling by 31% (P < 0.001). The mean α_2-globulin level fell by 20% while no significant change occurred in the total protein or plasma albumin levels.

Table 3 shows the effect of aspirin on some clinical parameters in these patients. The change from placebo to aspirin

Table 2: Effect of aspirin on plasma proteins in 6 rheumatoid patients. Table shows means ± sd.

	Placebo 48 hrs.	Aspirin 1 week	Fall percent	P (Paired 't')
Kininogen (µg Bk Eq/ml)	9.2 ± 0.7	6.3 ± 0.8	31.5	<0.0005
Alpha-2 Globulin (G per cent)	0.82 ± 0.01	0.65 ± 0.16	20.4	<0.01
Total Protein (G per cent)	7.6 ± 0.5	7.5 ± 0.6	1.5	Not Sign.
Albumin (G per cent)	3.6 ± 0.3	3.4 ± 0.4	4.7	Not Sign.

Table 3: Effect of Aspirin on indices of disease activity in 6 rheumatoid patients. Table shows means ± sd.

		Placebo 48 hrs.	Aspirin 1 week	Percent change	P
Pain Score		3.7 ± 1.8	2.7 ± 1.5	-27.0	<0.05
Articular Index		21.8 ± 10.9	12.5 ± 4.5	-42.7	<0.05
Grip Strength (mm µg)	R	112 ± 48	118 ± 55	+ 5.4	NS
	L	105 ± 51	132 ± 49	+25.7	<0.01
Ring Size (mm)	R	275 ± 14	277 ± 19	+ 0.7	NS
	L	276 ± 17	272 ± 16	- 1.8	NS

therapy caused a marked reduction in both pain score and articular index and the change occurred more often than would be expected by chance (P < 0.05). Although the mean left hand grip strength had increased after 7 days of aspirin treatment (P < 0.01), neither ring size nor right hand grip strength had changed.

Like indomethacin, the aspirin exerted its action on the plasma kininogen level with remarkable rapidity following an oral dose. Figure (1) shows the plasma kininogen levels in three patients from the aspirin study one and two hours and 1 week after recommencing aspirin therapy. One hour after taking aspirin, the mean plasma kininogen level had fallen by 25%, after two hours the mean level had fallen only another 3%. After one week of aspirin the mean plasma kininogen level had fallen only another 5.6% to 65.6% of the initial raised value.

DISCUSSION

It has been suggested that the components of the kinin system present in synovial fluid are derived mainly from plasma (Jasani, Katori & Lewis, 1969). If this is true, then activation of the synovial kinin system, reported to occur in rheumatoid patients (Melmon et al., 1967; Keele & Eisen, 1970), should produce changes in systemic kininogen levels, possibly stimulating compensatory synthesis of kininogen.

When patients with active rheumatoid arthritis received placebo treatment for 48 hours in the present study, their mean venous plasma kininogen level rose to nearly twice the level in healthy subjects. When placebo was replaced by indomethacin or aspirin therapy, the mean plasma kininogen level fell by nearly half with the former drug and by about a third with the latter drug. The changes were remarkably rapid and commenced within minutes of ingesting the drugs. Our earlier studies showed that these changes are not simple methodological artefacts produced by the effects of the drugs on the kininogen assay (Zeitlin et al, in press). This is borne out by plasma protein measurements in the present study. Little or no change occurred in either total plasma protein or albumin. However, the α_2-globulin fraction of plasma contains kininogen, and in these patients was found to be influenced by the non-steroidal anti-inflammatory drugs in parallel with the changes in plasma kininogen.

Of the clinical indices which we have so far examined, the assessments of pain have so far proved to be the most sensitive to the changes from placebo to drug and back again, marked reduction in pain and a return to high levels of pain respectively occurring within 24 hours. Ferreira and his colleagues have shown that prostaglandins, with little pain-producing activity of their own,

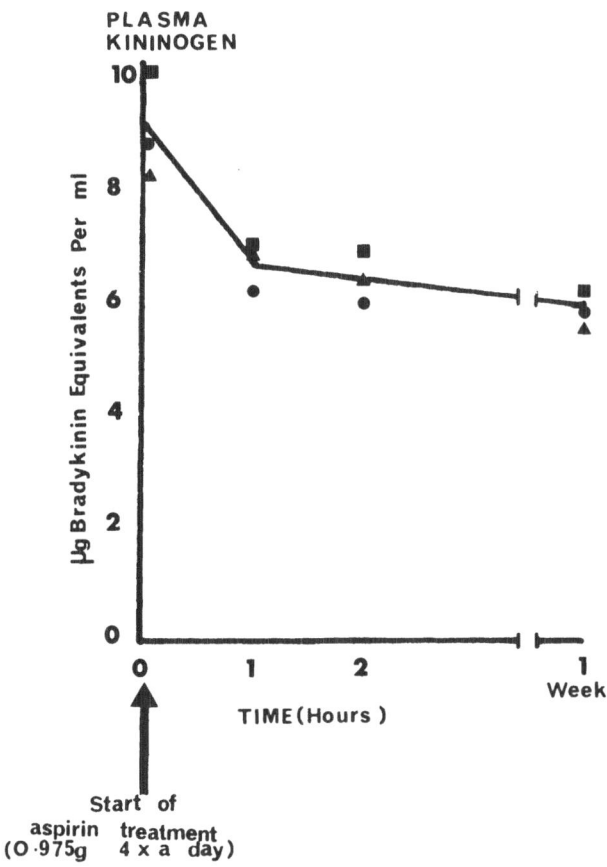

Fig. 1: The effect of aspirin on plasma kininogen in three rheumatoid patients.

powerfully potentiate the pain-producing ability of kinins (Ferreira & Vane, 1975).   Indomethacin and aspirin are both powerful inhibitors of prostaglandin synthesis (Vane, 1971).   The present studies indicate that in rheumatoid patients they are also capable of preventing the appearance of raised circulating levels of a kinin precursor in rheumatoid patients.

ACKNOWLEDGEMENTS

     The authors are grateful for support from Merck, Sharp & Dohme Ltd. P.M. Brooks is in receipt of an A.H. Robins Fellowship. Part of this research was supported by an MRC project research grant to I.J. Zeitlin. We wish to thank Sandoz Ltd. for a generous gift of synthetic bradykinin. Kininogen studies were carried out by J.N. Sharma in part fulfillment of requirements for Ph.D.

REFERENCES

Brocklehurst, W.E.; Zeitlin, I.J.; 1967: Determination of plasma kinin and kininogen levels in man. J. Physiol. (Lond), 1919, 417.

Brooks, P.M.; Dick, W.C.; Sharma, J.N.; Zeitlin, I.J., 1974; Changes in plasma kininogen levels associated with rheumatoid activity, Br. J. Clin. Pharmac., 1, 315P.

Emori, H.W.; Champion, G.D.; Bluestone, R.; Paulus, H.E., 1973; Simultaneous pharmacokinetics of indomethacin in serum and synovial fluid. Ann. Rheum. Dis., 32, 433.

Ferreira, S.H.; Vane, J.R.; 1975. Inhibition of prostaglandin biosynthesis and the mechanism of action on non-steriodal anti-inflammatory agents. In: "Future Trends in Inflammation:. Eds. G.P. Velp; D.A. Willoughby; J.P. Giroud P. 171, Piccin Medical Books.

Jasani, M.K.; Katori, M; Lewis, G.P.; 1969; Intracellular enzymes and kinin enzymes in synovial fluid in joint diseases. Ann. Rheum. Dis. 28, 497.

Keele, C.A.; Eisen, V. 1970: Plasma kinin formation in rheumatoid arthritis. In: "Bradykinin and related kinins" (Eds. F. Sicuteri, Rocha e Silva, N. Back) p. 471, Plenum, New York.

Lee, P.; Webb, J.; Anderson, J; Buchanan, W.W.; 1973; Method for assessing therapeutic potential of anti-inflammatory anti-rheumatic drugs in rheumatoid arthritis. Br. med. J., 2, 685.

Melmon, K.L.; Webster, M.E.; Godfinger, S.E.; Seegmiller, J.E., 1967: Presence of a kinin in inflammatory synovial effusion from arthritides of varying aetiologies. Arth. Rheum., 10, 13.

Ritchie, D.M.; Boyle, J.A.; McInnes, J.M.; Jasani, M.K.; Dalakos, T.G.; Grieveson, P.; Buchanan, W.W.; 1973: Clinical studies with an articular index for the assessment of joint tenderness in patients with rheumatoid arthritis. Q. J. Med., 37(NS., 393)

Vane, J.R.; 1971: Inhibition of prostaglandin synthesis as a mechanism of action for aspirin-like drugs. Nature New Biol., 231, 232.

Webster, M.E.; Maling, H.M.; 1970: Evidence for and against the kinins as endogenous mediators of arthritis. In: "Bradykinin and related kinins" (Eds. F. Sicuteri: M. Rocha e Silva: N. Back) p. 493, Plenum: New York.

Zeitlin, I.J.; Sharma, J.N.; Brooks, P.M.; Dick, W.C.: In Press. An effect of indomethacin on raised plasma kininogen levels in rheumatoid patients. In: "Chemistry and Biology of the Kallikrein-Kinin System." (Eds: J.J. Pisano & K.F. Austen) U.S. Govt. Printing Office: Washington.

THE CLEAVAGE OF A METHIONYL-LYSYL-BRADYKININ-LIKE PEPTIDE FROM

KININOGEN BY A PROTEASE OF HUMAN NEUTROPHIL LEUKOCYTE LYSOSOMES*

Henry Z. Movat**, Flavio M. Habal*** and David R.L. Macmorine

Division of Experimental Pathology, Department of Pathology, and Institute of Immunology, University of Toronto, Medical Sciences Building, Toronto, Ontario M5S 1A8, Canada

Polymorphonuclear (PMN) leukocytes are essential for the tissue and vascular injury associated with formation and deposition of antigen-antibody complexes (1). There are several mechanisms by which phlogistic agents derived from PMN-leukocyte lysosomes may act. Some act directly, other indirectly by generating vaso-active substances from certain protein substrates. Rabbit leuko-cytes contain cationic proteins which can act directly on the micro-circulation or by releasing vasoactive amines from mast cells (2). These same cells contain acid cathepsins which can generate "leuko-kinins" from "leukokininogen" at acid pH (3). The acid protease can degrade also basement membrane (4). Basement membrane, elastin and cartilage matrix can be degraded also by a protease of human PMN-leukocytes at neutral pH (5), and collagen by a collagenase (6). By acting on the 3rd and 5th component complement lysates of human PMN-leukocytes can cleave anaphylatoxin-like substances (7, 8). Our own studies indicate that lysates of PMN-leukocyte lysosomes contain a protease capable of cleaving a kinin-like peptide from highly purified kininogen (9). The enzymes were obtained either by fractionating cell lysates or by interacting the cells with antigen-antibody complexes. In the latter case the hydrolases were released into the ambient fluid, and in the

* The studies reported in this paper were supported by the Medical Research Council of Canada (MT-1251), the Ontario Heart Foundation and the J.P. Bickell Foundation.
** Holder of an Associateship of the Medical Research Council of Canada.
*** Postdoctoral Fellow supported by the Ontario Heart Foundation.

cell pellet the phagocytosing and degranulating cells were identified ultrastructurally as neutrophil leukocytes. Subsequently,
the enzyme was obtained in partially purified form (10) and in a
brief communication we reported on the properties of the highly
purified protease with kininogenase activity (11), concluding
that it is probably the same protease which degrades elastin,
basement membrane and cartilage proteoglycan (5).

This publication deals with the physico-chemical and biological properties of the highly purified enzyme and with the nature
of peptide generated from kininogen.

Materials and Methods

Granulocytes were isolated from ACD-plasma as described
before (9). Up to 4 units (2000 ml) of blood was processed in
one experiment. The leukocytes were adjusted to 2×10^8 cells
per ml and incubated in Tyrode-gelatin (0.1% gelatin) for 30 minutes
with an equal volume of antigen-antibody precipitates (bovine serum
albumin - rabbit anti-bovine serum albumin; 0.25 mg antibody N per
ml). To enhance enzyme release 10 μg/ml cytochalasin B was added
to the reaction mixture (9).

Kininogens were prepared as described in detail before (12)
with minor modifications (13).

The lysosomal lysate was fractionated on SP-Sephadex C-50
as outlined elsewhere (14), except that the equilibrating buffer
contained 0.2 M NaCl and the protease was eluted by increasing
the NaCl concentration stepwise as shown in Figure 1. Active
pools from several runs were passed through a 5 x 90 cm column of
Sephadex G-75 equilibrated with 0.1 M phosphate buffer, pH 6.0,
containing 0.15 M NaCl. Fractions with kininogenase and alanine
esterase activity were pooled, concentrated and passed once more
through an SP-Sephadex column. The buffer was 0.1 M phosphate
(pH 6.0) and elution was carried out with a gradient between
0.25 and 0.4 M NaCl.

Various analytical and other procedures were done as described
in the literature: cationic disc gel electrophoresis (15), disc
gel electrophoresis in SDS or sodium dodecyl sulfate (16), gel
filtration through Sepharose 6B in 5.0 M guanidine HCl (17),
sucrose density gradient ultracentrifugation (18), isoelectric
focusing (19), bioassay of kinin on the estrous rat uterus (12,19),
caseinolysis (20), hemoglobinolysis (21), esterolysis (22), and
assays for β-glucuronidase (23) and lactic dehydrogenase (24).

Antibody was produced in rabbits against the highly purified
protease.

Results and Discussion

The data presented in Table 1 show that incubation of leukocytes with buffer for one hour releases no kinin-generating activity and lysosomal hydrolases or the cytoplasmic marker lactic
dehydrogenase (LDH). However, incubation with immune precipitates
is associated with release of β-glucuronidase, neutral protease
(hemoglobinase) and kinin-forming activity, but there is no leakage
of the cytoplasmic marker LDH. When the cells are lysed all enzymes are demonstrable, including LDH. However, there is less
kinin-generating activity than in the samples in which the cells
were incubated with the immune complexes. As shown before (9)
this is due to a kinin inactivating enzyme in the cell sap.
This kininase is detectable in the 16,000 g supernatant. When
the cells were disrupted in sucrose and fractionated as described
before (9), most of the hydrolytic and kinin-forming activity
was in the granule or lysosomal fraction, whereas the cytoplasmic
marker LDH was recovered in the 16,000 g supernatant. Upon
incubation with cytochalasin B the release of hydrolases and of
kinin-generating activity was almost doubled.

The lysosomal lysate was subjected to cation exchange chromatography on SP-Sephadex. As shown in Figure 1 most of the kinin-
cleaving and alanine esterase activity bound firmly to the strong
cation exchanger, eluting with high concentrations of NaCl.
Upon gel filtration through Sephadex G-75 the kinin-forming,
caseinolytic and esterolytic activities eluted in an overlapping
peak, with the approximate void volume of soy bean trypsin inhibitor (10, 11). Further purification by rechromatography on SP-
Sephadex yielded an enzyme consisting of five bands by cationic
disc gel electrophoresis (Fig. 2). When the enzyme was eluted
with a very shallow gradient the bands migrating slowest towards
the cathode eluted first and those migrating fastest eluted last,
indicating a charge heterogeneity (11, 25). The charge heterogeneity could be demonstrated also by isoelectric focusing, a
crude enzyme preparation focusing between pH 6.0 and 11.5 and
the highly purified protease between 10 and 11.8. Despite this
heterogeneity the enzyme behaved as a homogeneous protein by SDS-
disc gel electrophoresis, gel filtration in aqueous buffer or in
the dissociating agent guanidine HCl, by ultracentrifugation (2.7S)
and by immunoelectrophoresis.

The discrepancy between some findings indicating heterogeneity
and other data suggesting homogeneity was solved by the method of
Hedrick and Smith (26), which distinguishes between size isomers,
charge isomers and unrelated proteins. As shown in Figure 3 when
charge isomers are subjected to electrophoresis in gels of increasing acrylamide concentrations a family of parallel lines is
obtained when gel concentration versus relative mobility is plotted.
Size isomeric proteins converge and unrelated proteins intersect.

H.Z. MOVAT, F.M. HABAL, AND D.R.L. MACMORINE

Table 1. Kinin-forming, hydrolase and lactic dehydrogenase activity of PMN-leukocyte fractions and of material released upon interaction of leukocytes and antigen-antibody precipitates

Sample	β-glucuronidase μg phenolphthalein/ hr/ml/sample	Protease μg acid soluble tyrosine-like material/hr/ml sample	Kinin μg/ml sample	Lactic dehydrogenase units/ml/sample
Cells + Ag-Ab	135	135	1.3	35
Cells + Tyrode	17	21	0	19
Cell lysate	362	188	0.68	5150
400g pellet	79	153	0.57	370
16,000g pellet	207	172	1.1	126
16,000g supernatant	55	19	0	5510

The final concentration of PMN-leukocytes was 10^8 ml. In the kinin assay 0.1 ml kininogen (2.05 mg protein) was incubated at 37° for 1 hour with 0.1 ml of the various samples and the reaction stopped by immersing the tubes for 10 minutes in boiling water. After dilution with de Jalon solution the reaction mixtures were tested on the estrous rat uterus standardized with synthetic bradykinin.

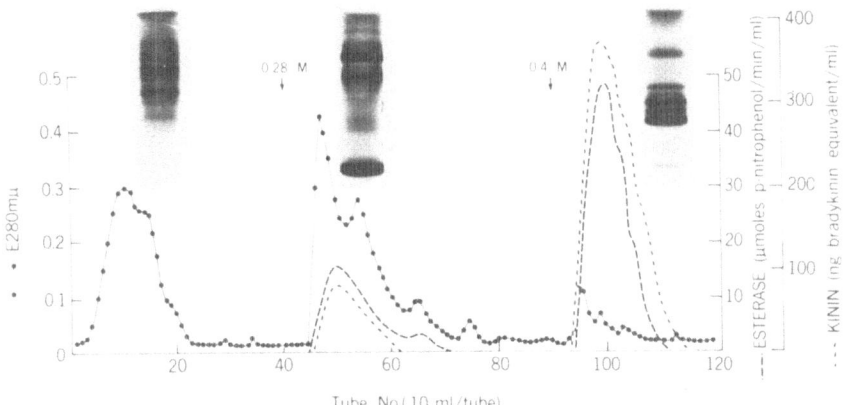

Figure 1. Cation exchange chromatography of 17.5 ml a lysosomal lysate (O.D. 280:118) of human neutrophil leukocytes on a 2.5 x 12 cm column of SP-Sephadex A-50. The lysate was dialysed against 0.01 M phosphate buffer, pH 6.0, containing 0.2 M NaCl. After elution of the excluded peak the NaCl concentration was raised to 0.28 M and then to 0.4 M. The latter eluted the bulk of the kinin-forming and alanine esterase activity.

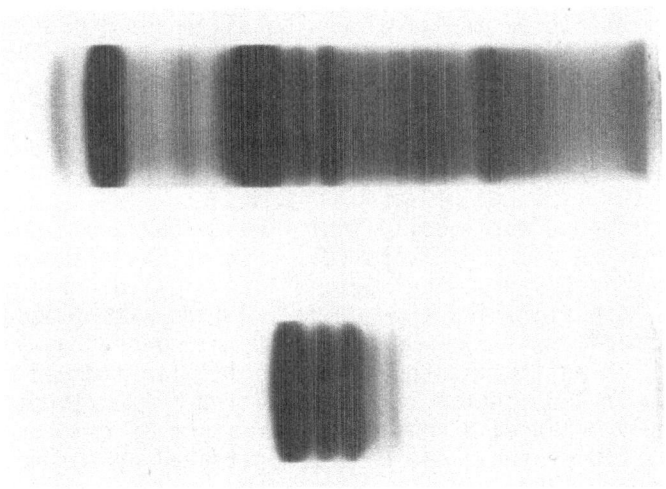

Figure 2. Cationic disc gel electrophoresis of lysosomal lysate (top) and of the purified neutral protease consisting of five bands (bottom). Cathode is to the left.

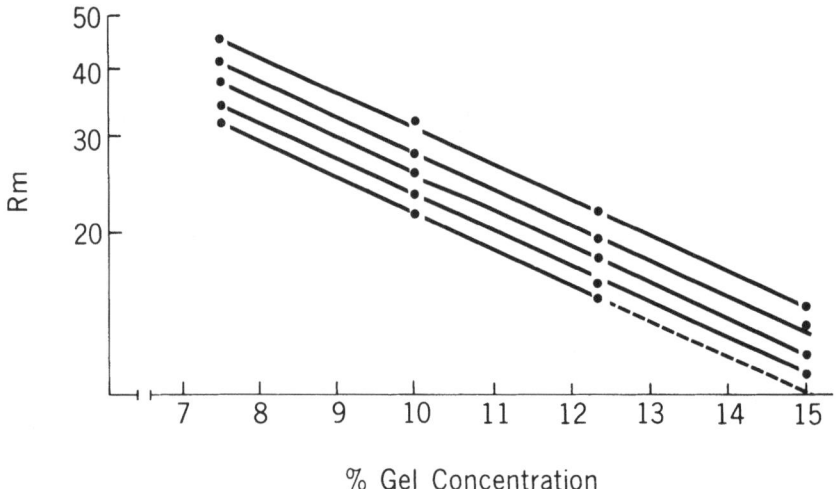

Figure 3. Plot of relative mobility of the five isozymes (similar to those shown in Figure 2) against gel concentration.

The molecular weight of the kininogenase was determined by SDS-disc gel electrophoresis and gel filtration in guanidine-Sepharose. However, in these dissociating agents the protease tended to undergo autolysis. In order to obtain accurate data the enzyme had to be inactivated with diisopropyl-fluorophosphate (DFP, 10^{-3}M). To be able to detect the inactivated protease during gel filtration in the presence of guanidine it was trace labelled with I^{125} (27). The molecular weight estimated by SDS acrylamide electrophoresis was about 27,000 and by gel filtration 28,000, both reduced and unreduced (Fig. 4).

The protease was readily inhibited by DFP and a number of chloromethyl ketone inhibitors (25). It has been shown that certain peptide chloromethyl ketones inhibit leukocyte elastase (5, 28). More significant were the findings with plasma proteinase inhibitors (25). Depending on the concentration of the inhibitor, α_1-antitrypsin and α_2-macroglobulin induced maximum inhibition in 1-5 minutes. The inhibition by antithrombin III was markedly enhanced by heparin. Formation of complexes between inhibitors and protease could be demonstrated by immunoelectrophoresis (Fig. 5).

Cleavage of kinin from kininogen at 37° occurred very rapidly (Fig. 6). The product of enzyme-substrate interaction, the peptide, was assayed on the estrous rat uterus. The contractions were not

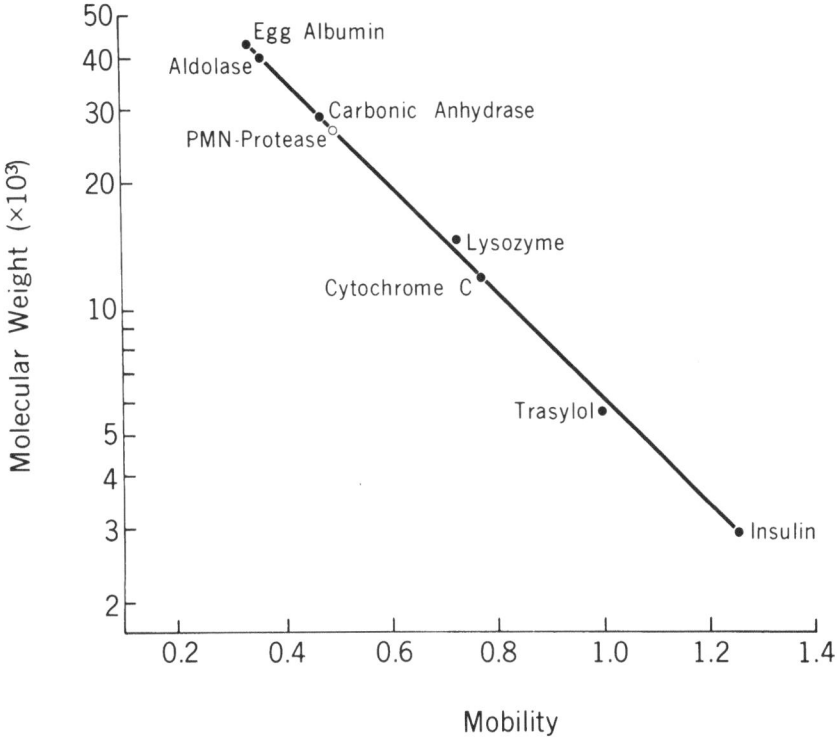

Figure 4. SDS disc gel electrophoresis. Plot of electrophoretic
mobility against molecular weight of PMN-protease and of marker
proteins.

inhibited by atropine or methysergide, but preincubation for 10
minutes with carboxypeptidase B (25 ng) completely inhibited the
contractions. Repeated applications of the spasmogen (within the
dose response range) caused no tachyphylaxis. To isolate the
peptide, partially purified kininogen (40 µg bradykinin equivalents)
and 10 ml lysosomal lysate were dialysed for 4 hours against 0.02M
ammonium formate, adjusted to pH 7.4 with ammonium hydroxide.
The two reactants were then incubated at 37° for 10 minutes; then
the pH was adjusted to 4.8 with formic acid and the tube immersed
for 10 minutes in boiling water. After centrifugation the supernatant was adjusted with distilled water to the conductivity of
0.02 M formate-formic acid, pH 4.8 and aliquots of 5-10 ml
applied to a CM-cellulose column equilibrated with the formate
buffer, pH 4.8, according to Habermann and Blennemann (29). After
washing with the equilibrating buffer and with 0.08 M formate,
the peptides were eluted with a linear gradient between 0.08 and

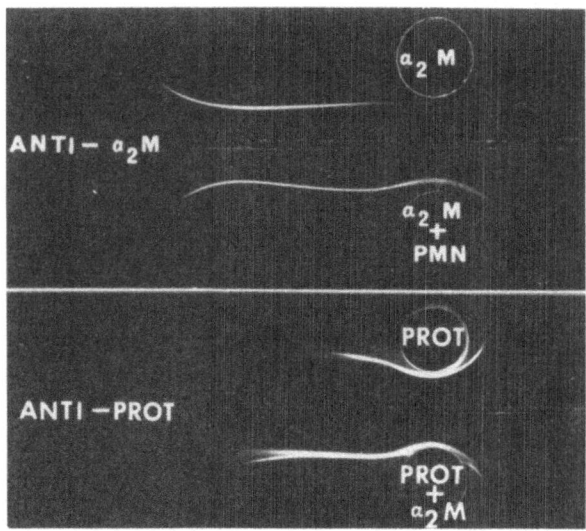

Figure 5.   Immunoelectrophoresis of α_2-macroglobulin (α_2M) and of
α_2-macroglobulin mixed with a PMN-lysosomal lysate (PMN), developed with antibody against the inhibitor.   Immunoelectrophoresis
of the isolated protease (PROT) and of the protease mixed with α_2-
macroglobulin, developed with antibody against the protease.

0.22 M formate.   Similar experiments were done by incubating the
kininogen and the crude protease in the presence of 10^{-4} M zinc
chloride or by incubating kininogen with highly purified protease.
Synthetic kinins were chromatographed on CM-cellulose columns
packed to the same height and with the same pressure head.   Two
columns were used, 1.5 x 15 and 1.4 x 8 cm respectively.   In
accordance with the data reported by Habermann and Blennemann (29)
the synthetic kinins eluted with a definite buffer concentration
as shown in Figure 7 (top).   Also in keeping with the findings
of these authors each kinin eluted slightly earlier with the smaller
column.   When the product of kininogen-crude enzyme preparation
was chromatographed most of the activity eluted in the position
of bradykinin (Fig. 7, bottom).   It is known that lysosomal lysates
contain an aminopeptidase (30).   Aminopeptidases cleave the lysine-
argine bond of meth-lys-bradykinin or lys-bradykinin (31).   This
is the most plausible explanation of the findings obtained with
the crude enzyme preparation, which yielded mainly a bradykinin-
like peptide.   When the aminopeptidase is blocked with salts of
heavy metals (32), or a purified kininogenase free of aminopepti-

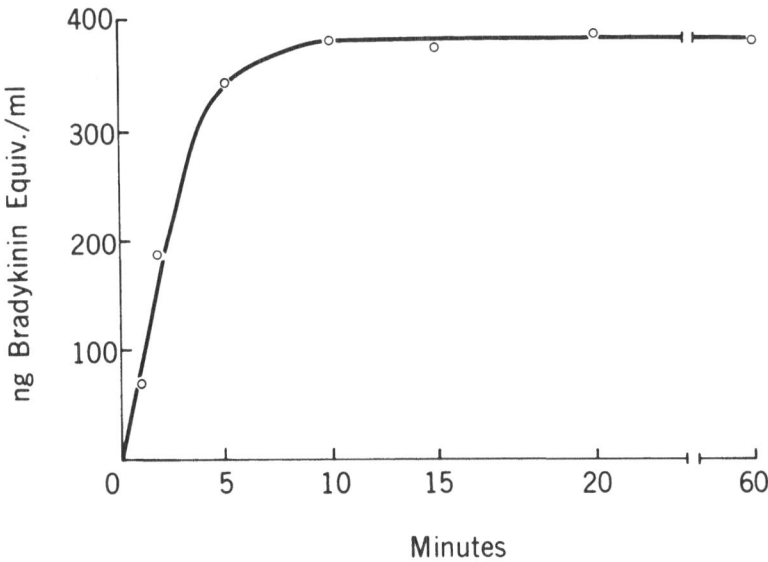

<u>Figure 6</u>. Time course of kinin-generation from HMW-kininogen
by the purified neutrophil protease (see text).

dase is used, a different peptide was generated. The peak shown
in Figure 7 bottom was pooled, concentrated by lyophilization and
1.0 ml applied to two interconnected columns (1.6 x 80 and 1.6 x
92 cm) of Sephadex G-15. The activity eluted with an elution
volume just slightly ahead of meth-lys-bradykinin (Fig. 8). Some
of the pharmacological characteristics (33) were similar, but not
identical to meth-lys-bradykinin. Assuming that trypsin converts
larger kinins to bradykinin, the material eluted from Sephadex
G-15 was treated with trypsin (50μg) and the trypsin inactivated
with excess lima bean trypsin inhibitor (100 μg). Comparing
the activity of the untreated and trypsinized preparations it was
found that when tested on the rat uterus the activity increased
4-5 fold after trypsinization, on the rat duodenum about 2 fold
and on the guinea pig ileum 10-15 fold. The effect of trypsinization was very rapid (Fig. 9). Trypsin incubated with lima bean
trypsin inhibitor did not induce contraction.

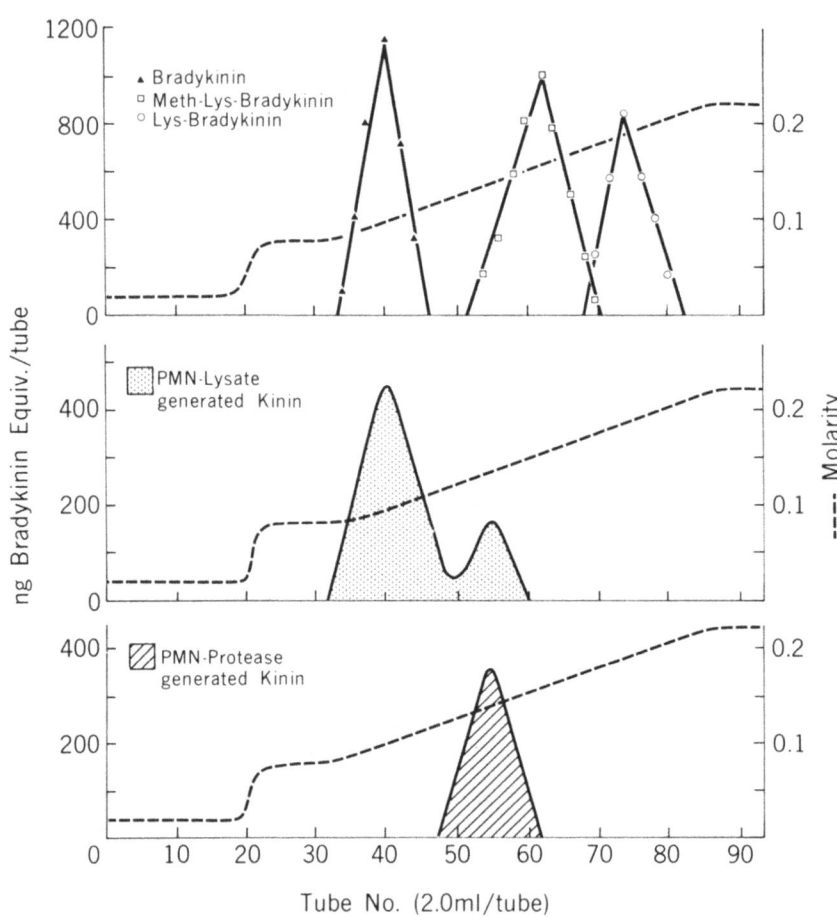

<u>Figure 7.</u> Chromatography of kinins on a 1.4 x 8 cm column of
CM-Sephadex equilibrated with 0.02 M formic acid-ammonium formate,
pH 4.8. The upper panel shows the elution pattern of synthetic
kinins, the middle panel that of the peptides generated by
incubating kininogen with a neutrophil leukocyte lysosomal lysate
and the lower panel the peptide formed when the kininogen is
incubated with the purified protease.

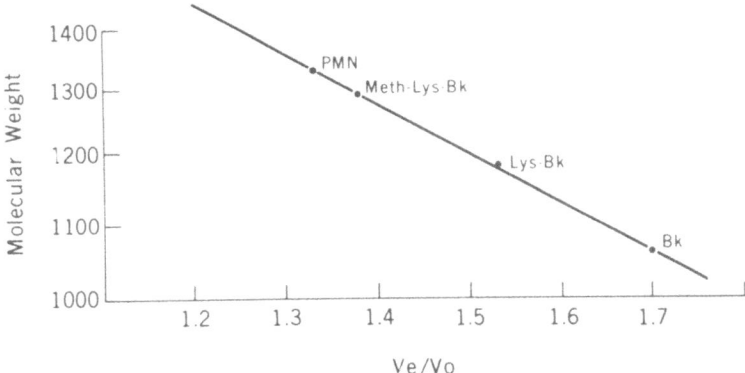

Figure 8. Gel filtration of the protease-generated kinin (Fig. 7, bottom) on two columns (1.6 x 80 and 1.6 x 92 cm) of Sephadex G-15 equilibrated with 0.2 M formate buffer, pH 4.0. The column was calibrated with synthetic kinins.

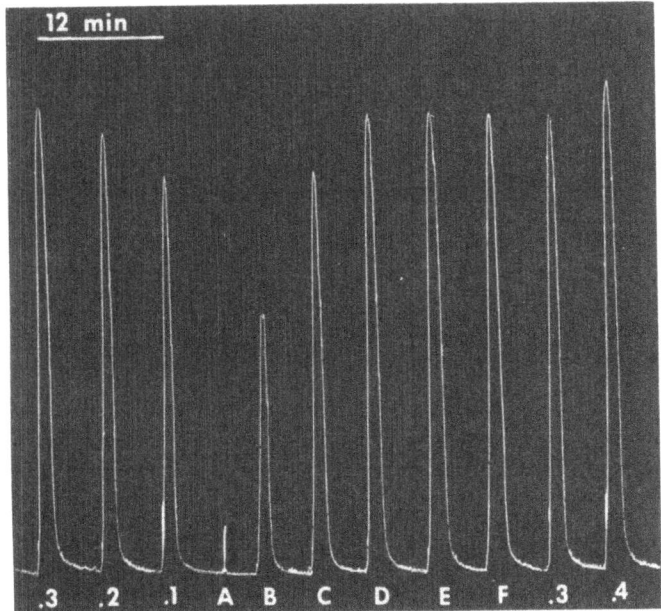

Figure 9. Kymograph tracing of estrous rat uterus. Numerals represent nanograms per ml of bradykinin applied to the bath. At A untreated sample obtained by Sephadex G-15 (Fig. 8) was applied to the bath. Samples were treated with trypsin; the trypsin neutralized with lima bean trypsin inhibitor and then applied to the bath. B-F represent samples trypsinized for 30 seconds, 1,2,4 and 8 minutes.

Concluding Remarks

Human neutrophil leukocytes contain a protease with kininogenase and alanine esterase activity. The enzyme consists of at
least 5 charge isomers, whose isoelectric point ranges between
pH 10 and 11.8. The molecular weight is about 27,000-28,000.
The enzyme cleaves kinin rapidly from kininogen at neutral pH.
The kinin has physico-chemical and pharmacological properties
similar to, but not identical to meth-lys-bradykinin.

Acknowledgements

The authors wish to thank Dr. D.M. Wrobel and Mrs. I. Macdonald
of the Canadian Red Cross for generous supplies of blood and plasma.
The skillful technical and secretarial assistance of Mrs. Otti
Freitag, Mrs. Anneliese Carre and Ms. Marica Michael are gratefully
acknowledged.

References

1. Movat, H.Z.: Allergic inflammation: The sequelae of antigen-
    antibody formation. Symposium on Pathways to Inflammation.
    Fed. Proc. 35, in press.

2. Ranadive, N.S. and Cochrane, C.G.: Isolation and characteri-
    zation of permeability factors from rabbit neutrophils.
    J. Exp. Med. 128: 605, 1968.

3. Greenbaum, L.M., Pakash, A., Semente, G. and Johnson, M.: The
    leukokinin system: its role in fluid accumulation in malig-
    nancy and inflammation. Agents and Actions 3: 332, 1973.

4. Cochrane, C.G. and Aikin, B.S.: Polymorphonuclear leukocytes in
    immunologic reactions: The destruction of basement membrane
    in vivo and in vitro. J. Exp. Med. 124: 733, 1966.

5. Janoff, A.: Human granulocyte elastase. Am. J. Path. 68:
    579, 1972.

6. Lazarus, G.S., Daniels, J.R. and Lian, J.: Granulocyte
    collagenase. Mechanism of collagen degradation. Am. J. Path.
    68: 565, 1972.

7. Taubman, S.G., Goldschmidt, P.R. and Lepow, I.H.: Effect of
    lysosomal enzymes from human leukocytes on human complement
    components. Fed. Proc. 29: 434, 1970.

8. Goldstein, I.M. and Weissmann, G.: Generation of C5-derived
    lysosomal enzyme releasing activity (C5a) by lysates of
    leukocyte lysosomes. J. Immunol. 113: 1583, 1974.

9. Movat, H.Z., Steinberg, S.G., Habal, F.M. and Ranadive, N.S.:
    Demonstration of a kinin-generating enzyme in the lysosomes
    of human polymorphonuclear leukocytes. Lab. Invest. 29: 669,
    1973.

10. Movat, H.Z.: Release of a kinin-forming enzyme from human
    polymorphonuclear leukocytes following interaction with
    immune complexes. In: Allergology, Proceedings of the VIII
    International Congress of Allergology, Yamamura, Y., ed.,
    Excerpta Medica, Amsterdam, 1974.

11. Movat, H.Z. and Habal, F.M.: Kininogenases of PMN-leukocyte
    lysosomes. In: Chemistry and Biology of the Kallikrein-Kinin
    System in Health and Disease. Pisano, J.J. and Austen, K.F.,
    eds., Fogarty Internat. Center Proc. No. 27, U.S. Gov. Printing
    Office, Washington, 1975.

12. Habal, F.M., Movat, H.Z. and Burrowes, C.E.: Isolation of two
    functionally different kininogens from human plasma. Separa-
    tion from proteinase inhibitors and interaction with plasma
    kallikrein. Biochem. Pharmacol. 23: 2291, 1974.

13. Habal, F.M. and Movat, H.Z.: Some physicocehmical and functional
    differences between low and high molecular weight kininogens
    of human plasma. In: Chemistry and Biology of the Kallikrein-
    Kinin System in Health and Disease. Pisano, J.J. and Austen,
    K.F., eds., Fogarty Internat. Center Proc. No. 27, U.S. Gov.
    Printing Office, Washington, 1975.

14. Movat, H.Z., Soltay, M.J., Fuller, P.J. and Ozge-Anwar, A.H.:
    The relationship between the plasma kinin system and the
    contact phase of blood coagulation in man. In: Vasopeptides,
    Chemistry, Pharmacology and Pathophysiology, Back, N. and
    Sicuteri, F., eds., Plenum Press, New York, 1972.

15. Reisfeld, R., Lewis, U. and Williams, D.: Disc gel electro-
    phoresis of basic proteins and peptides on polyacrylamide
    gels. Nature 195: 281, 1962.

16. Weber, K. and Osborn, M.: The reliability of molecular weight
    determination by dodecyl sulfate-polyacrylamide gel electro-
    phoresis. J. Biol. Chem. 244: 4406, 1969.

17. Fish, W.W., Mann, K. and Tanford, C.: The estimation of poly-
    peptide chain molecular weights by gel filtration in 6 M
    guanidine hydrochloride. J. Biol. Chem. 244: 4989, 1969.

18. Martin, R.G. and Ames, B.N.: A method for determining the
    sedimentation behaviour of enzymes: Application to protein
    mixtures. J. Biol. Chem. 236: 1372, 1961.

19. Movat, H.Z., Poon, M.-C. and Takeuchi, Y.: The kinin system
    of human plasma. I. Isolation of a low molecular weight
    activator of prekallikrein. Int. Arch. Allergy 40: 89, 1971.

20. Abiko, Y., Iwamoto, M., and Shimizu, M.: Plasminogen-plasmin
    system. I. Purification and properties of human plasminogen.
    J. Biochem. 64: 743, 1968.

21. Wasi, S., Murray, R.K., Macmorine, D.R.L. and Movat, H.Z.:
    The role of PMN-leukocyte lysosomes in tissue injury and
    inflammation. II. Studies on the proteolytic activity of PMN-
    leukocyte lysosomes of the rabbit. Brit. J. Exp. Path. 47:
    411, 1966.

22. Janoff, A.: Alanine p-nitrophenol elastase activity of human
    leucocyte granules. Biochem. J. 114: 157, 1969.

23. Fishman, W.H.: β-glucuronidase. In: Methods of Enzymatic
    Analysis, H.U. Bergmeyer, ed., Academic Press, New York, 1963.

24. Bergmeyer, H.U., Brent, E. and Hess, B.: Lactic dehydrogenase.
    In: Methods of Enzymatic Analysis, H.U. Bergmeyer, ed.,
    Academic Press, New York, 1963.

25. Movat, H.Z., Habal, F.M. and Macmorine, D.R.L.: The generation
    of a vasoactive peptide from kininogen by a protease of human
    neutrophil leukocyte lysosomes. Agents and Actions, in press.

26. Hedrick, J.L. and Smith, A.J.: Size and charge isomer separa-
    tion and estimation of molecular weights of proteins by disc
    gel electrophoresis. Arch. Biochem. Biophys. 126: 155, 1968.

27. Freeman, T.: Trace labelling with radioiodine. In: Handbook
    of Experimental Immunology, D.M. Weir, ed., Blackwell,
    Oxford, 1967.

28. Tuhy, P.M. and Powers, J.C.: Inhibition of human elastase
    by peptide chloromethyl ketones. FEBS Letters 50: 359, 1975.

29. Habermann, E. and Blennemann, G.: Uber Substrate und Reaktion-
    sprodukte der kininbildenden Enzyme Trypsin, Serum-und
    Pankreaskallikrein sowie von Crotalusgift. Naunyn-Schmied.
    Arch. Exp. Path. Pharm. 249: 357, 1964.

30. Folds, J.D., Welsh, I.R.H. and Spitznagel, J.K.: Neutral proteases confined to one class of lysosomes of human poly-morphonuclear leukocytes. Proc. Soc. Exp. Biol. Med. 139: 461, 1972.

31. Erdos, E.G., Nakajima, T., Oshima, G., Gecse, A. and Kato, J.: Kininases and their interactions with other systems, In: Chemistry and Biology of the Kallikrein-Kinin System in Health and Disease, Pisano, J.J. and Austen, K.F., eds., Fogarty Internat. Center Proc. No. 27, U.S. Gov. Printing Office, Washington, 1975.

32. Behal, F. and Folds, J.D.: Acrylamidase of neisseria cataralis. Arch. Biochem. Biophys. 121: 364, 1967.

33. Reiss, M.L., Okino, L. and Rocha e Silva, M.: Comparative pharmacological actions of bradykinin and related kinins of larger molecular weights. Biochem. Pharmacol. 20: 2935, 1971.

THE EFFECT OF WATER, SODIUM OVERLOADING AND DIURETICS UPON
URINARY KALLIKREIN

Croxatto, H.R., Huidobro, F., Rojas, M., Roblero, J.
and R. Albertini

Laboratorio de Fisiologia, Instituto de Ciencias
Biologicas, Universidad Catolica de Chile, Casilla
114-D, Santiago, Chile

Urinary kallikrein is significantly decreased in different
types of experimental (Croxatto and San Martin, 1970; Margolius
et al., 1972), clinical (Margolius,et al., 1972; Adetuyibi and
Mills, 1972; Greco et al., 1974) and spontaneous hypertension
(Porcelli et al., 1975). In contrast to the numerous reports
dealing with alterations in kallikrein excretion, there is still
meager information concerning the physiological role of the
kallikrein-kinin system in the kidney. Although renal kallikrein
appear to be directly related to sodium excretion (Marin-Grez and
Carretero, 1972; Adetuyibi and Mills, 1972), other data have been
published suggesting that not Na, but mineralocorticoids are the
primary factor regulating kallikrein excretion (Geller et al.,
1972; Pisano et al., 1974; Margolius,et al., 1974). Other
results indicate a functional relationship between kallikrein
and water excretion (Mills and Ward, 1975). In addition it has
been proposed that renal kallikrein, acting either locally in the
kidney (Pisano et al., 1974), and/or systemically (Croxatto, 1972
a,b) can be part of the vasodilator system.

Regarding the physiological role of the urinary kallikrein,
there is now strong evidence that the urinary enzyme is immunolo-
gically (Garcia et al., 1973) and biochemically indistinguishable
from renal kallikrein (Nustad and Pierce, 1975).

In order to obtain more information about the renal kallikrein-kinin system, experiments were designed to investigate kallikrein responses when the kidney excretory function is acutely
stimulated. This paper describes the effects of water, NaCl overloading, and of diuretic such as furosemide and acetazoleamide.

In uniform groups of rats, the excretory rate of kallikrein, water, sodium, and potassium were measured every 30 minutes for 2, 3 hours, immediately after gavage. In addition, at the end of some experiments in which the effects of furosemide were investigated the total amount of kallikrein in the kidneys was measured. The renal kallikrein values were compared to the total kallikrein excreted in the urine.

METHODS

Normal adult female rats (200-220 g b.w.) fed with a stock diet containing 0.03% NaCl were used. Food, but not water, was withheld for 14 h prior to the study. On the day of the experiment a group of 12 rats were placed in individual metabolic cages and submitted to double overloading as described previously (Rosas et al., 1962). This method provides regular diuresis in the period following the second overloading. In the beginning, all animals, excluding the normal hydrated control rats, received via a stomach tube a solution of 1 0/00 NaCl. Its volume was 2.5% of b.w. After 60 min a second hydration was performed giving either tap water or 2% NaCl solution according to the experimental procedure. In either case, the volume of the second load was 5% b.w. Diuretics were dissolved in saline and injected subcutaneously, at the same time of the second loading. The controls were injected with saline. In each protocol from the 12 rats, 6 were used as controls. The same rats were rarely used in more than one experiment.

Kallikrein, Na and K determinations (flame photometer) were carried out in the urine collected after both loads, but since the urine of the first period were found to have no conspicous differences between experimental and control groups, this paper deals only with the data obtained in the urine excreted after the second load. Kidney removal was carried out under bromethone anesthesia. The animals were bled by placing a polyethylene catheter in the carotid artery.

The following experiments were performed:

a) Effects of hyperhydration with tap water. Normal hydrated rats were used as controls. The experimental rats were double overloaded as described, and 1 hour after the first load, tap water was given by gavage. Urine was collected for 3 hours. 8 groups of 12 rats were included in the statistical analysis.

b) Effect of NaCl loading. A similar experiment as in (a) was adopted, but the controls had two hydrations: 1 0/00 NaCl solution and tap water (2.5 and 5% b.w., respectively). The experimental animals had as a second load a solution of 2% NaCl instead of water. The same number of animals as in (a) were included in this series.

c) Effect of furosemide (5 and 10 mg) on hyperhydrated rats. All the animals including controls were gavaged with NaCl 1 0/00 solution and then with water. The experimental rats (24) were injected subcutaneously with 5 mg furosemide dissolved in 0.5 ml saline at the same time as of the second hydration. The control rats were injected with saline. In another group, 12 rats were injected with 10 mg of furosemide (in 1 ml) and an identical number of rats were given with saline as controls. In these experiments the animals were sacrificed by bleeding under anesthesia, 2 hours after the injections. The kidneys were rapidly removed, cleaned and weighed, and then were dehydrated and extracted for kallikrein determination.

In another 12 animals, 5 mg of furosemide were injected once a day for 8 days. 12 control rats were injected with saline. On the 9th day the animals were placed in metabolic cages, and submitted to the double hyperhydration (1 0/00 NaCl solution and water). A dose of 10 mg of furosemide was administered to the experimental rats, but controls had only saline. The animals were sacrificed 120 min after the injections, in the way described, in order to evaluate the amount of kallikrein in the kidneys. In the first and second hours after the injections, kallikrein and several other parameters in the collected samples of urine were measured.

d) Effects of furosemide in 2% NaCl overloaded rats (24). A similar experiment as in (c) was carried out, but in the second load instead of water, the animals received a 2% NaCl solution.

e) Effects of acetazoleamide in hyperhydrated rats. The experimental design was similar to (c), but instead of furosemide, acetazoleamide was injected. In separate protocols, the effects of 5 and 20 mg were tested (5 and 3 groups, respectively).

f) Effect of acetazoleamide (5 mg) on 2% NaCl overloaded rats. The experiment was similar to (d), using a 2% NaCl solution instead of water; performed on 4 goups of rats.

KALLIKREIN DETERMINATION IN URINE AND RENAL TISSUE

Urine was dialyzed for 24 hours against distilled water (4°C) prior to kallikrein measurement. Two different biological methods were used:

a) Direct oxytocic effect (Croxatto and Noe, 1971). For this purpose, the effect upon isolated rat uterus, immersed in modified Tyrode solution, was evaluated using as the standard, pure bradykinin. The amount of the enzyme was expressed in ng of bradykinin (BR); and

b) Indirect method (Croxatto and Noe, 1971). This is a biological evaluation of the enzyme activity through its kininogenase
property which requires purified plasma kininogen II (Jacobson
and Krisz method, 1967) as substrate. Formed kinins after 2 min
of incubation were tested upon isolated cat jejunum (Croxatto
et al. 1974).

        Quantitative determinations of renal kallikrein were per-
formed using the method of Croxatto et al., (1974). The final
renal extracts were tested by using the same bioassays adopted for
urinary kallikrein determinations and the total amount of the enzyme
was expressed in ng of BR.

Drugs

        Furosemide HCl and acetazoleamide were dissolved in saline.
In the case of furosemide, the pH (7.4) was adjusted by the addition of 10% NaOH.

                              RESULTS

        Table I summarizes the results obtained on kallikrein, Na, K,
and water excretion at 60 and 120 min after the second load.

a) Water administration induces a significant increase in the kallikrein excretory rate in the first hour following the second load
(Table I). Even though the kallikrein concentration is much lower,
the total amount excreted in this period is about twice as much as
compared to the urine of non-hyperhydrated rats. In the urine
excreted during three hours by the latter group, a mean value of
85 ng BR per rat/hour was found. The hyperhydrated rats excreted
262 ± 66 ng BR in the first 60 min., and in the 120 min after the
second hydration, an accumulative amount of 436 ± 29 ng BR. In
the latter animals, the excretion of sodium was 27 ± 1.6 and
38.1 ± 2.8 uEq per rat, respectively which was significantly
higher than that observed in the control groups.

b) In the rats overloaded with 2% NaCl, the kallikrein excretion
were 83% and 69% more in 60 min and 120 min, respectively, when
compared to that obtained in controls hyperhydrated with water.
Obviously sodium excretion in the first group was considerably
higher; 25 and 72 fold more in 60 and 120 min, than in controls.
As can be seen in Table I, water excretion was less in the NaCl
overloaded rats.

c,d) In keeping with previous results in normally hydrated rats
(Croxatto et al., 1973), the administration of furosemide (5 mg)
in hyperhydrated rats induced a considerable increase of all the
urinary parameters investigated. Kallikrein excretion was 86%
greater in tap water loaded rats and 90% greater in NaCl loaded

Table 1.

Are indicated accumulative mean values and s.e. of kallikrein, Na, K and water excretion at 60 and 120 minutes
during the control diuresis period, in 9 different
experimental conditions. The differences between the
normally hydrated and the other 8 groups were statistically
significant (p < 0.001). (See text).

EXPERIMENTAL CONDITIONS	N° of GROUPS	KALLIKREIN in ng Br Eq		SODIUM in μEq		POTASSIUM in μEq		WATER in ml	
		60	120	60	120	60	120	60	120 min
1 NORMALLY HYDRATED	8	85±10	197±31	14±09	21±15	40±	65±38	.37±008	.71±22
2 HYPERHYDR.	8	262±66	436±29	27±16	38±28	326±5	46.4±5	6.56±36	1.6±.08
3 Na Cl LOADED	8	481±92	739±150	410±16	1516±459			3.6±.56	7.9±.5
4 HYPERHYDR. + FUROS. 5 mg	4	489±34	645±52	1042±73	1247±40	31±4	44±51	14.2±.9	19.3±1
5 NaCl LOADED + FUROS. 5 mg	4	915±130	1333±72	1602±	2727±107	158±12	235±19	14.7±1.5	20.5±2
6 HYPERHYDR. + ACETAZ.5mg	5	394±73	525±45	2471±20	388±24	90±5	135±9	10.7±.4	13.8±.3
7 Na Cl LOADED + ACETAZ.5mg	4	500±120	729±125	537±62	1570±170			3.4±.14	8±.21
8 HYPERHYDR. +ACETAZ. 20mg	3	58±39	754±83	370±18	796±18	158±9	319±15	10.9±2	6.9±3
9 HYPERHYDR. +FUROS. 10mg	2	609±39	732±62	977±53	1233±81	157±6	226±9	15.9±.3	21.3±.4

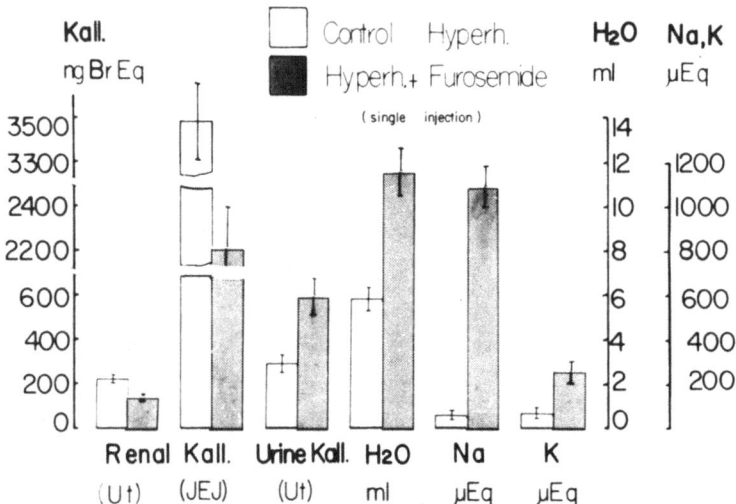

Figure 1.

    Columns indicate mean values (and S.E.) of renal kalli-
krein, and urinary excretion of kallikrein, water, sodium
and potassium in two groups of rats:
1) 12 control hyperhydrated rats;
2) 12 hyperhydrated similarly as 1 group plus 10 mg of
furosemide.

    Kallikrein in kidneys and in urine (2 hours after gavage),
is expressed in equiv. ng bradykinin. Kallikrein in the
kidneys was measured by the direct method (Ut) and by the
kininogenase activity (indirect method, JEJ). Urinary
kallikrein was measured by the direct method. (See text).

rats, in the first 60 min, as compared to the respective controls
(p< .001) Table 1, fig. 1. Furosemide exerts an additive action
over the effects of hyperhydration and NaCl loading. In furosemide treated animals overloaded with NaCl, kallikrein excretion
at the end of 120 min was 1333 ± 72 ng BR, very close to the
amount excreted in the same interval by hyperhydrate controls
(436 ± 29 ng BR) plus the amount excreted by NaCl loaded control
(739 ± 150 ng BR).

Kallikrein excretion was even higher in hyperhydrated rats
when the single dose of furosemide was elevated at 10 mg per rat,
but the difference with the 5 mg injected rats was significant
only in the first 60 min (p < 0.02). The kallikrein excretion
in rats treated with several doses of furosemide, as seen in fig.
2, reached a peak of 1618 ± 110 ng BR at 120 min and the excreted
Na and K also showed the highest figures. Comparing these results
to that obtained in controls, the mean values are significantly
higher (p < 0.001).

The average of the total kallikrein in the 2 kidneys of the
rats, 120 min after a single injection of 10 mg of furosemide,
was 140 ± 55 ng BR as measured by direct oxytocic method, and
2262 ± 200 ng BR measured through the kininogenase effect upon
cat jejunum. In the controls the respective values were 217 ±
80 and 3447 ± 250 ng BR (Fig. 2). Since the differences between
the two groups of rats were statistically different (p < 0.001),
this experiment gives the evidence that furosemide decreases the
kallikrein content of the kidney. The significantly greater
amount (p < 0.001) of kallikrein in the urine of furosemide
treated rats far exceeded (3.55 times more) the amount which disappeared in the kidneys of these animals. A similar situation
was found in the experiments where furosemide was administered
for 9 days (Fig. 2). In the kidneys of the furosemide treated
rats, the kallikrein mean values were 150 ± 7 ng BR (direct
method) and 2602 ± 261 ng BR (kininogenase activity), and in
the control were 175 ± 10 and 3538 ± 233 ng BR, respectively
(p < 0.001). The greater amount of kallikrein excreted in the
urine exceeds 42 times the amount which has disappeared in the
kidneys of furosemide treated animals.

e) Acetazoleamide in the dose of 5 mg in hydrated rats induces
significant increases in sodium and potassium (p < 0.001) and
water excretion (p < 0.005) and a moderate increase in urinary
kallikrein (525 ± 45 ng BR in 120 min) which was not statistically
significant (p = 0.1). With the same dose in rats loaded with 2%
NaCl, practically no change was observed within the 120 min.
However, 20 mg of acetazoleamide, in 3 experiments upon hyperhydrated animals significantly enhanced (p < 0.001) the excretion of
kallikrein and the other parameters in the urine. Kallikrein

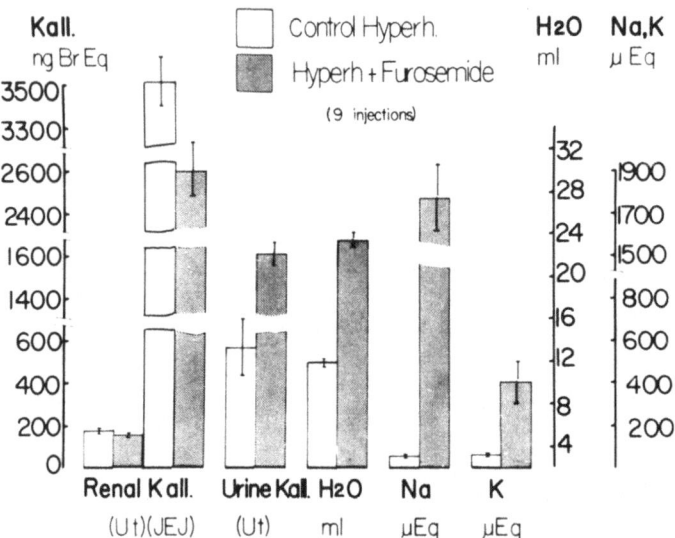

Figure 2.

The explanation is similar to Fig. 1. The difference was
the treatment of rats prior to hyperhydration: Group 1,
12 control rats were injected with 0,5 ml NaCl .9% subc.
once a day for 8 days; and Group 2, 12 rats, were similarly
injected but instead of saline, were given with 5 mg of
furosemide. The day when hyperhydration was performed
the rats of this group received 10 mg of furosemide.

excreted under the effect of 20 mg of acetazoleamide at the end of 120 min (754 ± 83 ng BR) is similar to that induced by 10 mg of furosemide (732 ± 62 ng BR) in the same type of experiment, but under furosemide, the sodium and potassium excretions were 2.6-fold more and 1.4-fold less, respectively, than under acetazoleamide.

DISCUSSION

The results show that the several factors which stimulate diuresis increase the urinary kallikrein excretory rate. In the normal hydrated rat, kallikrein is more concentrated in the urine, but if the total excreted volume is considered, there is always an enhancement of kallikrein excretion in the urine under water or NaCl diuresis. When the same volumes of water or 2% NaCl solution are given, there is consistently greater kallikrein excretion in the latter case. This indicates that the sodium load evokes a greater effect upon the enzyme excretion than the water itself. Possibly the sodium load sums its effect to the water load. It is difficult to reconcile these results with those published by Margolius, et al., 1974. These authors described a stimulatory effect of a low sodium diet upon kallikrein excretion in rats and in humans. It may be assumed that under long term dietary conditions, other regulatory mechanisms, probably depending on sodium retaining steroids, have more time to intervene and to change kallikrein turn over. In acute water and sodium over-loading experiments such as those described here, where results are recorded within a few hours, it is possible that other re-gulatory factors can be involved, depending on changes in blood volume and intrarenal circulation, or other mechanisms. Our results do not support the conclusion obtained by Mills and Ward (1975) in rabbits. According to them, the positive correlation of kallikrein excretion with sodium excretion found in previous experiments (Adetuyibi and Mills, 1972) may be only secondary to the positive relationship of kallikrein excretion with urinary volume. In the present experiments kallikrein excreted under the 2% NaCl load is significantly greater than that excreted under hyperhydration, notwithstanding that in the NaCl loaded rats the urine volume is smaller. Apparently both water and NaCl which suddenly produce an activation of kidney excretory function, pro-mote an acceleration on the kallikrein excretory rate. In the same line are the effects of diuretics particularly of furosemide which contributes to raise even more the amount of kallikrein in the urine. In the case of furosemide plus hyperhydration, the marked increase in the volume can account for the greater enzyme excretion. However, the urine volumes were similar in both groups, water and NaCl loaded, and the amount of urinary kalli-krein in the NaCl loaded group was twice as much as that excreted by hyperhydrated rats. Therefore, the results clearly indicate that sodium has a decisive role.

Assuming that urinary kallikrein is produced by the kidney and comparing the amount of renal kallikrein with the amount excreted in the urine (120 min), it is necessary to admit that furosemide in the kidney brings about a complex process which accelerates kallikrein synthesis and excretion. The decrease in kallikrein content in renal tissue, although statistically significant in the animals chronically treated with furosemide, is rather small when compared to the marked additional amounts of the enzyme which appear in the urine after diuretic administration. It is interesting that within a few hours kallikrein can appear in the urine an amount which is much greater than the total enzyme stored in both kidneys. One could be tempted to accept that an important fraction is coming directly from the blood, but it has been shown by Roblero et al., 1973; 1974 that an isolated kidney perfused with a solution which does not contain kallikrein or its precursor can release considerable amounts of this enzyme in the perfusate and in the urine. It is possible that the kidney may contain an inactive kallikrein precursor in storage.

Comparing the effects of acetazoleamide (20 mg) and furosemide (5 mg), it was observed that both promote similar increases in urinary kallikrein although the water diuresis, natriuresis and kalliuresis evoked by them are significantly diverse. Nevertheless, collectively, the data show that the highest values of kallikrein excretion were associated with the highest values of sodium excretion. It is striking that the great acceleration of kallikrein excretion in furosemide treated rats coexists with a rather small depletion of the enzyme stored in the kidneys, which is only conceivable with a very rapid synthesis which can cope with the excretory demands. This very rapid synthesis provides additional insights in evaluating the renal kallikrein-kinin system involvement in the excretory function of the kidney.

SUMMARY

The effects of acute administration of either water or 2% NaCl solution via a stomach tube and injections of diuretics, furosemide (5, 10 mg) and acetazoleamide (5, 20 mg per rat), in adult rats upon urinary kallikrein (Kal), Na and K, were studied.

Hyperhydration with water (5% b.w.) produced an 121% increase and 2% NaCl overloading (5% b.w.) 275% increase in urinary Kal within 120 min after gavage, when compared with the excretion of non hyperhydrated rats.

Furosemide 5 mg in hyperhydrated animals produced in the same period an excretion of 645 ± 52 ng BR of Kal, which is 147% higher to that excreted by the hyperhydrated controls. The same dose of furosemide in 2% NaCl loaded rats, produced an excretion of Kal equivalent to 1333 ± 72 ng BR which is 180% greater than in controls similarly loaded. Acetazoleamide 20 mg and furosemide 5 mg produced similar excretions of Kal even though natriuresis is greater and kalliuresis is lesser in furosemide injected rats.

Evaluation of total kidney Kal has shown that a single (10 mg) or a series of furosemide injections (8 days 5 mg + 1 day 10 mg), brings about a significant (p < 0.001) decrease in renal Kal, but the increase of Kal excreted in the urine (120 min) is 3.5 times more (under a single injection) and 42 times more (under 9 injections) than the amount which disappears from the kidneys. Apparently furosemide not only stimulates Kal excretion, but also Kal synthesis in the kidney. The results support the concept that the Kal system would be involved in excretory functions dealing both with sodium and water excretion.

REFERENCES

1. Adetuyibi, A., and I.H. Mills. Relationship between urinary kallikrein and renal function, hypertension and excretion of sodium and water in man. Lancet, II 203-207 (1972).

2. Croxatto, H.R., and M. San Martin. Kallikrein-like activity in the urine of renal hypertensive rats. Experientia, 26: 1216-1217 (1970).

3. Croxatto, H.R., and G. Noe. Kallikrein like enzyme in purified renal extracts containing renin. Commentarii Pontif. Acad. Scient. 40: 1 (1971).

4. Croxatto, H.R. Rinon y sistema calicreina-cininas. Medicina (B. Aires) 72 (Supl. I) 18: 29 (1972,a)

5. Croxatto, H.R. Calicreina versus renina? Rev. Med. de Chile, 100: 708-717 (1972,b).

6. Croxatto, H.R., J. Roblero, R. Garcia, J. Corthorn and M.L. San Martin. Effect of furosemide upon urinary kallikrein excretion. Agents and Actions, 3: 267-274 (1973).

7. Croxatto, H.R., R. Albertini, J. Roblero and J. Corthorn. Renal kallikrein (kininogenase activity) in hypertensive rats. Acta Physiol. Lat. 24: 439-442 (1974).

8. Garcia, R.L., J. Roblero, and H.R. Croxatto. Antibodies of rat urinary kallikrein, preparation and specificity. Acta physiol. Latinoam. 23: 149-151 (1973).

9. Geller, R.G., H.S. Margolius, J. Pisano, and H.R. Keiser. Effects of mineralocorticoids altered sodium intake and adrenalectomy on urinary kallikrein in rats. Circulation Res. 31: 857-861 (1972).

10. Greco, A.V., G. Porcelli, H.R. Croxatto, G. Fedeli and G. Ghirlanda. Ipertensione arteriosa e callicreina urinaria. Minerva Medica, 65: 3058 (1974).

11. Jacobsen, S. and M. Krisz. Some data on two purified kininogens from human plasma. Br. J. of Pharmac. Chemother. 29: 25-36 (1967).

12. Margolius, H.S., R. Geller, W. De Jong, J.J. Pisano and A. Sjoerdsma. Altered urinary kallikrein excretion in rats with hypertension. Circulation Res. 30: 358-362 (1972).

13. Margolius, H.S., D. Horwitz, R.G. Geller, R.W. Alexander, J.R. Gill Jr., J.J. Pisano and H.R. Keiser. Urinary excretion in normal man. Relationship to sodium intake and sodium retaining steroids. Circulation Res. 35: 812-819 (1974).

14. Marin-Grez, M., P. Cottone and O.A. Carretero. Evidence for an involvement of kinins in regulation of sodium excretion. Am. J. Physiol. 223: 794-796 (1972).

15. Mills, I.H. and P.E. Ward. The relationship between kallikrein and water excretion and the conditional relationship between kallikrein and sodium excretion. J. Physiol. 246: 695-707 (1975).

16. Nustad, K. and J. Pierce. Purification of rat urinary kallikrein and their specific antibody. Biochemistry (N.Y.) 13: 2312-2319 (1974).

17. Pisano, J.J., R. Geller, H.S. Margolius and H.S. Keiser. Urinary kallikrein in hypertensive rats. Acta Physiol. Latinoamer 24: 73-78 (1974).

18. Porcelli, G., G. Bianchi and H.R. Croxatto. Urinary kallikrein excretion in a spontaneously hypertensive strain of rats. Proc. Soc. of Exp. Biol. and Med. (in press) (1975).

19. Roblero, J.S., H.R. Croxatto, J. Corthorn, R. Garcia and E. De Vito. Kininogenase activity in urine and perfusion fluid of isolated rat kidney. Acta Physiol. Latinoamer 23: 154-156 (1973).

20. Roblero, J.S., H. R. Croxatto, R. Garcia and J. Corthorn. Kininogenase in urine produced by isolated perfused rat kidney. Experientia 30: 771-772 (1974).

21. Rosas, R., L. Barnafi, T. Pereda, and H.R. Croxatto. Effect of oxytocin structural changes on rat renal excretion of Na, K and water. Am. J. of Physiol. 202: 901 (1962).

LIST OF CONTRIBUTORS

Abraham, Z., Israel Institute for Biological Research, Tel-Aviv
    University, Medical School, Ness-Ziona, Israel

Albertini, R., Physiology Laboratory, Institute of Scientific
    Biology, Catholic University of Chile, Santiago, Chile

Altomonte, L., Center for the Study of Receptors Chemistry, National
    Research Council, Rome

Alzamora, F., Dept. of Physiology and Biophysics, Institute of
    Biological Sciences, Belo Horizonte, Brazil

Anselmi, B., Dept. of Clinical Pharmacology, University of
    Florence, Italy

Antonio, A., Dept. of Pharmacology, Faculty of Medicine, Ribeirao
    Preto, Sao Paulo, Brazil

Back, N., Dept. of Biochemical Pharmacology, School of Pharmacy
    State University of New York at Buffalo, USA

Baldoni, F., Dept. of Medicine, University of Rome, Italy

Beraldo, W.T., Dept. of Physiology and Morphology, Institute of
    Biological Sciences, Belo Horizonte, Brazil

Bertelli, A., Dept. of Pharmacology, University of Pisa, Italy

Berti, J.D., Dept. of Pharmacology and Protein Chemistry Laboratory
    Faculty of Medicine, Ribeirao Preto, Sao Paulo, Brazil

Bhoola, K.D., Dept. of Pharmacology, University of Bristol, Medical
    School, University Walk, Bristol, England

Branconi, F., Dept. of Obstetrics and Gynaecology, University of
    Florence, Italy

Brooks, P.M., Dept. of Pharmacology, University of Strathclyde,
    Glasgow, Scotland

Burrowes, C.E., Division of Experimental Pathology, Dept. of
    Pathology, University of Toronto, Canada

Caciagli, F., Dept. of Pharmacology, University of Pisa, Italy

Camargo, A.C.M., Dept. of Pharmacology and Protein Chemistry
Laboratory, Faculty of Medicine, Ribeirao Preto, Sao Paulo,
Brazil

Castania, A., Dept. of Pharmacology, School of Medicine of Ribeirao
Preto, Sao Paulo, Brazil

Catanzaro, O.L., Dept. of Physiology and Biophysics, Federal
University of Minas Gerais, Belo Horizonte, Brazil

Chiarini, P., Dept. of Medicine, University of Florence, Italy

Chiu, A.T., The Papanicolaou Cancer Research Institute, Miami,
Florida, USA

Chung, A., The Papanicolaou Cancer Research Institute, Miami,
Florida, USA

Cicilini, M., Dept. of Pharmacology and Protein Chemistry Laboratory,
Faculty of Medicine, Ribeirao Preto, Sao Paulo, Brazil

Corrado, A.P., Dept. of Pharmacology and Surgery, Faculty of
Medicine of Ribeirao Preto, Sao Paulo, Brazil

Corti, F., Dept. of Medicine, University of Florence, Italy

Croxatto, H.R., Physiology Laboratory, Institute of Scientific ·
Biology, Catholic University of Chile. Santiago, Chile

Curradi, C., Dept. of Clinical Pharmacology, University of Florence,
Italy

Day, A.R., The Papanicolaou Cancer Research Institute, Miami,
Florida, USA

De Almeida, A.P., Dept. of Pharmacology, Faculty of Medicine,
Ribeirao Preto, Sao Paulo, Brazil

Del Bianco, P.L., Dept. of Clinical Pharmacology, University of
Florence, Italy

De Saint Pierre, G., Dept. of Cardiology, Main Regional Hospital
S.M. Nuova, Florence, Italy

Dick, W.C., Dept. of Pharmacology, University of Strathclyde,
Glasgow, Scotland

Diniz, C.R., Dept. of Biochemistry, Faculty of Medicine, University of Sao Paulo, Ribeirao Preto, Sao Paulo, Brazil

Dorer, F.E., The Papanicolaou Cancer Research Institute, Miami, Florida and the Cleveland Veterans Hospital, Cleveland, Ohio USA

Edery, H., Israel Institute for Biological Research, Tel-Aviv University, Medical School, Ness-Ziona, Israel

Ehret, W., Institute of Clinical Chemistry and Clinical Biochemistry, University of Munich, Germany

Erspamer, V., Dept. of Pharmacology, University of Rome, Italy

Faldi, P., Dept. of Obstetrics and Gynaecology, University of Florence, Italy

Fanciullacci, M., Dept. of Clinical Pharmacology, University of Florence, Italy

Felix, A.M., The Papanicolaou Cancer Research Institute, Miami, Florida, USA

Fiedler, F., Institute of Clinical Chemistry and Clinical Biochemistry, University of Munich, Germany

Figueiredo, A.F.S., Dept. of Biochemistry, Faculty of Medicine, University of Sao Paulo, Ribeirao Preto, Sao Paulo, Brazil

Förg-Brey, B., Institute of Clinical Chemistry and Clinical Biochemistry, University of Munich, Germany

Franchi, G., Dept. of Clinical Pharmacology, University of Florence, Italy

Fritz, H., Institute of Clinical Chemistry and Clinical Biochemistry, University of Munich, Germany

Fujii, S., Dept. of Enzyme Physiology, Institute for Enzyme Research, School of Medicine, Tokushima University, Japan

Galletti, R., Dept. of Medicine, University of Florence, Italy

Galli, P., Dept. of Clinical Pharmacology, University of Florence, Italy

Gecse, A., Institute of Pathophysiology, University Medical School of Szeged, Hungary

Giroux, E.L., Merrel International Research Center, Strasbourg, France

Gomes, J.C., Dept. of Pharmacology, Faculty of Medicine of Ribeirao Preto, University of Sao Paulo, Ribeirao Preto, Sao Paulo, Brazil

Greco, A., Center for the Study of Receptors Chemistry, National Research Council, Rome, Italy

Greenbaum, L.M., Dept. of Pharmacology, College of Physicians and Surgeons, Columbia University, New York, USA

Grellet, M., Dept. of Pharmacology and Surgery, Faculty of Medicine of Ribeirao Preto, Sao Paulo, Brazil

Guimaraes, J.A., Section on Physiological Chemistry, Hypertension-Endocrine Branch, National Heart and Lung Institute, Bethesda, Maryland, USA

Habal, F.M., Division of Experimental Pathology, Dept. of Pathology, University of Toronto, Canada

Haberland, G.L., Bayer AG., Wuppertal-Elberfeld, Germany

Han, Y.N., Institute for Protein Research, Osaka University, Japan

Hashimoto, K., Dept. of Biochemical Pharmacology, State University of New York at Buffalo, USA

Heap, P.F., Dept. of Pharmacology, The Medical School, University of Bristol, England

Heneine, I.F., Dept. of Physiology and Biophysics, Federal University of Minas Gerais, Brazil

Hial, V., Section on Physiological Chemistry, Hypertension-Endocrine Branch, National Heart and Lung Institute, Bethesda, Maryland, USA

Hojima, Y., Lab. of Physiological Chemistry, Sciences University of Tokyo, Japan

Hirschauer, C., Institute of Clinical Chemistry and Clinical Bio-chemistry, University of Munich, Germany

Horowitz, J.D., Dept. of Medicine, University of Melbourne, Australia

Huidrobro, R., Physiology Laboratory, Institute of Scientific Biology
     Catholic University of Chile, Santiago, Chile

Iwanaga, S., Institute of Protein Research, Osaka University, Japan

Kato, H., Institute for Protein Research, Osaka University, Japan

Kizuki, K., Lab. of Physiological Chemistry, Sciences University
     of Tokyo, Japan

Koppelmann, L.E., Dept. of Pathology and Surgery, Westwood and
     Harbor General Hospital Campuses, School of Medicine, Los
     Angeles and Torrance, California, USA

Kohn, R.M., Department of Medicine, Buffalo General Hospital,
     Buffalo, New York USA

Kutzbach, C., Bayer A.G., Elberfeld, Germany

Lacombe, O.L., Dept. of Biochemistry, Faculty of Medicine,
     University of Sao Paulo, Ribeirao Preto, Sao Paulo, Brazil

Lauar, N.S., Dept. of Physiology and Biophysics, Federal University
     of Minas Gerais, Brazil

Lemmi, C.A.E., Dept. of Pathology and Surgery, Westwood and Harbor
     General Hospital Campuses, School of Medicine, Los Angeles
     and Torrance, California, USA

Lemon, J.C., Dept. of Pharmacology, The Medical School, University
     of Bristol, England

Lemon, M., Institute of Clinical Chemistry and Clinical Biochemistry,
     University of Munich, Germany

Li, H.C., Dept. of Biochemical Pharmacology, School of Pharmacy,
     State University of New York and the Roswell Park Memorial
     Institute, Buffalo, New York USA

Macmorine, D.R.L., Division of Experimental Pathology, Dept. of
     Pathology, University of Toronto, Ontario, Canada

Mair, G., Institute of Clinical Chemistry and Clinical Biochemistry,
     University of Munich, Germany

Mann, K. Dept. of Medicine, University of Munich, Germany

Mares-Guia, M., Dept. of Biochemistry, Faculty of Medicine, University of Ribeirao Preto, Sao Paulo, Brazil

Marlborough, D.I., Papanicolaou Cancer Research Institute, Miami, Florida, USA

Mashford, M.L., Dept. of Medicine, University of Melbourne, Australia

Mason, B., Lister Institute of Preventive Medicine, London, England

Matassi, L., Dept. of Medicine, University of Florence, Italy

McLimans, W.B., Dept. of Biochemical Pharmacology, School of Pharmacy, State University of N.Y. and the Roswell Park Memorial Institute, Buffalo, N.Y. USA

Monetti, M.G., Dept. of Clinical Pharmacology, University of Florence, Italy

Moore, T.C., Dept. of Pathology and Surgery, Westwood and Harbor General Hospital Campuses, School of Medicine, Los Angeles and Torrance, California, USA

Morato, M., Dept. of Pharmacology, Faculty of Medicine, Ribeirao Preto, Sao Paulo, Brazil

Moriwaki, C., Lab. of Physiological Chemistry, Sciences University of Tokyo, Japan

Moriya, H., Lab. of Physiological,Chemistry, Sciences University of Tokyo, Japan

Movat H.Z., Division of Experimental Pathology, Dept. of Pathology, University of Toronto, Canada

Nakajima, T., Dept. of Oral Surgery, School of Dentistry, Niigata University, Niigata City, Japan

Nava, G., Dept. of Clinical Pharmacology, University of Florence, Italy

Nuzzaci, G., Dept. of Cardiovascular Disease, University of Florence, Italy

Palm, S., Institute of Clinical Chemistry and Clinical Biochemistry, University of Munich, Germany

Pedata, F., Dept. of Clinical Pharmacology, University of Florence, Italy

Pela, I., Dept. of Clinical Pharmacology, University of Rome, Italy

Peruzzi, G., Dept. of Medicine, University of Rome, Italy

Pierce, J.V., Section on Physiological Chemistry, Hypertension-Endocrine Branch, National Heart and Lung Institute, Bethesda, Maryland, USA

Pisano, J.J., Section of Physiological Chemistry, Hypertension-Endocrine Branch, National Heart and Lung Institute, Bethesda, Maryland, USA

Porcelli, G., Institute of Chemistry, Faculty of Medicine, Catholic University, Rome, Italy

Poeter, D.D., Department of Pathology and Surgery, Westwood and Harbor General Hospital Campuses, School of Medicine, Los Angeles and Torrance, California, USA

Ranieri, M., Center for the Study of Receptors Chemistry, National Research Council, Rome, Italy

Ribeiro, R.T.N., Dept. of Pharmacology and Surgery, Faculty of Medicine, Ribeirao Preto, Sao Paulo, Brazil

Roblero, J., Physiology Laboratory, Institute of Scientific Biology, Catholic University of Chile, Santiago, Chile

Rocha E Silva, M., Dept. of Pharmacology, Faculty of Medicine, Ribeirao Preto, Sao Paulo, Brazil

Rojas, M., Physiology Laboratory, Institute of Scientific Biology, Catholic University of Chile, Santiago, Chile

Rossoni, R.B., Dept. of Physiology and Biophysics, Federal University of Minas Gerais, Brazil

Rothschild, A.M., Dept. of Pharmacology, School of Medicine, Ribeirao Preto, Sao Paulo, Brazil

Ryan, J.W., The Papanicolaou Cancer Research Institute, Miami, Florida, USA

Ryan, U.S., The Papanicolaou Cancer Research Institute, Miami, Florida, USA

Sangiorgi, M., Dept. of Medicine, University of Rome, Italy

Schachter, M., University of Alberta, Edmonton, Canada

Schill, W.B., Dept. of Dermatology, University of Munich, Germany

Schinetti, M.L., Dept. of Pharmacology, University of Pisa, Italy

Schmidt-Kastner, G., Bayer A.G., Elberfeld, Germany

Schnells, G., Bayer A.G., Wuppertal-Elberfeld, Germany

Schultz, D.R., Papanicolaou Cancer Research Institute, Miami, Florida, and the Cleveland Veterans Hospital, Cleveland, Ohio, USA

Semprini, A., Dept. of Medicine, University of Rome, Italy

Seravalli, G., Dept. of Obstetrics and Gynaecology, University of Florence, Italy

Sharma, J.N., Dept. of Pharmacology, University of Strathclyde, Glasgow, Scotland

Sicuteri, F., Dept. of Clinical Pharmacology, University of Florence, Italy

Steger, R., Dept. of Biochemical Pharmacology, School of Pharmacy, State University of New York at Buffalo, USA

Suzuki, T., Institute for Protein Research, Osaka University, Japan

Svendsen, L.S., Pentapharm Ltd., Basel, Switzerland

Szekeres, L., Institute of Pathophysiology, University Medical School of Szeged, Hungary

Tallarida, G., Dept. of Medicine, University of Rome, Italy

Tschesche, H., Institute of Organic Chemistry, Technical University of Munich, Germany

Vargaftig, B.B., Merrell International Research Center, Strasbourg, France

Vecchiett, L., Civil Hospital of Penne, Italy

Vogt, W., Max-Planck-Institute of Experimental Medicine, Dept. of Biochemical Pharmacology, Gottingen, Germany

Wallner, O., Dept. of Gynaecology and Obstetrics, University of Munich, Germany

Wanka, J., Buffalo General Hospital, Buffalo, New York, USA

Webster, M.E., Section on Physiological Chemistry, Hypertension-Endocrine Branch, National Heart and Lung Institute, Bethesda, Maryland, USA

Weinberg, J., Dept. of Biochemistry, Faculty of Medicine, University of Sao Paulo, Ribeirao Preto, Sao Paulo, Brazil

Werle, E., Institute of Clinical Chemistry and Clinical Biochemistry, University of Munich, Germany

Wilkens, H.J., Dept. of Biochemical Pharmacology, State University of New York at Buffalo, USA

Zeitlin, I.J., Dept. of Pharmacology, University of Strathclyde, Glasgow, Scotland

Zsilinszky, E., Institute of Pathophysiology, University Medical School of Szeged, Hungary

AUTHOR INDEX

(Underscored numbers indicate complete papers in this volume.)

SUBJECT INDEX

Acetazolamide, effect on urinary
  kallikrein excretion, 306
Acetylcholine, depletion of submandibular secretory granules,
  62
Acetyl salicylic acid
  effect on
    clostripain kinin release,
    101
    kininogen levels, 339,341
  inhibition of kallikrein
    activation, 197
Acid protease, from fibroblasts
  191-196
  cysteine activation 192
  isolation, 192
  kinetics, 194
  molecular weight, 193
  pH profile, 193
  purification, 192
  subcellular localization, 194
Acute myocardial infarction
  kininase in, 255
  kininogen I in, 250,254
  kininogen II in, 251,254
  kininogen total in, 249,253
  prekallikrein in, 248,253
Alpha 1-antitrypsin
  inhibition of plasmin, 29
  purification, 27
Alpha 2-macroglobulin
  chromatography, 282
  complex with kallikrein, 281,
  283-284
    functional properties, 283-
    284

Angina pectoris
  kininase in, 251
  kininogen I in, 250
  kininogen II in, 251
  kininogen total in, 249
  prekallikrein in, 248
Angiotensin converting enzyme
  endothelial cell in culture,
  217-226
  subcellular site of, 235-243
Antithrombin III
  inhibition of
    plasma kallikrein, 30
    plasmin, 29
  purification by
    isoelectric focusing, 27
Arthritis, rheumatoid
  kininogen levels, 335-343
  aspirin, effect on, 339, 341
  indomethacin, effect on, 337
  placebo, effect on, 339
Asthenozoospermia, treatment with
  hog pancreatic kallikrein,
  274-276
Atropine, inhibition of
  acetylcholine-induced salivation, 63
  bradykinin-induced salivation,
  86,87
Ballotini, adsorption of surface
  factor, 54,55
Bothrops jararaca venom, 2
Bradykinin, 2,5-13,43-51,81-95,
  103-107, 117, 118, 301-314
  action on mammalian heart,
  117, 118

391